World Protein Resources

World Protein Resources

Allen Jones

M T P
Medical and Technical Publishing Co Ltd

Published by

MTP
Medical and Technical Publishing Co. Ltd.,
St. Leonard's House,
St. Leonardgate,
Lancaster, England.

Printed by The Garden City Press Limited,
Letchworth, Hertfordshire SG6 1JS.

ISBN 0 85200104 5

Contents

			page
	PREFACE		vii
PART 1	INTRODUCTION TO PROTEINS		
	1	General Comment	3
	2	Protein chemistry	5
	3	Proteins in diet	17
	4	Vitamins	31
	5	Minerals	35
	6	Allergy, addiction, preference and prejudice	43
	7	Mixtures and compounds	47
	8	Preservation	50
	9	Canning	55
PART 2	ANIMAL PROTEINS		
	10	Meat	63
	11	Birds and poultry	97
	12	Dairy protein	107
	13	Fish	119
PART 3	VEGETABLE PROTEINS		
	14	Cereals	155
	15	Fresh vegetables	161
	16	Oilseeds	167

17   Pulses   183
18   Dehydrated vegetables in feed   186
19   Vegetable genetics   197
20   Monoculture   200
21   Infestation   203
22   Green leaf protein   209

PART 4   MICROBIAL PROTEINS
23   Algae   219
24   Fungi   223
25   Yeasts   228
26   Bacteria   248
27   Oil   257

PART 5   PROTEIN ECONOMICS
28   Variations in production, distribution and
     consumption   265
29   Agricultural outputs   275
30   Industrial protein   280
31   World protein supply and demand   289
32   Speculation   309
33   Natural situations (selected countries)   319
34   Future proteins   362
INDEX   375

Preface

Protein is the origin, foundation and essential component of life and of human activity. It is an emotive subject and any claim, statement or opinion is sensitive to attack from experts and others who have a restricted experience or are subjects of commercial or political pressure. Many of the facts, opinions and forecasts are disputed and may be disproved in due course. As presented, they are true as far as is known but may represent little more than majority impression at the time of writing. Changes in the seventies are rapid, drastic and mainly unanticipated. At any time there could be a comprehensively influential discovery or incident which could alter the entire pattern of protein supply and demand.

Scientific and academic statements in this book may be criticised by purists but it is to be appreciated that the book is intended for universal appreciation. Statements are written to be understood within the context. If the author offends by slightly bending the rules of scientific presentation, or by making a claim which might not prove absolutely accurate if all factors are analysed, he makes no apology. When everybody in the world has a full belly and a contented mind there will be time to argue about details. At present, we need an extra 20 million tons of protein per year. If this book helps to find it the author will be happy.

The author is grateful to many workers for the information. Many of the tables are without identification, being collations. Where a source of information is identified the author accepts no responsibility for its accuracy.

Part I

Introduction to Proteins

Chapter 1

General Comment

Protein is an essential component in diet. The greatest single problem in the world today is inefficient distribution of protein foods, without which human beings are reduced in health including mental health. Some of the inefficiency in distribution is deliberate and intended to inflate prices, but it must be accepted that most of the failure to benefit from available protein foods arises from ignorance and incompetence at all levels from the consumer to the administrative organisations. Political interference with the potential pattern of protein production and distribution is notably inhibitive.

Consumers are, in general, ignorant of protein technology and there is a background of preference and prejudice which limits patterns of consumption. Notable perhaps is the emphasis on flesh protein with the invalid impression that only fish and meat provide 'good' protein. The eating of flesh is primeval, dating from the hunting and scavenging period of man's development. It is directly related to the killer instinct and has therefore become subject to regional and sectarian habits, preferences, traditions, ceremonies and convictions. Throughout the development of man these social controls have influenced technological progress and have caused unnecessary famines. Many of the present restricting factors in diet can be related to social problems which no longer exist in the society concerned. Likewise, many of the handling techniques for flesh protein today were common in prehistoric times. There is a need to educate all concerned with protein and to eradicate attitudes and activities which prevent effective utilisation of available protein, which will be shown to be much more than is needed to feed the world population.

It is necessary to differentiate between protein needed for survival and that needed for health, and to accept that the details of demand may be dictated more by social considerations than by basic body needs. The human body needs a comprehensive balance of amino acids and, since we are still discovering facts about diet, it is better to over-estimate requirements rather than work to calculated statistics.

The function of consumed protein is to manufacture body tissue and to take part in body chemical reactions. It is obviously desirable that the consumed protein has a similar composition to the protein pattern of the consumer, so that the probability of deficiency is reduced. On the other hand, possible amino-acid deficiencies in one protein source can be compensated by mixing with another protein source of different amino-acid deficiency, giving a complete pattern of amino acids which is as good as and can be better than a single protein source with a full pattern.

Satisfaction of personal demands in terms of type and condition of food is a factor in mental health. Full benefit will not be gained if eating is with revulsion and there is some evidence that bodies become attuned to diets so that unfamiliar food groups may take time to be accepted (in the chemical sense) by the digestion chemistry. On the other hand, bodies have sufficient flexibility of chemical performance to adapt to new conditions. New conditions have arisen in the world by urbanisation, which divorced man from his fresh-food supply, and by overpopulation associated with national boundaries, which prevented hungry man from moving to pastures anew. When man now meets unsatisfactory diet it is more difficult for him to change it.

With the current system of distribution and production, world agriculture can not be relied upon to feed the world. In fact, there could now be sufficient disruption of ecological and social balances for agriculture to be incapable of meeting requirements even if production was maximised and distribution was efficiently organised. There is now an urgent need to find protein sources which do not rely on climates and which can, in effect, introduce protein foods which escape the confused pattern of social and religious prejudice. Most potential is seen in microbial protein, which can be manufactured by industrial techniques and which is too new in its recent form to be condemned on religious grounds.

Chapter 2

Protein Chemistry

As the 'primeval soup' cooled it allowed the formation of water and similar simple chemicals. Most of these clouded the atmosphere to reduce levels of ultraviolet radiation. As temperatures dropped and destructive radiation declined there were more chemicals manufactured and retained in the 'soup' or in the space above. Further improvement in the conditions allowed reaction between very large molecules, including those using the peculiar ability of carbon to link with more carbon in a chain or network. A range of large molecules developed around formaldehyde, water and ammonia, with additions as dictated by accidental contact under conditions which encouraged the sharing of energy patterns. Some energy structures had the ability to link together as polymers without significant damage to the structures of the small molecules which acted as mononers. An infinite number of such very large molecules resulted from the various patterns in which monomers combined. Variation was by type of monomers, number of monomers and by the layout of the monomers in the final structure. Having a complicated energy structure the large molecules were (to a greater or lesser degree according to the individual energy patterns) able to re-organise or change with the uptake or release of energy. They could also, to a greater or lesser degree, disintegrate to component members and reform as new materials. Hence there developed a variety of intricate reactions with energy transfer and reformation as operating systems, leading to accidents of availability and conditions which allowed self-generation. Such self-generation required exceedingly varied and complex reactions, some involving energy transfer and others relying on reformation. Without going into detail, carbohydrates provided the facility for energy transfer in organisms whilst proteins provided the facility for reformation to construct required tissues but could also take up, carry and release energy.

Thus organisms developed according to available chemicals and conditions of reaction. As each organism type was generated it was characterised by an individual collection of chemical reactions involving specific chemicals. Such chemicals were, however, mildly unstable and could be modified by circumstances, to become not completely unlike the original but sufficiently changed to be individual. Consequently, although like organisms use like chemistry each individual has very slight personal chemical modifications which, for example, interfere with skin grafting even between members of a family.

POLYMERS

Polymers have very high molecular weights, as indicated by the table:

	Mol wt.		*Mol wt.*		*Mol wt.*
Water	18.0	Dextrose	198.11	Amylose	10 000–80 000
Ethyl alcohol	46.05	Sucrose	342.18	Casein	15 000–375 000
Benzene	78.05	Glycerin	92.06	Pectin	Approx. 270 000
				Cellulose	Approx. 570 000
				Silk protein	Approx. 150 000

The point to appreciate is that when molecular weights are high they are far from exact and are better regarded as ranges about an average, likely to be varied in the average and in the divergence from the average. Natural substances of high molecular weight in organisms are working members and their construction depends on the prevailing situation in the constant traffic in energy and the constant reformation of tissue. Rarely is such a molecule constant in structure for any length of time, although some body chemicals have apparent stability when their main function is storage, as for example ferritin storing iron.

The molecular weight limit, below which polymerisation is unlikely and above which polymerisation is probably the only practical construction method, is 1200 to 1500. There are molecules based on repeated units and with molecular weights below 1500 but these are not polymers in the academic sense but can be monomers bringing blocks of repeated units into a polymeric structure. For example saccharides are not polymers to a defining chemist, but are chains of CHOH units which can be united to become polysaccharides of high molecular weight, whereby the substance satisfies the academic definition of polymers with the mentioned cyclic repeated unit. In general, high polymers have molecular weights above 10 000. Polymeric saccharides are found in almost all plants whilst proteinic polymers are associated with animals but are also in almost all plants even if only in small doses.

The frontier between plants and animals is not as distinct as might be thought but there is difference in the chemical modifications used by the two main sectors of organisms in their development. Biological functions are performed in plants, according to their place in the scale of development, by various polymers such as pectins, gums, mucilages and various complexities of lignins and celluloses. Polysaccharides are stored as starches which reconvert as required. Inulin and a few other polymers are also found as storage systems. Chlorophyll, which some purists define as essential to identify plants, has association with protein polymers.

Proteins are polymers using a repeating unit of —NH—CH(R)—CO—, which differs from most natural repeating units in that there is a link through a nitrogen atom whereas other natural polymers link mainly through direct carbon–carbon systems or use oxygen as a linking atom. Cellulose, for example, has a cyclic repeating unit in which oxygen is one link in the ring and also the link between units. The affinity of vegetable and animal substances can be illustrated by studying chitin, which has a repeating unit almost identical to that of cellulose but an —OH group in the cellulose cycle becomes an —NHR group in chitin. Such a small difference in structure can have considerable influence on the characteristics of the substance and its performance. In the case of proteins the characteristics of the polymer depend on the nature of the group R, which can in theory be any element or group capable of resting on a CH group otherwise connected to an NH and a CO group.

Polysaccharide polymers are the main theme in plants whilst protein polymers perform much the same tasks and functions in animals. In muscle tissue there are four main proteins of initial interest:

Myogen—molecular weight approx. 81 000 and therefore soluble in water
Globulin—molecular weight approx. 160 000
Myosin—molecular weight approx. 1 000 000
Stroma proteins

The connective tissue, which relates to lignins in plants, is collagen, a protein in animal muscle. Further up the molecular scale is keratin, which is the basis for hair and horn and can be related to the cellulose which is the insoluble tough fraction in plant structures. Haemoglobin is the protein which is responsible for the red colour in blood. It is loosely related to the green colour in plants, although the connection is ill-defined, has a molecular weight of approx. 69 000 and has a molecular design suitable for temporary oxidation. Also found in the blood is fibrinogen which can be converted by the enzyme thrombin to fibrin, in which condition it is not soluble and forms a clot. Further within the theme of plants and animals, glycogen in animals stores energy in much the same way that starch functions in plants. Fats comprise another chemical family containing fatty acids and capable of absorbing or reacting with hydrophobic chemicals whereas carbohydrates and lower proteins are associated with hydrophilic chemicals.

In general, but with exceptions which infuriate academic purists, variations of carbohydrates are within the limits of a standardised molecular structure. Fats and proteins, on the other hand, exhibit variation of groups within the structure and can be loosely identified by the fatty or amino acids used in their composition. When some seeds ripen they lose starch in favour of fats, and in animals there is a similar exchange mechanism converting carbohydrates into fats. Until recently, it was thought that the pattern of fats in an organism was an unalterable characteristic but it has now been shown possible to breed meat containing vegetable fats. There is the opinion that protein patterns might also be modified but it must be appreciated that any such change could only be introduced during the final period of an animal's life. If the fats and proteins are to function correctly during the active development of the animal they must function according to the characteristic patterns of that animal species, not according to the wishes of the eventual consumer.

AMINO ACIDS

Protein polymers are built from amino-acid monomers, of which about twenty are important in this present context. Of these, some can be synthesised by body chemistry and the others need to be supplied as amino acids in diet. Amino acids which need to be supplied as such are described as essential, those which can be self-manufactured as non-essential. As will be seen in the section on diet, the differentiation is not exact because one amino acid can replace another under special con-

* *

ditions, or can be of sufficient value in the diet to be highly desirable if not essential. The normal list of *essential* amino acids for humans is:

Arginine, cystine, histidine, isoleucine, leucine, lysine, methionine, phenylalanine, threonine, tryptophane, tyrosine, valine.

In theory and in academic terms the list should have only eight members but histidine and arginine are included because they maintain the nitrogen balance; cystine and tyrosine are included because they can in part replace methionine and phenylalanine. This leaves six amino acids to be classified as *non-essential*, namely:

Alanine, aspartic acid, glutamic acid, glycine, proline, serine.

Given a satisfactory content of dietary nitrogen, a healthy human body need not be supplied with the non-essential amino acids. On the other hand, one is never quite certain of the reaction mechanics of proteins and it might be presumptuous to declare the listed non-essential amino acids as not needed, particularly since some protein reactions are specific to occasions and involve trace quantities.

Glycine has been of considerable interest to research workers because it has a simple formula, NH_2CH_2COOH, and can be investigated in relation to its polymers to provide some insight into polymerisation mechanics. Two glycine molecules react to give diketopiperazine—

$$2NH_2CH_2COOH \rightarrow \begin{matrix} NH-CH_2 \\ | \quad\quad | \\ OC \quad CO \\ | \quad\quad | \\ CH_2-NH \end{matrix} + 2H_2O$$

—which is a cyclic compound, earlier considered to be the repeated unit in an association polymer (lots of diketopiperazine molecules binding together through strong secondary valency forces). Then came the examination of higher combinations of glycine, in which the ratio between end-groups and mass proved that there were chains of glycine molecules simply strung together, not assembled in units of cyclic twin-molecules. The high molecular weight is obtained by condensation reactions, in the case of glycine—

$$NH_2CH_2COOH \quad NH_2CH_2COOH \quad NH_2CH_2COOH$$
$$H \quad HOH \quad HOH \quad OH$$

—to give the protein chain of —NH—CH(R)—CO— in which R is hydrogen (H). Glycine, with hydrogen as the effective radical (R), is the simple amino acid. When the effective radical is more complicated the structure and reaction pattern is less clear, particularly in mixtures.

The interesting amino acids are:

Arginine

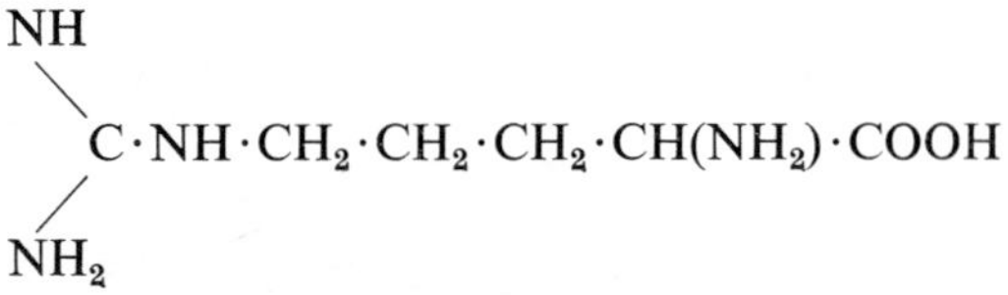

$$\begin{array}{c}
NH \\
\diagdown \\
\quad C \cdot NH \cdot CH_2 \cdot CH_2 \cdot CH_2 \cdot CH(NH_2) \cdot COOH \\
\diagup \\
NH_2
\end{array}$$

Arginine is widely distributed and plays some part in the production of urea as an excretory product.

Cystine

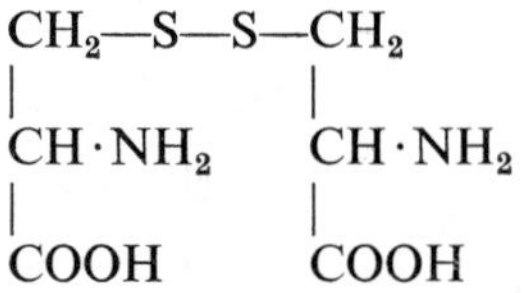

$$\begin{array}{ll}
CH_2-S-S-CH_2 \\
| \qquad\qquad | \\
CH \cdot NH_2 \quad CH \cdot NH_2 \\
| \qquad\qquad | \\
COOH \qquad COOH
\end{array}$$

Cystine breaks down in the body to two molecules of cysteine (HS—CH$_2$ · CH(NH$_2$) · COOH). It is the most common sulphur-containing amino acid and is associated with skeletal and connective tissue.

Histidine

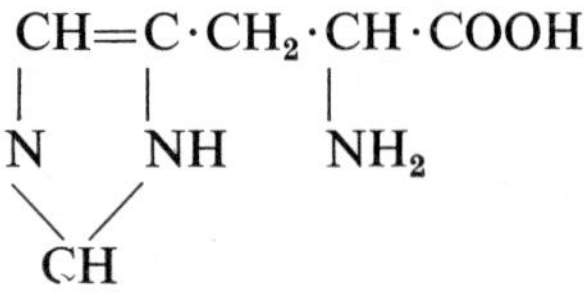

$$\begin{array}{c}
CH=C \cdot CH_2 \cdot CH \cdot COOH \\
| \quad\; | \qquad\quad | \\
N \quad NH \quad\; NH_2 \\
\diagdown \; \diagup \\
CH
\end{array}$$

Histidine appears to play some vital part in tissue construction and is reputed to cure ulcers when injected. There is an interesting relationship to histamine, a base formed by bacterial breakdown of histidine. Histamine encourages the flow of gastric juices.

Isoleucine

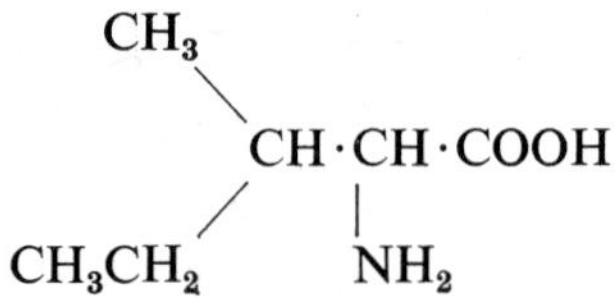

$$\begin{array}{c}
CH_3 \\
\diagdown \\
\qquad CH \cdot CH \cdot COOH \\
\diagup \qquad\quad | \\
CH_3CH_2 \qquad NH_2
\end{array}$$

Leucine CH_3
$\diagdown$
$\quad\quad CH \cdot CH_2 \cdot CH \cdot COOH$
$\diagup \qquad\qquad |$
$CH_3 \qquad\quad NH_2$

Lysine $CH_2 \cdot (CH_2)_3 \cdot CH \cdot COOH$
$\quad\quad |\qquad\qquad\quad |$
$\quad\quad NH_2 \qquad\qquad NH_2$

Lysine will be shown in later chapters to be probably the most important amino acid to study, in that it is usually noted for its absence in deficient diets.

Methionine $CH_3 \cdot S \cdot CH_2CH_2 \cdot CH \cdot COOH$
$\qquad\qquad\qquad\qquad\qquad |$
$\qquad\qquad\qquad\qquad\quad NH_2$

Methionine is affiliated to cystine in that it carries sulphur. Like lysine, it is frequently lacking in diets.

Phenylalanine $C_6H_5 \cdot CH_2 \cdot CH \cdot COOH$
$\qquad\qquad\qquad\qquad\qquad |$
$\qquad\qquad\qquad\qquad\quad NH_2$

Alanine $CH_3 \cdot CH \cdot COOH$
$\qquad\qquad\quad |$
$\qquad\qquad NH_2$

The human body can manage to synthesise alanine but finds it impossible to add the phenyl group. Hence alanine is non-essential but phenylalanine is essential.

Threonine $COOH$
$\qquad\qquad |$
$\qquad\quad CH \cdot NH_2$
$\qquad\qquad |$
$\qquad\quad CHOH$
$\qquad\qquad |$
$\qquad\quad CH_3$

Threonine is particularly essential in blood proteins.

Tryptophane

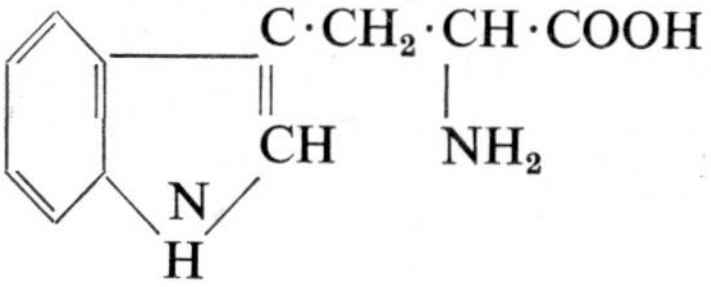

Tryptophane has influence on rates of growth in animals.

Tyrosine

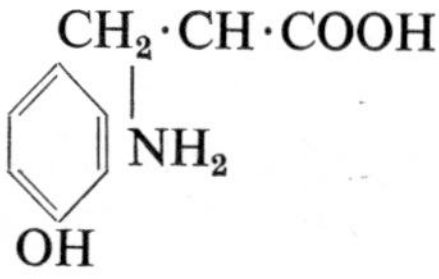

Tyrosine is the least soluble of the amino acids. It is concerned with the body manufacture of adrenaline and thyroxine.

Valine

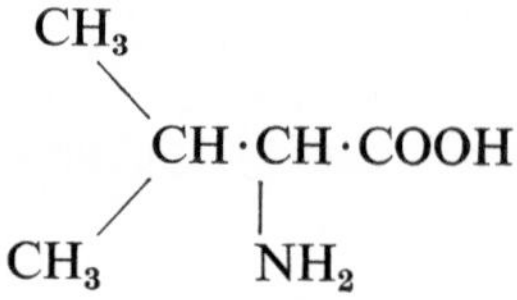

Aspartic acid

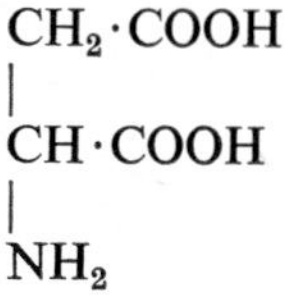

Glutamic acid

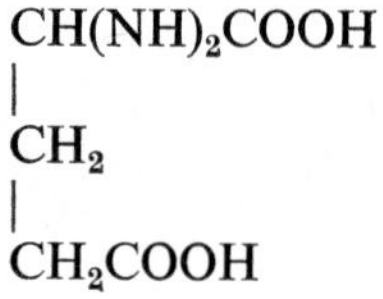

Proline

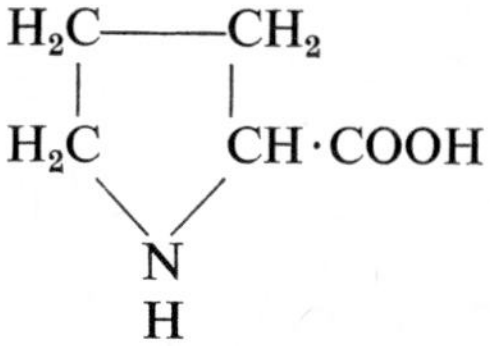

Serine

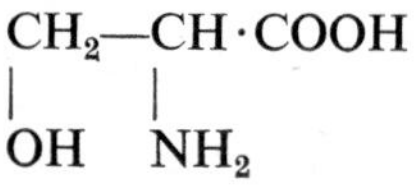

The amino acids, vital though they be, are only a part of the chemical network. Nitrogen is a vital element and is frequently associated in reaction, as for instance in adenine compounds.

Adenine is a component in the nucleic acid part of nucleoproteins and adenylpyrophosphate. Adenine plus D-ribose is a nucleoside which is part of plant nucleic acid. With phosphoric acid added the result is a nucleotide existing in muscle or adenylic acid in plant nucleic acid. Adenyl pyrophosphate breaks down in muscle to adenylic acid and phosphoric acid, the adenylic acid then taking up the phosphate group from phosphagen to reform adenyl pyrophosphate.

Adrenaline is another chemical of interest in that it increases blood pressure and increases the sugar content of blood. The characteristics of meat are therefore influenced by the mental state of the animal before killing. Insulin gives a reversed reaction, lowering the sugar content of blood. Agmatine, a component of fish spawn, also lowers blood sugar and has some chemical affinity to arginine, the amino acid with influence on urea production. It is important to appreciate that there is a link between body reactions and emotion, hormones being activated by stress and likely to interfere with body chemistry. It is also important to isolate animals according to their body chemistry. As a simple example of the individuality of species, allantoin is an end-product of purine metabolism, uric acid being broken down by the enzyme uricase. Most animals have uricase and therefore excrete allantoin but men and apes do not. Protein chemistry also includes many unwelcome products. Alloxantin is a mild poison found in soya, vetches and beets, reasonably deadly to cold-blooded animals but little more than a marketing inhibition in the supply of vegetation for human or animal feed. More serious are the arrow poisons proteins, which are toxic in very small proportions.

This brief introduction to proteins is not intended to replace the voluminous accounts of research into proteins but to indicate to the reader that protein chemistry is far from simple and that much is yet to be discovered. It is certain that more of the available information will be used in future, not only in the effort to produce perfect meat and vegetables but also in the manipulation of the chemistry of organisms to satisfy market demands.

FIBRE PROTEINS

Protein fibres are classified in two main groups:

those which occur in nature on animals
those which are manufactured from protein raw materials, mainly vegetable.

Wool, hair and fur are largely composed of a special group of proteins known as keratins. Keratins differ, but are all characterised by high cystine content. The protein structure depends on a sulphur–sulphur cross-link and most of the desirable properties of the fibres are due to this cystine disulphide linkage. There are also acidic and basic amino acids, which is why the fibres will accept acid or alkali dyes. The cystine contents of selected fibres are:

% of keratin content as cystine	
Human hair	16.0
Chimpanzee hair	15.5
Pig hair	13.9
Sheep wool	13.6
Hen feathers	8.7
Human finger nails	12.9
Cow horn	12.4
Rhinoceros horn	8.9
Human skin	3.5

Silks contain no cystine but are characterised by high contents of fibroin and sericin proteins. The 15–25% sericin is removed when silk is degummed. More than 80% of the amino acids in silk are low in molecular weight (glycine, alanine and serine).

The fibres which are manufactured from non-fibre proteins include those from zein, groundnuts and casein. Fibres can be produced from

Fibre proteins—collated statistics

Fibre (% of total protein)

Amino acid	Spider silk	Silk	Wool	Casein	Ground-nut	Soya	Zein	Gliadin	Collagen	Gelatin	Egg albumen	Insulin	Edestin
Alanine	23.4	26.4	4.1	3.5	3.0	4.1	9.8	2.0	9.1	8.7	2.2	4.6	4.3
Aspartic acid	—	3.0	7.3	6.7	15.0	3.9	3.4	0.8	3.4	3.4	8.1	5.7	12.0
Arginine	5.2	1.1	8.6	3.9	13.1	5.8	1.6	2.6	8.1	8.7	5.7	3.0	16.7
Cystine	—	—	11.8	0.4	1.6	1.0	0.9	2.4	—	0.2	1.8	12.5	1.4
Glycine	35.1	43.8	6.5	1.9	—	0.2	—	0.0	25.9	25.5	—	4.3	3.8
Glutamic acid	11.7	2.0	16.0	22.0	21.1	19.5	36.6	43.7	5.9	5.8	16.1	18.6	20.7
Histidine	—	0.5	0.7	3.2	2.3	2.3	0.8	3.3	0.9	2.9	1.5	4.9	2.9
Isoleucine	—	1.4	—	5.3	—	4.0	4.3	} 6.6	} 5.4	} 7.1	} 10.7	} 15.7	} 12.1
Leucine	—	0.8	9.7	10.6	6.5	8.4	15.4						
Lysine	—	0.9	2.5	8.3	3.3	5.4	0.0	0.7	5.9	5.9	5.0	2.4	2.4
Methionine	3.7	—	0.4	3.5	1.2	2.0	2.3	2.0	—	—	5.2	—	2.4
Proline	—	1.5	7.2	10.5	5.3	3.9	9.0	13.2	14.6	19.7	4.2	2.6	3.6
Phenylalanine	—	1.5	1.6	6.5	4.7	5.3	7.6	2.4	4.0	1.4	5.1	8.1	5.9
Serine	—	12.6	9.5	5.9	6.4	6.0	1.0	0.1	3.1	3.3	—	5.2	6.3
Threonine	—	1.5	6.6	4.5	2.9	4.0	2.2	—	2.3	1.4	4.0	2.1	3.9
Tyrosine	8.2	10.6	6.1	6.3	6.0	4.3	5.9	3.0	0.0	0.0	1.2	13.0	4.3
Tryptophane	—	—	0.7	1.4	1.2	1.5	0.2	1.1	0.0	0.0	2.2	—	1.5
Valine	—	3.2	5.5	6.0	3.4	4.5	9.8	2.0	9.1	8.7		4.6	4.3

NOTE: Zein is an incomplete protein derived from maize. Gliadin is from wheat and rye, being evident in gluten flours. Collagen is a connective tissue in animals. In water, collagen swells and loses ammonia to become gelatin. Insulin is a hormone secreted by the pancreas. Edestin is a first-class protein from hempseed.

soya, whey proteins, blood proteins—in fact from any protein capable of solution, extrusion and precipitation. There is a direct technical link between regenerated protein fibres and imitation meats formed by manipulation of protein isolates or concentrates. It is far from impossible that many discarded animal protein fractions will be manipulated for feed or food purposes.

Chapter 3

Proteins in Diet

Each species of organism has its own pattern of requirement of diet. That of man was laid down when he was a nomadic scavenger, not particularly suited to the violent combat which would have encouraged him to become a carnivore. His construction was sufficiently flexible for him to find a rich and varied diet under or above water, in trees or up cliff faces, and underground if need be. His freedom of movement introduced more new proteins than were enjoyed by lesser animals and he was able to develop a highly-integrated body chemistry with intelligence and reason at an advanced level. This body chemistry was generated by, and subsequently depended upon, fairly frequent feeding on mixed proteins as found in nomadic scavenging. Carnivores developed digestive systems suited to infrequent overfeeding on flesh protein. Herbivores developed digestions which could handle high bulks of food containing little nutrition per mouthful. Man's development was related to a diet which included a little of everything frequently provided in its most attractive and beneficial form. The mixture contained proteins for tissue building (and for energy if carbohydrates were in short supply) plus a very wide range of other chemicals, many of which had direct association with the proteins as eaten.

When man became a farmer he selected his crops and animals according to the local climate, picking the ones which gave maximum yield for minimum effort. Animals served a dual purpose in that they worked before they were slaughtered. They were, therefore, large strong animals sufficiently docile and stupid to carry loads or pull sledges at more-or-less the walking speed of man. Also, the animals lived on food rejected by man. This favoured the keeping of ruminants which could consume masses of fibrous vegetation. Plants were also dual-purpose in that they provided an edible fraction, which could probably be stored after sun-dehydration, and an inedible fraction of value in housebuilding or the bedding down of men and beasts. Consequent emphasis was on carbohydrate foods which provided grain for storage and straw for bedding down and building. The inevitable norm in agriculture was a grain crop partly for human consumption and partly for support-feeding of animals. This provided a reasonable diet of whole grain and meat, and it can be presumed that man continued to scavenge and hunt in his spare time.

The original date of man is still disputed but at about 2 000 000 B.C. he ate natural vegetation, small game and a fair proportion of discard left by carnivores. At about 400 000 B.C. he graduated to larger game but was still mainly a scavenging animal. Circa 12 000 B.C. he invented bows and arrows, and began to hunt in organised packs. In 9000 B.C., according to the refuse he left at Shanidar, he began to eat more sheep than goats and the proportion of yearling sheep increased from 25% to 60%. The evidence indicates that he was then rearing domestic sheep and killing off the young as required. Southwards to Jarmo, there is evidence that in 6750 B.C. man was using sickles on cultivated wheat. For the record, the wheat was from two strains—emmer and einkorn—which were the originals for the present range. Maize and cattle became part of the picture about 5000 B.C., to be joined in 3500 B.C. by pigs, rice and poultry. The events of importance were the recognition of fire as an agent for making tough meat into tender steaks, the invention of bows and arrows which brought more game into killing range, and the domestication of food sources.

There is no doubt that European diet in the Middle Ages was superior to modern European diet, and can be accepted as responsible for the dynamic activity and population growth of the period. The notable agricultural development was triennial rotation with its extra output of fresh vegetables. All levels of society had more than their needs of first-class protein from cereals and dairy products. In the environment of plenty, diets were planned, as exampled by the records of Champagne leper colonies. Each inmate had a daily ration of three loaves, one cake and one measure of peas. Above the basic rations of bread, oil, salt and onions, there was meat on three days of the week, eggs or herrings on the other days. There are many similar records of excellent diet, and it is interesting to note that expenditure on food by the highest levels of society was only twice that by the lowest levels of society. Most of the expenditure was on food of quality, there being sufficient output for rejection of inferior material, and there being no significant marketing organisation to confuse the buyer. Purchase was of familiar food of high quality.

Records from Trets school show a daily breakdown of:

Calories—2000 plus, mostly from rye bread
Protein—90 g
Fat—65 g
Carbohydrate—475 g
Iron—10 mg
Calcium—400 mg
Phosphorus—2300 mg
Vitamin A—1700 i.u.
      B—10 mg

The school at Trets served meat on 217 days of the year including mutton on 160 days. Eggs were served on 109 days.

With regard to the Middle Ages, it might be mentioned that the period of plenty in Europe was followed by uncontrolled inflation, devaluation of currencies, and a final economic recession leading to bankruptcy in 1343 and 1346 of the leading banks.

With the development of trade, farm production patterns became more specialised and local diets became more related to local crops and animals. A district carrying herds of mammals would develop dairy products whilst an area covered with beans would invent interesting local dishes based on beans. A community near water would learn the art of salting or drying fish, and probably ate fish seven days a week. The world population became fragmented into isolated groups, each of which developed a culture of consumption according to local crops, local storage skill and local climate as an influence on agriculture. One community might protect its animal herds by the imposition of taboos, whilst another community might indulge in an annual 'killing-off' ceremony to save storage grain over the winter. There is some evidence that differences between racial groups arise mainly from variations in diet. The development of trade also brought some mixing of diet by the inclusion of imported food but this concerned only a minor fraction of the population. There was a split in society between primary food producers, eating simple and unvaried meals derived from their own land and labour, and non-productive consumers who diluted local diet with imported food. Then, there was a third class of consumer—the man who lived near agricultural districts but remained a hunter or scavenger, often hunting the reared livestock and scavenging the cultivated grain. The communal need for protection resulted in semi-urbanised communities, bringing legislated social structures and an increased proportion of non-producers in the community. Enclosure reduced the quality of diet but there is no evidence that there was widespread protein deficiency. As a rule in such societies the land was farmed by owner-occupiers and their wives used idle time to grow fresh vegetables.

Protein deficiencies became evident after the introduction of factory processing of food. This brought a demand for reliable mass production of crops, as a rule only possible by large-area cultivation. It was found economic to farm land through managers or through owner-occupiers who would not use land for purposes other than the main farm business. Labour was brought into the fields and was fed little more than a survival diet. There was inevitable protein deficiency caused by over-emphasis on one type of vegetation in diet, not to be confused with other types of deficiency yet to be examined. Much of the protein gap in the world concerns areas where this type of deficiency is evident and where it is vital to introduce new diet.

Factory processing, which initiated mass farming, was made essential by the urbanisation arising from industrial development. Urbanisation is the concentration of people around pockets of raw material or energy, away from their sources of food. An urban community can only exist if it is furnished with a distribution system backed by a storage system supplied by a delivery service using standardised products. For such a chain it is necessary to have factory processing of food and to restrict diet to foods which can be processed and stored and supplied through the distribution system. Low-income consumers are restricted to this deficient diet but high-income consumers can usually find alternative foods carrying higher prices because they do not fit into the system of process–store–sell. For example, fresh liquid milk is a luxury not consumed by the majority of the world's urban population. It is consumed, however, by affluent urban populations who have sufficient purchasing power to justify the establishment of a distribution system for a luxury product. In effect, evidence of urban protein deficiency can be seen wherever there is lack of spending power, either of individuals or of communities, and this deficiency is characterised by low protein intake, not over-emphasis on one deficient protein type. The need in this situation is to improve eating habits by reducing the effective cost of good food (and possibly increasing the cost of poor foods).

Malnutrition varies in character between the impoverished workers in the carbohydrate-rich maize or sugar areas, the low-income districts of industrial cities, the worker compounds where people exist on minimum provision of food, and the affluent regions where diet is unsatisfactory because eating habits are influenced by social activities (including over-consumption of alcoholic drink) and mother's favour bottle-feeding instead of breast-feeding. Although the provision of a satisfactory diet is dictated mainly by the characteristics of the consumer, it must allow for rectification of previous damage to body chemistry and body structure through neglect, particularly neglect during the formative years of development. Furthermore, it needs adjustment to the emotional situation and particularly to the mental stress level at the time of con-sumption. In practice this means using stated requirement levels as absolute minimum values, and overfeeding with substances known to be easy to digest. Then it becomes necessary to remove stresses and to educate the individual so that subsequent diet maintains good health. Above all else, malnutrition is a human problem and not a simple matter of providing a satisfactory amino-acid balance in quantities sufficient to satisfy energy demands and to repair tissue wear and tear.

PROTEIN AS ENERGY

The generalisation regarding energy supply is that a body, according to its characteristics and situation, requires a calculated number of calories, these being nutrition calories equivalent to the energy needed to heat one litre of water through one degree Centigrade, or 1000 times the academic scientific heat calorie. For the record, 1 litre of water weighs 2 lb 3 oz and 1 °C = 1.8 °F. Continuing the generalisation:

1 g of carbohydrate provides 4 calories
1 g of fat provides 9 calories
1 g of protein provides 4 calories

How much of the potential energy value is derived depends on the cooking. A ¼ lb of boiled fish should give about 72 calories from its protein, 10 from the fat and nothing from the carbohydrate because solubles from the protein–carbohydrate fraction are lost in the water. If the fish is fried the solubles are retained and it should give 85 calories from the protein, 22.5 from the held carbohydrate and at least 120 from the augmented fat. Boiled fish adds up to only 82 calories whilst the fried version offers about 227.5. On the other hand, if a constitution rejects the fried food it is likely to derive no energy from the final vomit. If the body concerned needs a high energy intake it will use the protein mainly as an energy-source and little will be used for tissue or body chemistry operation. If, on the other hand, the previous diet is rich in carbohydrate and therefore of energy the protein can be devoted mainly to tissue and body chemistry operation. It is not possible to state exactly what the protein requirements are, although a figure can be given as an approximate requirement alongside adequate carbohydrate and fat, presuming that the body is in fair condition.

To be effective, food needs to be absorbed. It serves no purpose whilst in the digestive tract, which is no more than a tube which passes through the body and is open at both ends. Digestion is the breaking down process by enzymes in the tract, the end-products being capable of being absorbed. Once the breakdown products have passed through the walls of the tract they are subject to the complications of body chemistry.

The mouth is used to apply physical forces to rupture eaten tissue and open the mass for subsequent action by digestive juices. Protein digestion starts in the stomach where the addition of pepsin in hydrochloric acid partly breaks down the protein polymers. On reaching the small intestine the damaged polymers are broken down into their amino acids, which are absorbed. Broadly, the mouth provides initial physical rupture and the stomach starts the breakdown process. The small intestine completes the breakdown and claims the amino acid monomers for reconstitution within the body. The remains pass to the large intestine and are expelled with a content of unused chemicals from the tract, about twenty-four hours after the original meal. A healthy body furnished with good teeth should be able to absorb up to 92% of edible protein. Various tables exist concerning the advised daily allowance of protein; the following is a fair cross-section of the advice:

	Grammes dry weight first-class protein/day
Children—	40 during the first year
	60 from 2 to 6 years
	80 from 7 to 10 years
	100 from 11 to 14 years
Adolescents—	100 to 140 according to size and activity; as a rule more for boys than for girls

Grammes dry weight first-class protein/day		
Adults—	40 to 50 when inactive	
	60 to 80 when engaged in light work	
	80 to 90 when engaged in average work	
	90 to 100 when engaged in heavy work	
	100 to 150 when engaged in very heavy work	
Pregnant women—	About 100 with more in the late stages of pregnancy and when nursing	

This presumes a satisfactory supply of calories, which in itself is a subject of dispute since low-calorie diets have been found to be associated with long life. It could prove valid that energy gained from protein encourages a longer life than energy gained from carbohydrate. The approximations in the table do not take into account the protein needed to rectify faults in body chemistry which may have resulted from previous malnutrition, failures of digestive systems to absorb or digestive juices which are less effective due to previous neglect. Nor does it take into account cooking losses arising from ignorance. The protein needed to bring bodies back to functional efficiency is variable and a subject of medical concern. With the majority of the world population needing attention to diet the only practical approach is to overfeed with a protein which has been selected for its amino acid pattern.

Preservation techniques other than deep freezing are destructive by definition. They are intended to inactivate contained organisms and enzymes which cause deterioration and, since the chemicals to be inactivated are similar to the required protein chemicals there is inevitable damage to the protein substance. In fact, preservation technology mainly concerns methods of controlling destructive processes so that the maximum proportion of undesirables are damaged whilst the minimum of desirables are undamaged. This is very difficult when both materials are proteinic within the same range of molecular weights. With liquids such as milk it is possible to use very fine temperature control on thin films of liquid, as for example UHT processing which damages very little of the milk protein. With solids it is almost impossible to introduce short-term high-temperature techniques and there is damage to all components in long-term lower-temperature cycles. Fortunately for the canning industry, most solid protein needs cooking and it is practical to preserve by cooking in a sealed container. The damage during preservation is no more than that which would occur by cooking the original fresh protein and, in fact, the damage from controlled cooking is likely to be considerably less than that produced by the average housewife-cook.

AMINO-ACID CONTENTS

The amino-acid compositions of the proteins in foods of similar type are not identical but are sufficiently alike for rough classification. Since foods also contain non-protein nitrogen, again fairly constant in proportion for a food group, it is possible to express amino acids in terms of nitrogen rather than in terms of weight or volume of food. This avoids the complications of water and fat content and it allows common examination of fresh, preserved and cooked versions of the same food. As will be seen later there are weaknesses in the calculation of amino-acid content by total nitrogen for foods by groups.

In an affluent society, which can be defined as one in which diet is selected by preference and not by compulsion, roughly half the consumed protein is from animal sources. Roughly a third comes from cereals and the rest is derived from mixed foods. The main variation is vegetarian diet which in some cases means more dairy products and less meat in the fraction derived from animals. A true vegetarian diet appears to follow no common pattern but it can be presumed that it obtains most of the protein from cereals and pulses with compensating amino acids from green leaf and nuts. Fruits can be ignored in protein examination. Masai tribesmen in East Africa have lived entirely on a diet of roast sheep, fresh milk and fresh cattle blood, plus a little fresh fruit. They rarely died from heart failure and frequently walked 100 kilometres in one day without concern. In sharp contrast, some Polynesians live mainly on taro and fish with a fair addition of fresh fruit. The Indians who cannot eat meat rely on rice and chapati made from wheat, with protein derived from dairy products and vegetables. Dahl made from chick peas is important. In Latin America the mixture is mainly maize, cheese and black beans. In Japan the basics are rice, fish and soya, with seaweed and a few other unusual foods providing the essential traces. In the United States of America a meal is incomplete without meat.

The figures in the table are indicative only and cannot replace analysis of food as supplied or in the condition of consumption. It is particularly important to appreciate that high-lysine cereals have been developed and that the groups listed as pulses, green vegetables, nuts and root crops, have many members. The ranges listed are simply intended to give some idea of the orders. Not all the amino acids as listed are available for digestion. As will be seen later phytic acid has to be considered and some proteins are not effectively broken down in the initial chewing for later rupture in the stomach. Taking arginine as an example, wool has about the same potential content as cereals and oilseeds but it is not

---

United Kingdom. Food purchases 1969

Average expenditure £2 per person per week (£1.84 rural to £2.16 urban).
Breakdown in percentages of total:
  Meat 30
  Dairy products 17
  Cereal products 15
  Vegetables 10
  Fruit 8

Quantities in ounces per person per week (Add 4.4 eggs and 4.89 pints of milk per person per week).

Meat (47% of meat purchases were of carcase meat)

Beef and veal	7.70	
Mutton and lamb	5.30	
Pork	2.80	
Liver	0.80	
Other offal	0.50	
Total carcase meat	15.80	
Poultry	4.60	(of which 3.5 was from birds of weight less than 4 lb)
Uncooked ham and bacon	5.10	
Cooked ham and bacon	0.94	
Corned beef	0.58	
Other canned meat	1.85	
Pork sausage	2.40	
Beef sausage	1.30	
Meat pies	0.77	
Quick-frozen meat products	0.51	

Fish	5.46	(of which 0.6 was quick-frozen)

Dairy products

Cheese	3.15	(of which 0.35 was processed)
Butter	6.15	
Margarine	2.80	(total fats including butter and margarine were 11.8%)

Sugar	16.4

Vegetables

Potatoes	49.0
Greens	9.0
Frozen peas	1.1
Tinned beans	3.6
Salads	1.0
Onions	2.8

Fruit (6% of purchases were fresh)

Oranges	3.8
Bananas	3.4
Apples	6.7
Tomatoes	4.1
Canned	4.9
Dried fruit and nuts	1.2

3—WPR * *

g/g nitrogen in food

Possible amino acid	Meat	Fish	Human milk	Cow milk	Eggs	Whole flour	White flour	Rice (white)	Oats	Maize	Barley	Nuts	Pulses	Green vegetables	Root crops
Arginine	0.41	0.36	0.21	0.23	0.40	0.23	0.21	0.50	0.41	0.31	0.31	0.6–0.9	0.3–0.6	0.3–0.5	0.2–0.4
Cystine	0.08	0.07	0.12	0.05	0.13	0.13	0.14	0.10	0.11	0.13	0.13	0.1–0.2	0.06	0.1	
Histidine	0.20	0.13	0.14	0.17	0.16	0.13	0.13	0.14	0.12	0.15	0.12	0.12–0.15	0.1–0.2	0.1	0.09
Isoleucine	0.32	0.32	0.35	0.39	0.36	0.24	0.23	0.29	0.29	0.25	0.24	0.2–0.4	0.3–0.4	0.18–0.3	0.2–0.3
Leucine	0.49	0.47	0.59	0.62	0.56	0.40	0.44	0.51	0.44	0.75	0.43	0.4–0.45	0.45–0.5	0.25–0.4	0.2–0.4
Lysine	0.51	0.56	0.39	0.49	0.42	0.17	0.12	0.19	0.23	0.19	0.21	0.15–0.25	0.3–0.5	0.2–0.35	0.2–0.3
Methionine	0.15	0.18	0.13	0.15	0.19	0.10	0.10	0.13	0.09	0.13	0.09	0.05–0.35	0.03–0.08	0.05–0.15	0.03–0.1
Phenylalanine	0.26	0.23	0.25	0.32	0.33	0.29	0.34	0.30	0.31	0.31	0.31	0.2–0.35	0.2–0.4	0.15–0.3	0.1–0.3
Threonine	0.28	0.28	0.28	0.29	0.33	0.18	0.18	0.24	0.21	0.26	0.23	0.15–0.25	0.15–0.3	0.15–0.3	0.15–0.25
Tryptophane	0.08	0.06	0.10	0.09	0.11	0.08	0.08	0.09	0.08	0.05	0.09	0.05–0.15	0.06–0.08	0.05–0.1	0.05–0.08
Tyrosine	0.21	0.19	0.30	0.35	0.27	0.20	0.21	0.31	0.24	0.24	0.22	0.2–0.25	0.2–0.3	0.1–0.2	0.15–0.2
Valine	0.33	0.33	0.39	0.44	0.45	0.27	0.26	0.41	0.34	0.35	0.31	0.3–0.5	0.3–0.4	0.2–0.35	0.2–0.35
Alanine	0.39	0.38	0.24	0.23		0.21	0.20		0.32	0.62	0.28	0.18	0.16		0.26
Aspartic acid	0.57	0.59	0.58	0.51	0.67	0.31	0.26	0.28	0.26	0.77	0.37	0.4–0.9	0.4–0.55		1.0
Glycine	0.96	0.88	1.24	1.39	0.77	1.73	2.09	0.67	1.15	0.96	1.28	1.2–1.3	0.8–2.0		1.5
Glutamic acid	0.28	0.38	0.14	0.12	0.24	0.24	0.21	0.41	0.26	0.19	0.27	0.3–0.6	0.2–0.3		0.12
Proline	0.26	0.33	0.30	0.36	0.48	0.63	0.73	0.28	0.36	0.52	0.58	0.3–0.4	0.3		0.16
Serine	0.26	0.33	0.30	0.36	0.48	0.30	0.29	0.31	0.21	0.26	0.23	0.4–0.6	0.36		0.17

available. In the table amino acids are listed as fractions of nitrogen contents and it is reasonably simple to discover the nitrogen content of foods as supplied. It is not simple to list such nitrogen contents because the value depends on water content and the proportions of fat, bone, denatured cellulose and any other non-protein. Where protein nitrogen can be divorced from non-protein nitrogen it is practical to multiply the protein nitrogen content by 6.25 to give a protein content. In dairy products it is practical to multiply total nitrogen by 6.38 to give a total protein content and in cereals the total nitrogen should be multiplied by 5.7. As a rule of thumb in most foods the protein content can be taken as 6.25 times the total nitrogen content.

Part of the protein content may be lost in juices running out of the food and certainly protein is lost in soaking or boiling. How much of each protein is lost depends on its solubility and its availability to the water used for soaking and boiling. The intention in cooking is to process the protein so that the digestive system can find soluble protein in the mash reaching the enzymes. An earlier example pointed out that the boiling of fish was likely to lose 15% of the soluble protein. Apart from direct loss of solubles in cooking water, several foods take up water on boiling to give a new final weight and consequently new protein content. Oatmeal multiplies its weight ten times when it becomes porridge and the nitrogen content drops from 2% to 0.2%. When peas are examined the following could apply:

Condition of peas	Weight edible percentage of bought weight	Water percentage	Nitrogen percentage
Fresh raw	37	78.5	0.92
Fresh boiled for 20 minutes	37	80.0	0.80
Dried raw	100	13.3	3.45
Dried soaked 24 hours then boiled for 2 hours	270	70.3	1.11
Split dried	100	12.1	3.54
Split dried soaked 24 hours then boiled for 2 hours	250	67.3	1.33
Canned	100	72.7	0.94

This example shows not only the need to consider the condition of the food when defining the protein content, but also shows the need to relate bought weight to water content and useful weight. If the nitrogen figures are converted to percentages of protein (multiply by 6.25), the dried peas are seen to have about 22% protein before soaking and boiling and 7–8% after. The fresh peas start at nearly 6% and show much the same value after industrial cooking for canning. Household cooking, however, reduces the protein of fresh peas to 5% despite a very slight change in water percentage. With regard to peas it should be added that dehydration converts some of the tissue to a form which is insensitive to water and the protein of dried peas is less available than the protein content of fresh peas.

The uptake of water in boiling has been mentioned and it is obvious that compositions will alter by dehydration in dry-heat cooking. Frying, which in this context can also mean basting, brings a new factor into the calculations—the uptake of fat. In general, proteins are not taken up by fats and the influence of fats on final protein contents is a combination of high-temperature destruction of food components and a change in overall weight after fat has been taken up by the food. Other than up to 0.03% in margarine and up to 0.15% in suet, the nitrogen content of fats can be taken as nil. Fried steak is likely to show a 20% reduction of water content when compared with the original meat, very little change in the protein content but a 60% increase in the available calories. On the other hand the frying of sheep liver is likely to increase its proportional protein by 6% and to double the available calories.

PROTEIN SWEETENERS

There is worldwide excessive consumption of sugar, mostly in urban diet. To provide sweetness without sugar there have been produced a number of synthetic chemicals which offer the necessary stimulation of taste buds. Four such synthetics are familiar:

	Known since	Sweetness times that of sugar
Saccharin (benzoyl sulphonic imide)	1879	500
Dulcin (*para*phenetolecarbamide)	1883	250
Cyclamate (cyclohexylsulphamic acid)	1937	30
P-4000	1946	4100

P-4000 is probably the sweetest synthetic product so far perfected. It is known as Verkade's compound and is derived from dinitrochloro-benzene and an alkali propoxide, resulting in one form of 2-amino-4-nitropropoxybenzene. In 1951, both Dulcin and P-4000 were declared unsafe for humans and the market was left to saccharine and cyclamate. With overlap, saccharine developed as tablets for personal use in tea and coffee whilst cyclamate developed in jams and other prepared foods. About the period 1969–70 the sugar industry and others applied pressure which resulted in a poor image for saccharine and cyclamate. Notably, when rats were fed on 5% saccharine, 35% of them developed tumours. Later, 25% of the rats developed uterine tumours. In another test, when rats were fed on 7.5% saccharine they developed bladder tumours.

The development of tumours with this diet would be almost inevitable. The intake of saccharine equates to a human consuming 500 to 1000 bottles of soft drinks per day, or towards 2 tons of saccharine during a human lifetime. Any body chemistry is likely to reject overdoses of this order, and a tumour is typical rejection.

More recently, amino-acid sweeteners have been synthesised, the claim being that they are 200 times sweeter than sugar. The product is aspartyl phenylalanine methyl ester, filed for acceptance under the name of Aspartame. It is manufactured from aspartic acid, which is amino succinic acid, a common non-essential natural amino acid, reacted with phenylalanine. Phenylalanine is also a natural amino acid, also known as alpha-amino-beta-phenylpropionic acid. Both raw materials can be synthesised but it is probably easier to extract them from protein breakdown products.

More recently it has been realised that the sweetness of ripe fruit may not be entirely due to sugars. The protein in a West African berry, *Thaumatococcus danielli*, has about 1000 times the sweetness of sugar and is thought to be very rich in methionine. Another plant in West Africa of interest is *Dioscoreophyllum cumminsii*, this yielding a protein of perhaps 3000 times the sweetness of sugar.

One interesting discovery is Miraculin, a glycoprotein which is not sweet-tasting but can convert sour foods into sweet foods as far as the tongue is concerned. A long and fascinating list of new products which relate to non-sugar sweetness can be expected. These will certainly include chalcone derivatives from food processing waste. Neohesperidin dihydrochalcone is probably the sweetest, at 1000 times the sweetness of sugar. Hesperetin dihydrochalcone or naringin dihydrochalcone, at 100 times the sweetness of sugar, may have the most commercial potential since they can be produced from waste citrus peel.

There are two probabilities to be appreciated. It could be shown that the tumours in rats, when the rats were overfed with saccharine, were due to the impurity toluene *ortho*sulphonamide. If so, the saccharine industry may yet grow at the rates predicted during previous periods of enthusiasm. The other probability is that sweetness may yet prove to be a result of a deficiency, not the result of a presence. Thaumatin and monellin, the sweet proteins extracted from African plants, both lack histidine.

Chapter 4

Vitamins

Diet provides protein polymers which are broken down during digestion for the purpose of reconstitution. The body therefore builds protein polymers as required but the final proteins cannot, however, function in body chemistry without catalytic agents or associates. These promotional chemicals may be inorganic but most body functions rely on complex organic chemicals which are the vitamins.

The conception of vitamins, as a fifth essential group in diet alongside protein, fat, carbohydrate and minerals, dates from about 1912 and it is not surprising that much is yet to be learnt. In 1915 the vitamins were divided into the A fraction to cover those soluble in fat and the B fraction to cover the water-soluble. As more were revealed they were given further letters of identification. As far as possible, each vitamin has been related to its deficiency indications but, since one bodily complaint is likely to arouse several others the relationship is vague and can be deceptive. Also, although workers try to define specified vitamins as individual substances they are in fact dealing with chemical events which might occur with many chemicals. Hence, it is safer to discuss vitamin-activity, which means ability of a chemical or mixture of chemicals to make a reaction occur.

Vitamin A
Vitamin A is fat-soluble and is derived from animal fat, notably offal fat and dairy fat. However, vegetables supply carotene, which is similar to vitamin A and is converted to vitamin A in the body. In green

vegetables the carotene content is greater as the vegetable gets darker in green colour, indicating some relationship to chlorophyll. Deficiency can occur if diets consist mainly of carbohydrates. Excess vitamin A in the diet can also produce unpleasant results.

Vitamin B

The vitamin B group is extensive, comprising many water-soluble complexes which are frequently found together. They are particularly concerned with the release of energy from carbohydrates but also are essential components in protein reactions and tissue building. The close relationship to amino acids is illustrated by the fact that niacin can be manufactured in bodies from tryptophane, an amino acid, and deficiency of niacin is only of consequence if tryptophane is also missing.

Vitamin C

In the early 1930s, vitamin C was identified as hexuronic acid. It is now known as ascorbic acid and appears to be important as an oxygen carrier. Vitamins A and B are fairly widely spread amongst foods but vitamin C is found in significant quantities only in fresh vegetables and fruit. It is easy to destroy by heating, exposure to light and dehydration (for storage). Solubility in water is high, which means loss in soaking or cooking and the probability of vitamin C reaching the digestive system is low but intake can be supported with tablets or fresh fruit juice. This vitamin is not stored in the body for significant periods and daily excess is lost in urine, but even so, indications of deficiency may not appear for several months.

Vitamin D

Vitamin D is of most importance in the body chemistry of children, particularly in the processing of calcium and phosphorus for bones. As vitamin D it exists in fish and dairy fats but not elsewhere to any useful extent. It can be alternated with a number of chemicals which develop vitamin D activity when subjected to ultraviolet light radiation. The range includes components in skin, which means that bodies can manufacture their own vitamin D if exposed to sunlight. Irradiated ergosterol is a source, the radiation producing at least five isomers, of which two which are mixed are known as calciferol and this has vitamin D activity. More activity comes from irradiated 7-dehydrocholesterol, which is a component of skin. Being fat-soluble, vitamin D can be stored in the body. Deficiency produces soft bones and decay in teeth whereas excess produces general sickness and can lead to death if continued.

Vitamin E

Reproductive functions in animals appear to need vitamin E, which is fat-soluble and found to be at least four different substances of similar chemical structure. The richest source is cereal germ but green leaf can provide a source. The body function appears to be protection of fats and fat-soluble components of fats against oxygen. Deficiency is observed less in humans than in other animals. In cattle it can lead to degeneration of muscles and heart failure and, in poultry to poor hatching of eggs and muscle failure in those which hatch. The importance of vitamin E in the reproduction of animals has been shown following extensive work on rats where deficiency results in sterile males and females.

Detailed examination of all vitamins and their close relatives is not necessary in the present context but *vitamin K* requires some attention. There are at least two forms, one existing in green leaf and the other being formed by micro-organisms. Vitamin K is essential for the formation in the liver of prothrombin, which helps to clot blood and healthy humans can gain sufficient vitamin K from bacteria in their intestines. A newly-born infant has no bacteria in its intestines and is fed on relatively bacteria-free milk, which has very little vitamin K, therefore up to 1% of new infants are slightly deficient in vitamin K and may bleed to excess if cut if vitamin K is not administered. Absorption of vitamin K relies on the presence of bile salts and people suffering from obstructive jaundice, which robs the body of bile salts, may need vitamin K. One of the richest sources is putrid fish but most deterioration bacteria thriving on protein are likely to provide it. Evidently poultry also need vitamin K in their diet.

In recent years, partly because vitamins are too confusing to be classified according to the alphabet, chemicals which catalyse or control body reactions have been given names rather than letters. Vitamin A potency is expressed with differentiation between the actual vitamin and carotene. One international unit of vitamin A is 0.3 microgrammes but there are many carotenoids of varying potency and an adjustment is needed according to the mixture. The carotene content of dairy products and liver can be included with vitamin A because the concentration is low.

Thiamine estimates vary according to the extraction method and are expressed as mg/100 or on a basis of 3 mg thiamine to 1000 i.u. whilst riboflavine is invariably expressed as mg/100 g.

Nicotinic acid includes nicotinamide, co-enzymes and bound forms which make results unreliable. Expression is in terms of mg nicotinic acid/100 g.

Ascorbic acid includes the reduced and the oxidised versions but since the conversion is frequent and easy the expression is of mg/100 g including all ascorbic acid.

Vitamin D estimates use 0.025 microgrammes $\mu(g)$ of vitamin as one international unit. Pantothenic acid is found mainly as a co-enzyme and has to be released before expression as mg/100 g.

Vitamin B6 exists as pyridoxine, pyridoxal, pyridoxamine, various phosphates and some conjugated forms. Expression is as mg/100 g.

Biotin occurs in strongly-bound forms and it is almost impossible to be accurate in estimation. Expression is in terms of μg/100 g. The same is true of folic acid and of vitamin B12.

The tocopherols include four main fat-soluble anti-oxidants and are expressed as mg/100 g.

The estimates for ascorbic acid, thiamine and riboflavine are altered by cooking. Nicotinic acid, vitamin A and D, are more stable under heat but may be lost in cooking water or lost fat. The influence of cooking on other vitamins is not yet fully evaluated but it follows the general pattern of destruction by heat and loss into cooking fluids, these losses varying according to the stability of the vitamin and the conditions of cooking. They can include total loss, as for example of folic acid in fruit when cooked, or can in fact be counted as a gain, as for example of thiamine, riboflavine and nicotinic acid when beef is grilled and consequently loses weight, giving the vitamin content more significance.

Chapter 5

Minerals

Protein reactions are influenced more by minerals than is widely appreciated. There is a valid theory that body chemistry became defined in early marine ancestors and that body fluids need to have roughly the mineral composition of original seawaters. This is supported by the fact that the sodium chloride content of body fluid is self-adjusting to a common norm of about 0.9%, and any variation from this norm brings muscular trouble. Most of the protein reactions originated in the mineral-rich environments of early cell formation and the association of proteins with minerals is inevitable.

Sodium

Adults need approximately 4 g sodium chloride a day and any excess is lost in urine and sweat. Common salt is used as a preservative which limits the pattern of micro-organic attack to halophilic microbes. Such microbes are much safer in the diet than are many other microbial groups, and excess salt in diet is no problem for a healthy body. However, the sodium need not be supplied as sodium chloride and, for example, sodium acetate is used in meat preservation as the acetate inhibits a wider selection of microbial populations. Sodium benzoate is also used as a preservative in some countries but it is thought to have some adverse influence on protein reactions, probably from the benzoate. The bicarbonate of sodium is common in food processing and is used to rectify temporary disturbances of chemical equilibrium in the digestive tract. Sodium bisulphite is used in preservation and in carbohydrate processing. The fact that sodium salts are soluble is used extensively to introduce curative chemicals to the blood stream. It also encourages instant reaction from body sensory organs, as for instance when sodium benzosulphimide (saccharin) is used as a sweetening agent and when sodium citrate is used to give sharpness to flavour in soft drinks and some cheeses.

The safest sodium salts are the various carbonates but these reduce acidity in food compounds (acidity discourages microbial attack), therefore most of the sodium provided is as the chloride. In general, sodium is used as a carrier of substances needed by the body and its direct participation in body chemistry is minor. The gluconate is used to prevent precipitation of iron in alkali solutions. The glutamate, which is a salt of an amino acid, is used to blend flavours in food without adding its own flavour contribution. The nitrite is used to pickle meat but is suspected of producing some damage to body chemistry. The permanganate is absorbed rapidly and can be an antidote for certain toxins such as morphine, curare or phosphorus. The phosphate is used in baking powders and cheese manufacture, as is the pyrophosphate.

This list should suffice to indicate the vast range of sources of sodium, making it unlikely that sodium deficiency can be caused by failure of supply. In addition to the supply of sodium which arises from deliberate inclusion in diet, a further source is derived from the use of soluble salts in washing equipment used by industry. To some extent the body ensures its salt supply by having sensory systems which react favourably to saline flavours.

Potassium

Potassium chloride in the body differs from sodium chloride in that it is held by cells and is not lost as sweat. The retention of potassium is essential and is related to protein operations. Potassium deficiency is common in cases of kwashiorkor, which is a protein deficiency. Fresh meat and fish are not rich in sodium but are rich in potassium and are therefore effective against kwashiorkor, whilst simple balancing of the amino-acid intake may be less effective. The sodium–potassium balance is important to bodily health.

Potassium is frequently regarded as an alternative to sodium, having the same virtue of producing soluble salts, and is frequently considered to be conducive to good health of animals as it is known to be vital for vegetable growth and reproduction. The bicarbonate is used in baking powders to replace the sodium salt or yeast. The bisulphate is used in food preservation, as is the metabisulphite. The nitrate is used for pickling meat and the phosphate is used to improve food value. As with sodium there is no famine of sources but potassium deficiency can occur in societies denied flesh protein and compounded foods which are likely to carry potassium.

Calcium

Calcium like the phosphate is needed for bones and teeth. The problem is that calcium salts are generally not soluble and the calcium in food may not pass from digestion into body chemistry. Proteins and vitamin D help absorption and it is beneficial to supply the calcium alongside protein, as in dairy products and fish, but fats and phytic acid reduce absorption, as do many chemicals producing insoluble calcium salts, notably magnesium sulphate (Epsom salts).

The calcium and magnesium salts of phytic acid are insoluble and if a supplied protein contains too much phytic acid the insoluble salts are deposited in the stomach, with no consequent absorption of the calcium or the phosphorus in the phytic acid. Phytates are extremely stable and pass through digestion carrying their minerals and any other potential nutrition. Phytic acid is an organo-phosphorus compound found in protein foods, notably in cereals, pulses and nuts. It is common to express phytic-acid content in terms of phytic-acid phosphorus as a percentage of total phosphorus, giving a reduction factor for estimation of the useful phosphorus or, alternatively, of the quantity of phosphorus which needs saturation and precipitation by calcium addition during processing.

Phytic-acid phosphorus as percent of total phosphorus			
Brown Bread	55	Soya	31
White Bread	15	Brazil nuts	86
Whole flour	70	Groundnuts	57
White flour	30	Copra	81
Raw oatmeal	70	Raw beans	70–85
Polished rice	61	Boiled beans	5
Rye	72	Raw peas	11
Boiled potato	20	Dried peas	80
Raw turnip and swede	Nil	Canned peas	17

Raw root crops are not the only foods with nil percentage phytic-acid phosphorus. Unfortunately, the foods showing nil are mainly low-protein foods.

Calcium deficiency, whether by insufficient supply or limited absorption, forces the body to extract supplies from the bone structure, leading to failure of the parathyroid gland and failure of the blood to clot. Calcium bromide is used in food preservation as is the chloride. The carbonate is commonly used as an extender and organic calcium salts are fairly common as food additives. The phosphate, frequently in the form of bone meal, is a common mineral supplement particularly in cattle foods. The saccharate has application in preserving and dehydration of milk.

Phosphorus

Phosphorus is not only required with calcium for bone and teeth. As an active participant in body chemistry it influences the rate of extraction of energy from food and it helps to maintain constancy in body fluids. Even with half the available phosphorus unusable because phytic acid produces insoluble phytates it is rare for phosphorus deficiency to arise from inadequate supply, although cattle grazing on poor pasture can show deficiency which needs compensation. It is now fairly common for purified chalk to be added to cereals to compensate for phytic acid, e.g. approx. 0.33% for wheat flour. Previously, it was thought that phosphorus depreciation could be overcome by the provision of inorganic phosphates and that this provided phosphate would increase body energy. A notable example was the German issue of phosphate beverage to soldiers in the 1914–1918 war but following the production of many phosphate-rich energy-giving drinks in subsequent history, it is now known that the provision of supplementary phosphorus does not improve human ability to work or resist exposure.

Iron

Iron deficiency is common, the body needing about 4.5 g per day with significant loss in faeces and bleeding. The main function of iron is in haemoglobin, which uses iron to carry oxygen in the blood.* Two-thirds of body iron is in the blood, each corpuscle lasting about six weeks, after which the iron is used for manufacture of new corpuscles. Some iron is held in reserve in body tissue at a constant level, mainly as ferritin which is a complex protein. Phytic acid inhibits absorption of iron but proteins help absorption, giving a situation similar to that of

---

* Haemoglobin and its relationship to oxygen are of notable importance in the marketing of meat, purchase being mainly related to colour. The conditioning of meat for sale is with the intention of producing exactly the shade of red which housewives consider to represent excellent quality.

calcium. Deficiency of phosphorus or vitamin B6 results in over-absorption of iron but this is rare. However over-absorption did occur in one Bantu society which lived mainly on maize—thereby lacking phosphorus because it was depreciated by phytic acid—and overboiled their food in iron-rich water in rusty vessels. Their iron intake was therefore at least ten times the normal value. There have also been reports of over-absorption of iron from equivalent overdosage of medical ferrous sulphate, but as a general rule, over-absorption is unlikely in a healthy body.

Although up to 20% of contained iron can be extracted by digestion from fresh meat, only about 10% is likely to be extracted from a mixed diet. Contrary to expectation, iron absorption from consumed haemoglobin is low but iron absorption from consumed ferritin is high. Absorption is variable according to:

1. The condition of the body, particularly the level of stored iron in the ferritin and the balance of chemical influences in the blood (including the carbon monoxide content which reduces the efficiency of haemoglobin).
2. Anaemia, which produces an increased absorption of inorganic iron from diet.
3. The chemical combination of the iron in foods and the degree to which the combinations can be broken down in digestion.
4. Phytic acid levels in the diet and the associated level of calcium.
5. Vitamin C, which helps absorption and thereby makes green leaf a valuable source.
6. Protein content, as protein helps absorption.
7. Vitamin B6, or pyridoxin, which restricts absorption and prevents over-absorption.
8. Iron contents of water and cooking vessels used for the food.

Most chemical elements are known to play some part in body chemistry, even if the quantities involved are very small. Calcium, phosphorus and iron dominate the chemistry but they need other elements in their reactions, e.g. magnesium, which is stored as phosphate in bones and is found in blood. The total requirement is small but if it is removed there is early death and there are indications of some vital catalytic influence from magnesium on the iron activity. Fluorine is another element needed in small concentration, mainly by the teeth. Cobalt is a component of vitamin B12 and is concerned as a trace influence on blood carrying efficiency and protein formation for tissue. Iodine is essential for the thyroid gland and is reasonably specific in its function. Zinc, on the other hand, appears to have a comprehensive controlling function and could be catalytic in enzyme reactions.

Sulphur is a component of several enzymes and is derived from proteins in food, more from animal protein than from vegetable protein. It is also found in the vitamins thiamine and biotin, and in insulin, which regulates the sugar content of blood. There is some evidence that onions act as general tonics in diet through their sulphur content.

Doses of metals need not be heavy for them to have influence on body chemistry. Over a century ago it was known that a little zinc was needed for aspergillus to grow well and more recently there has been evidence that very small concentrations of mercury can produce pink disease in children after the absorption of the metal from teething powders. The influence of galvanised waste and mercurial seed dressing on soil compositions is worthy of consideration. It is highly probable that individual bodies differ in their sensitivities and it may prove difficult to relate essential requirements of metals from overdoses. Also, many plants and animals can concentrate metals far beyond requirements or levels normal to their environments. Lead and mercury will concentrate in some woods and cadmium is concentrated by some shellfish. In theory, according to some references, children of humans can concentrate lead in their bones and suffer very little until some other factor causes bodily damage.

Metal-dependent enzymes are important in correct body function. They appear to be highly-specialised chains of amino acids with the metals located in a specific geometric pattern. Many toxins are simply substances for which no such complex molecule exists, which means that the body cannot digest and convert. Other toxins appear to be those which replace the metal in such enzymes, making them useless in the patterns of reaction. The enzymes relating to plasma proteins are associated with calcium, iron and magnesium, whilst protein regeneration is associated with zinc, chromium, nickel and manganese. Manganese is known to inhibit certain aspects of immunity in blood, giving weight to the theory that cups of tea are excellent invalid diet.

Zinc is proving to be more important than was thought. It has association with deoxyribose nucleic acid and ribose nucleic acid. Zinc has been well known in the treatment of skin and surface flesh damage for a long time, although the reasons have never been clear. Platelets and red cells in blood are rich in zinc and most high-molecular weight proteins contain zinc. There could be a specific zinc-containing protein which is concerned with building protein. If so, zinc has importance in studies of malnutrition.

Amongst the enzymes and vitamins which are associated with metals are:

	Metal	*Function Area*
Alcohol dehydrogenase	Zinc	Liver
Alkaline phosphatase	Zinc	Cell formation
Arginase	Manganese and cadmium	Liver
Ascorbic acid	Copper	Teeth, bone and skin
Carbonic anhydrase	Zinc	Lungs
Ceruloplasmin	Copper	
Choline esterase	Calcium	Nerves
Creatin kinase	Magnesium	Muscles
Deoxyribonuclease	Magnesium and Manganese	General
Lactate dehydrogenase	Iron	
Phosphorylase	Magnesium	
Pyruvate kinase	Magnesium	

The one metal which does not appear to have a relationship in enzymes is lead, although there may yet prove to be a link with zoolipase, a fat enzyme.

RADIOACTIVITY

The most serious potential contamination of protein food is not chemical but is radioactivity. A single particle of plutonium, for example one micron in diameter, can lodge in lung tissue and cause cancer. Plutonium 239 has a half-life of 24 000 years. Normal evolution processes had more-or-less cleared the surface of the earth of plutonium before man arrived, but new exposures have come with the recent development of nuclear fission. The radioactivity calculated to cause cancer is of the order of 0.3 picocuries. Bomb tests have released activity to about 300 000 curies of plutonium 239, sufficient to induce cancer in 3×10^{17} lungs. Plutonium 238 is less deadly in that its half-life is only 90 years. Release of plutonium 238 from test explosions has been only 10 000 curies but another 17 000 curies were introduced by a satellite powered by plutonium and allowed to burn out in our atmosphere during 1961. At least two similar satellites have fallen into, or have been pushed into, seawater. Many more have disintegrated outside the atmosphere but within reach of future gravitational pulls.

If plutonium-containing food is eaten it is probable that the particles will pass through the body rapidly. If taken into lungs, however, particles lodge for about one year before moving into lymph lodes near the spine. By then a single particle will have delivered over 100 000 times the safe dose to near-by tissue. The toxicity situation resembles that of snake venom, which is also relatively harmless when eaten by persons without stomach ulcers but is deadly if absorbed or injected. As far as plutonium is concerned, there is still ignorance of the rate of absorption through skin, and of organic chemical reactions which combine the plutonium to form substances capable of passing through the stomach walls. Lead metal is also harmless when eaten but is capable of reacting to form toxic complexes.

Chapter 6

Allergy, Addiction, Preference and Prejudice

With over 3500 million human bodies, each one of which manufactures its own version of an integrated mixture of thousands of proteins under many different circumstances of diet and activity, it is not unusual that some proteins have peculiar constructions. As a rule, the aberrations are of little consequence because they relate to potential reactions outside the pattern of normal body energy derivation and tissue building. Occasional structural alterations open the foreign polymers to attack from chemicals which do not attack standard body polymers. As a result, the foreign polymer refuses to function as it should and it may produce a toxic reaction. Allergy is the hypersensitivity of an organism when falsified body chemicals meet the specific substances which can produce reaction which is not normal for the organism. Each individual organism has a pattern of sensitivity but this is not regarded as allergy if it produces no discomfort or damage. Also, because body chemistry is so complex any body function or tissue can be influenced and any chemical can provide the unfortunate stimulus.

There is an indistinct demarcation line between allergy and poisoning. Allergy in theory concerns a minority of the population whilst poisoning concerns the majority. Both show graduation of reaction which defeats attempts to produce statistics. Both concern protein reactions, partly because protein reactions dominate in body chemistry but also because reaction products containing nitrogen are more likely to be toxins than are products of reactions involving only carbon, hydrogen and oxygen.

The familiar forms of allergy are those which irritate delicate membranes and those which manifest as gastric disorder and associated blood poisoning. In fact, it covers a much wider range and any chemical which does not exist as a normal component in the original new-born infant can cause allergy, although it may not be apparent. Obviously, if a newly-born body reacts to one of its own essential components it will not survive to become adult. This may sound like a long explanation of a relatively simple aspect of life but it is important to differentiate between allergy and aversion or antagonism, which can also produce the symptoms of allergy. True allergy is chemical and can be avoided by removing the source of trouble. Aversion or antagonism is an emotional reaction and is much more complicated.

As mentioned, allergy is personal reaction to toxicity and it can be:

Acute—Single exposure or short-term dose
Chronic—Repeated exposure or long-term dose
Local—Producing reaction at the point of contact
Systemic—Producing reaction elsewhere than the point of contact

Absorption is entry of the offensive chemical into body fluids, notably the blood. It can be through skin, tract lining, membranes or the air sacs of the lungs. Irritation by absorption through the skin mainly concerns washing liquids and solvents used directly on the skin, including cosmetics components. Irritation of the tract lining arises mainly from absorption of water-soluble chemicals, which is why raw egg-white can cause allergy when cooked egg-white produces no reaction. The lungs may be irritated by absorption of a wide range of dusts and fumes, the average adult breathing about 10 cubic metres of air during a working shift when lung contamination is most common. Absorption susceptibility and rates change during the lifetime of the individual and are influenced by many factors. Obesity encourages reaction to solvents, amino-acid deficiency encourages general reaction and indulgence in alcoholic drink also encourages reaction. Systemic reaction occurs after the unwelcome chemical has been absorbed into the blood and distributed. Notable in this context are chemicals which prevent the haemoglobin from carrying oxygen, brain tissue being the most sensitive to oxygen starvation and therefore the first to show results.

An allergic body, probably by inheritance, produces reagins in the blood and deposits them in a specific locality, in effect producing a modified local tissue. When an allergen arrives it unites with the reagin and produces a product of the histamine type. This product affects local tissue, as for example by increasing the permeability of walls of blood vessels to give hives or by irritating the insides of muscle fibres to produce spasms. Allergy may be to a single chemical or to a range of substances which contain similar chemicals. A body may, for example, be allergic to a single identifiable water-soluble protein found only in one shellfish or may be allergic to all pollens or to all feathers. Allergy, therefore, indicates the presence in the body of an unwelcome chemical. Given fully comprehensive analysis most bodies would also show deficiencies, the majority of which would not be of sufficient importance to initiate ill-health but could influence emotional reactions. The mental structure of animals is capable of letting it be known that a requirement exists, but may not be capable of defining the requirement. Standard practice for a body is to answer the request by providing mixed food in the hope that whatever is required is within the mixture. It is reasonably common for the required substance not to be in the supplied food mixture or for the body to be incapable of absorbing it. Hence, the specific hunger continues and can be manifested as a yearning for some specified substance which need have no similarity to the substance needed. Since the hunger is not satisfied, it continues and the body continues to answer appeals by feeding the wrong substance to excess. This is addiction, which is widely mistaken for weak will-power and consequently treated by entirely wrong methods. If addiction is recognised as indication of an unidentified need, it will be appreciated how it can be used in marketing techniques.

Addiction is a sickness but preference is a right. The manipulation of addiction to sell products is immoral and can be justifiably criticised as can be the manipulation of preference. Provided a diet carries the correct mixture of components it matters little how the components are presented, and before the advent of marketing techniques preference depended on the character of the consumer who may have conformed to the wishes of the majority for a safe diet or could have been more selective. However, marketing techniques, based on a study of the character of the consumer, have recently led to manipulation of preference through publicity and the creation of myths and impressions. For example, protein needs in diet can be met by meat or some alternative. There is a widespread preference for meat and those selling bean protein extract capitalise upon this when they texturise the vegetable to imitate meat. Alternatively, fear of early death in a character can be used to profit by the publicised relationship of fatty meat to heart failure, bringing preference for vegetable protein. Conversely, microbial protein can be put forward as mass-produced health food with a hypothetical link between oil derivatives and cancer. The technical attributes of a product have little bearing on preference. Preference depends on the image held by the consumer, partly drawn from past experience but strong influenced by hearsay and the circumstances of visual contact.

Prejudice, on the other hand, is not dominated by character but is an outcome of individual social history. Frequently, as is the case with most religious prejudice, the history reaches back into the period of formation of the society when it was motivated by situations which no longer exist. Early domestic animals were needed more for their pulling power than for their edible protein and objections against the eating of meat were encouraged by tribal law, rather than for reasons such as the fact that excess meat could be a problem in movement or could drain stocks of stored vegetation. The balance of humans to kept animals had to be maintained by regulations enforced by religious laws. Also, with regard to meat, superstition in primitive people made killing an emotive experience and religious leaders used killing events to further their own importance by the imposition of legislation. Other legislation was introduced to standardise food treatment in a social group, partly to prevent unfair consumption but also to ensure that storage and cooking habits which were known to maintain good health would be common to all storing and cooking of food. Also, legislation was laid down relative to eating, partly to prevent private consumption of extra rations but also to cement communal good-will by making eating a social event.

In short, prejudice in diet is a major component of culture and whilst people have pride in their origins they will have prejudice in diet. It is in general harmless, although extreme vegetarianism with ignorance can lead to serious deficiencies and it can be difficult to feed starving communities against an inhibiting wall of prejudice. As a rule, although marketing attempts the manipulation of preferences it accepts prejudice and to some extent encourages it and converts it into areas of preference. Prejudice is thus deeply rooted in culture whilst preference is transitory and available for adjustment.

Chapter 7

Mixtures and Compounds

Urbanisation can be shown to be one cause of reduced variety in diet, and to be the primary cause of food preservation. The divorce of man from fresh food made it essential to establish processing–distributing organisations to provide at least the basic foods. It was desirable, but not always practical, to establish sister organisations to bring in any fresh food which would travel to consumers without excessive spoilage. The first stage was simple preservation based on precooking and enclosure in airtight containers. The subsequent stage was premixing, partly to widen the market but also to allow processing companies to profit from low-cost raw materials. Further stages took more responsibility away from the housewife-cook, the ultimate being modern convenience foods which are precalculated, premixed, precooked, etc., so that the housewife-cook has simply to heat to the required table temperature (predetermined and printed on the package). Recently, it has been realised that much of the malnutrition in famine areas is due to unsatisfactory handling of the food followed by poor cooking. Levels of health and welfare could be vastly improved by introducing factory-cooked meals but, for reasons not clear, projects do not appear to develop.

Reasons for mixing and compounding can be listed as:

1. To allow processing by techniques beyond the ability of house-wives.
2. To reduce product cost by bulk buying and a reduced degree of discard.

3. To reduce product cost by dilution.
4. To offer a balanced meal.
5. To introduce a new food into established market sectors or to introduce an established food into new market sectors.
6. To avoid contamination, infection and infestation.
7. To convert the food into a form suitable for storage and travel.

The compositions are mainly invented by the processing company. To avoid air pockets in solid foods it is common to mix the solids with liquids (or gels which are liquid at the time of compounding and filling). This gives rise to fish in oil or sauce, fruit in syrup, meat in gravy, etc. To a limited extent, air can be removed by granulation and compression of solids but the standard procedure is to discover a compatible liquid in which the solid can be delivered. The liquid fraction of a mixture is almost essential to distribute the applied heat when cooking is used as the preservation technique. As a general rule, such heating is only sufficient to kill contained organisms which could cause trouble under the anticipated conditions of storage and travel. If an organism in the food is unlikely to cause trouble, or would cause trouble only if the food reached improbably high temperatures, then it is liable to be ignored in processing, being given insufficient heat treatment for destruction before passing through to the consumer. Obviously, no manufacturer will risk his market by shipping dangerous microbes with his product but there is no point in using excess heat for the sake of harmless microbes. To kill all known germs, which are protein, would necessitate using sufficient heat to destroy protein, which would spoil the product. Hence, the heat input is only that required to inactivate unwelcome microbes and it is essential that heat-treated protein foods are not stored at elevated temperatures, in which thermophilic microbes might develop.

The development of infections is inhibited by the inclusion of chemicals, notably halogen and nitrogen derivatives. It is further inhibited by adjustment of acidity, the pH value dictating which groups of microbes are capable of thriving. In brief, the protein in a compound is preserved by:

1. Reducing the oxygen content to an absolute practical minimum.
2. Adding inorganic chemicals.
3. Heating any microbes which are likely to survive the airless chemical environment and still be capable of damage to consumers.

In general, processing and compounding in bulk preserves more of the quality of the protein food than does normal household cooking. There is some danger of excess mineral addition and it is not unusual for compounds to suffer the wrong storage and handling, leading to deterioration within containers but as a rule, any deterioration is obvious although it need not be so.

Chapter 8

Preservation

The early populations of the land mass stretching across Europe and Asia developed many local preservation systems. In the extreme north it was common to freeze meat and there is an unconfirmed rumour that an unfortunate Siberian mammoth was edible after countless years locked in supercooled ice. In the hotter climates there was widespread use of spices and in the intermediate climates there was use of sun drying.

HERBS AND SPICES

Spices are known to have been used to preserve human flesh in mummies, in association with dehydration and waxing. Most of the spice technology of ancient times was, however, concerned with food preservation and the masking of unpleasant flavours in food which had high food value but low flavour acceptance. Notably this concerned Asiatic tropical food, which needed a fungicide, but European consumers needed strongly-flavoured chemical preservatives to mask offensive odours and to allow preservation of meat over hard winters. In the twelfth and thirteenth centuries most European farmers killed off meat other than breeding stock, ate very well during the autumn through a succession of pagan and christian festivals, then endured unavoidable fasting until the new lambs were born. The lambs born dead initiated a further succession of festivals, suitably associated with fish supplies as soon as boats were able to brave the local seas. Spices allowed the carrying over of killed meat, and were consequently much sought after. Pepper was sold by the number of corns and a sack of pepper was worth the life of a man. A pocketful of ginger was worth a sheep and a pocketful of mace was worth half a cow. Cloves were particularly valuable, containing eugenol which is still recognised as a powerful antiseptic. Eugenol is 4-allyl-2-methoxyphenol and is the effective component in cloves, cinnamon and bay.

Ginger contains citral, which is also to be found in lemon grass. It also contains borneol, which is a component of camphor, and phellandrene. The virtue of ginger is its attractive combination of flavours, which will hide unpalativity in almost any protein.

Mace is the outside of nutmeg seeds and contains pinene, which is one of the substances in pine products used as insecticides and antiseptics. There is also phellandrene, a monocyclic terpene found in many preserving strongly-flavoured vegetables including eucalyptus and some mints. Phellandrene is one of the effective components in peppers. Mustard relies mainly on a lethal-sounding mixture of sulphur derivatives and allyl cyanide, which is listed as highly toxic.

There is biblical reference to myrrh, which is an antiseptic gum or resin. Academic myrrh is from *Commiphora myrrha* but any vegetable with myr in its identification, including nutmeg (*Myristica fragrans*), is likely to deliver a product which has been, is or will be described as myrrh.

Spices function as preservatives because they contain toxins of sufficient power to inhibit micro-organisms. There is a reasonably-delicate balance between sufficient spice to preserve and sufficient spice to cause damage to consumers. The incidence of cancer amongst curry-eaters is high, although this does not by necessity mean that curry causes cancer. The foundation of a curry powder is *Curcuma longa*, a rhizome which is also responsible for turmeric and saffron. In the mixture is turmerol, about which little appears to be known. There is also valerianic acid, which is one of the many aliphatic combinations of $C_5H_{10}O_2$. One can also find capronic acid, or butylacetic acid in disguise, and phellandrene.

There is strong opinion that traces of toxins, as provided by spicy preservatives, are essential to good health. Ancient Egyptians purged their bodies every month to clean out infections taken with the food. It could well be that periodic intakes of toxins are valuable to seek and destroy traces of dormant infections in body tissues, and that the modern search for purity in food is a serious mistake.

Herbs, which are associates of spices, are inferior preservatives but are excellent maskers of flavour. They also have historic recognition of curative properties, and occasional mystical influences. The recognised curative properties include: *Basil*—cures indigestion and repels flies; *Bay*—takes the pain out of rheumatism (and reveals the identity of lovers to maidens on St. Valentine day); *Borage*—cures almost any complaint but notably benefits the lungs and the kidneys. The Greeks used it to induce forgetfulness when taken with wine; *Camomile*—cures indigestion, toothache and nightmares; *Chervil*—cleans the blood and cures bruises; *Chives*—are antidotes for some poisons, or were some 2000 years ago in China; *Fennel*—slims down fat people. Cures inflamed eyes and smooths skin; *Hyssop*—helps to digest fat. Cures nasal congestion; *Marjoram*—cures hay fever and bruises; *Mint*—cures almost any complaint and improves the complexion; *Parsley*—cures indigestion and rheumatism; *Rosemary*—cures headaches and nervous tension. Greek students wore rosemary crowns during examinations; *Sage*—is a universal cure for all ills; *Savory*—takes the pain out of stings; *Tarragon*—is a general medicant; *Thyme*—is antiseptic.

The curative powers of herbs have scientific recognition, particularly with regard to a few such as thyme. Thyme contains thymol (isopropyl metacresol) which is known to be effective as an antiseptic in gargles and mouth washes.

Broadly, the spices are important to protein foods in that they preserve by the introduction of toxins which are effective against bacteria and fungi. The herbs are important to proteins in that they mask flavours and convert unpalatable protein into delighting food. Collectively, and without strict definition of function, they extend the range of protein foods which can be used by man.

DEHYDRATION

If sufficient moisture is extracted from a tissue, micro-organisms find it impossible to thrive and insects seek more-attractive diet. In a relative humidity below about 70%, such a dehydrated tissue will have a long storage life if isolated from rodents and birds. Hence, dehydration developed as a storage technique along the arid corridor between wet tropics and wet temperate regions. History is concentrated around ancient Egypt and grain but the technique was familiar for other products. Followers of Genghis Khan sun-dried milk from their mares, reconstituting the lightweight powder when needed to wash down the raw meat pounded to tender perfection under a saddle during a full day of travel. Turkey has a historic Tarhana, which is sun-dried soured milk previously mixed with flour and assorted vegetables, and which is the origin of modern dehydrated soup powders. The tarhana was convenient to carry and could be converted to excellent soup by boiling a few minutes.

CANNING

Short-term extra storage life for food is possible by cooking to destroy contained enzymes and frequently to provide a hard baked skin on the outside of the food. The extra shelf life can be improved by providing a deliberate outer skin, as for example by covering with baked pastry or clay or wax. In the 1790s, French armies were fighting in most parts of Europe and were being destroyed, not by human enemies but by the deficiencies of a diet of smoked fish, salted meat and insanitary cereal compounds. The French government offered 12 000 francs for a preservation system for food and Nicolas Appert decided to win the prize. Knowing nothing about enzymes, but having long experience of food and fermentation, he took 14 years to invent food cooked in sealed bottles.

In 1809, Appert used his prize money to start a canning operation. In 1847, mass-production of cans became common and by the time of the American civil war both sides could use canned food as a means of maintaining fighting fitness.

REFRIGERATION

It could be that 50 000-year-old steaks were cut from a discovered frozen mammoth, and were enjoyed by the discoverers. It is more probable that, in the temperatures involved the meat would suffer toughening from a rapid chill, apart from toughening of the meat from the effort needed by the living mammoth to survive in a barren cold place.

It is well known that the Romans had cold stores using snow and ice brought down from the mountains in straw packages. In post-Roman Europe it was fairly common for rich landowners to have a private cold store. This was, as a rule, brick-built with an air-gap between the walls and with a single small door. Over the winter period, snow would be packed in the store and stamped down hard. A relatively small volume of cavity would be left to hold the master's delights. It is said that a temperature of zero to 5 °C was maintained through the summer and until new snow could be introduced.

In the early nineteenth century there were sufficient domestic wooden insulated ice-boxes for an industry to exist relative to the supply of ice. The ice was cut in winter and stored in warehouses through the summer. In the mid-nineteenth century there was the invention of mechanical refrigeration, which helped the ice-merchants to reduce storage volumes. During the 1920s small refrigeration units were developed, leading to domestic refrigerators. In due course, this led to the design of high-efficiency small-volume deep freezing boxes, mainly to serve the ice cream industry but responsible for the subsequent development of home freezers.

Chapter 9

Canning

Tin cans were designed to be functional—that is, to contain food for long periods without puncture or interaction of the can and the contents. Appearance and consumer convenience played little part in design and to a large extent the needs of those shipping and storing were ignored. Development was concentrated on rates of filling and handling by the supplier of the packaged product, leading to a very close relationship of the tinplate and food manufacturing industries but a very wide gap between the tinplate industry and the retailer or the ultimate consumer. Over the past twenty years there has been serious effort to close this gap between the tinplate industry and the ultimate consumer, bringing innovations such as the slimline can and tear-off systems of opening.

The traditional tinplate can with soldered seams is still the most common for low and medium-acid food, which means processed protein foods. Other than in the introduction of easy-release silicone lacquers for solid meat products there have been improvements only with regard to the can ends. These include integral forming by drawing and the use of ring-pulls or other tear-off systems. Aluminium tears better than steel whilst steel is more rigid than aluminium for the body. Hence, bi-metal systems are favoured but it is possible to have all-steel or all-aluminium tear-off systems. At the time of writing all-steel easy-opening cans are used for soups and meat products, all-aluminium easy-opening cans are used for pâté and shellfish.

It is probable that soldered seams will give way to thermoplastic bonded seams and that, subject to the price of tin metal, plastic seams will be associated with tin-free steel. Tin-free steel at present means steel with a chromium–chromium oxide coating down to one-millionth of an inch, rating against exposure being equivalent to a tin coating at least thirty times as thick. It is claimed that adhesion of lacquers is better to tin-free steel than to tinned steel but, of course, solder can not be used without a tin layer. There are developments of welded seams, mainly in beverage cans, but the significant development is probably drawn and ironed cans. For these, a cup is drawn from a blank with profiled wall thickness. Hence, whereas the wall of a standard can may be a uniform 6.5 thousandths of an inch (thou.), the wall of a drawn can could vary from 12 thou. at the base to 4.5 thou. at the wall and up to 7.5 thou. at the flange. The obvious next stage of development is the wedding of drawn-and-ironed cans to easy-opening ends.

CANNING SEQUENCE
A typical sequence in canning protein food is:

    Food preparation
    Filling
    Vacuum extraction of air and possible gas flushing
    Closing and sealing
    Heating to a controlled pattern
    Cooling at a fixed rate

The food is prepared in much the same way that an efficient house-wife might perform but discarded fractions are smaller and the use of machinery helps to reduce preparation loss. Filling may be manual or on sophisticated machinery, either with full premixing or by placing large solids in the cans and running liquid in. An air space of 6–9 mm above the food in the can is normal. Overfilling can expand the can during subsequent heating and underfilling is a waste of space. The rate of heat penetration subsequently depends on the solid : liquid ratio and the sizes of solid chunks or granules, making it vital to fill with a constant mixture and to ensure that air pockets are not left in the solids.

The common technique for vacuum extracting is to pass the can through a steam chamber for 10–40 mins, replacing the air in the can by steam. The can is then sealed and cooled, leaving a vacuum in the previous air space. Cans filled with hot foods may not need the air space and vacuum extraction. More recently, the slow passage of the can through a steam chamber has been replaced by steam injection using superheated steam, but this method does not remove air from the depths of the mass. Another system of extraction, useful for cold-sensitive products, is direct application of a vacuum derived from pumps, but the equipment for direct extraction is expensive and the process is slow although the technique has value in canning some meats.

After closure, the cans are heated to destroy microbes which are likely to develop in the food under anticipated conditions of storage and travel. For canned fruits, which are acid, heating may be in hot water only. For meats, fish and other proteins which are not acid it is necessary to use steam heating. It is common to cook protein in an autoclave at 110–125 °C (0.42–1.34 kg/cm² above atmospheric), from 20–90 mins. The steam pressure in the autoclave compensates for the pressure inside the cans as they heat up. Cooling must, therefore, be conducted with care to avoid damage to the cans as the pressure eases. The cans are cooled down to about 37 °C using chlorinated water as a precaution against inevitable but very infrequent leaking cans since cans cooled in river water have been known to carry infection to the consumers.

The most heat-resisting spore likely to be found in protein food, and likely to be a danger to consumers, is *Clostridium botulinum*. This bacterium is now accepted as a standard enemy to be destroyed in processing. Destruction is relative and is according to the heat input and the acidity, the heat resistance of cells and spores being lower in acid conditions. If a non-sporing bacterium such as *Aerobacter aerogenes* is heated to 55 °C its population would be reduced to 10% after 2 mins, to 1% after 4 mins, to 0.1% after 6 mins and so on. The time period to reduce the population to 10% is the decimal reduction time. For the sporing bacterium *Clostridium sporogenes* the decimal reduction time at 115 °C is about 3.5 mins, but this varies with the pH and chemical composition. Not only are the harmless microbes ignored in processing but the harmful microbes are not completely destroyed, although the traces remaining are unlikely to do damage to healthy bodies.

The influence of pH values on microbe survival results in division of canned foods into those above pH 4.5 and those below pH 4.5. Meat, fish, milk and a few vegetables are at pH 5.0 or higher, and need intensive heat treatment. Meat and vegetable mixtures are mainly in the pH 4.5 to pH 5.0 range and require less heat. Below pH 4.5 are the fruits, which are not protein foods, and below pH 3.7 are those products with added vinegar and citrus fruits. Bacteria which cause food poisons are unable to develop below pH 4.5 but a few fungi and the bacteria producing lactic acid can thrive below pH 4.5.

5—WPR   *   *

Heat is applied for the thermal death time, which is the period at the stated temperature for 12 decimal reductions to occur. Hence, the thermal death time for *Aerobacter aerogenes* at 55 °C is 24 mins and for *Clostridium sporogenes* at 115 °C is 42 mins. The vegetative cells of bacteria and fungi are destroyed at 100 °C for a few minutes, as in hospital sterilisation. Spores are more difficult and may take hours at 100 °C, calling for an acid medium so that death rates can be accelerated. Common wine yeasts are destroyed in seconds at 75 °C, contrasting strongly with some species of penicillium which can survive long periods even in an acid medium. Taking *Clostridium botulinum* as the main enemy in proteins, this shows a death time of 6.5 hours at 100 °C but only 2.7 mins at 120 °C. This is within the limitations of cooking meat without breakdown of the protein but there are occasional spore-formers which are more dangerous than the standard enemy. *Bacillus stearothermophilus* needs 30 mins at 121 °C and this heat treatment will spoil protein.

There can be problems in the satisfactory heating of the inner depths of a solid protein mass and it is not uncommon for the required temperature to be not reached in all locations within one hour in an autoclave at 115 °C. Canning technologists appear to have selected 121 °C as a temperature to be used in thermal discussions, which can become very complicated in their variation of temperatures and times, particularly when pH and lethal coefficients are involved. Most canning operations are likely to leave some thermophilic organisms in the product. These will not develop in anticipated circumstances but may develop in careless high-temperature storage. Nor do they develop in compounds with 3.5–4% sodium chloride and up to 20 p.p.m. nitrite. Nitrite with protein results in some unidentified complex which inhibits spores, and also reduces the heat input required to kill spores. However, some spoilage can be expected even with salty compounds with nitrite and this can be with or without gas formation. As a rule, spoilage arises from damage to the can and is with gas formation, although it can arise from unsatisfactory heat treatment and then is likely to be:

1. Flat sour spoilage from bacteria which manufacture acid but not gas from any carbohydrates in the compound.
2. Gassy spoilage from some bacteria but more probably from clostridia, the main evidence being a cheese or sour milk odour.
3. Putrefaction arising from clostridia breaking down compounds containing sulphur, the evidence being hydrogen sulphide gas. Fish

and meat may form volatile sulphur compounds without the attention of microbes.

The thermophilic bacteria which cause most of the spoilage in canned protein include:

Type of spoilage	Bacteria	Optimum temperature °C
Flat sour	*Bacillus stearothermophilus*	50–65
	Bacillus coagulans	28–40
Gassy	*Bacillus subtilis*	28–40
	Bacillus cereus	28–32
	Bacillus megagherium	28–35
	Bacillus macerans	28–40
	Bacillus polymyxa	28–35
	Clostridium thermosaccharolyticum	55–62
	Clostridium perfringens	35–37
	Clostrium butyricum	30–37
Putrefaction	*Clostridium sporogenes*	Approx. 37
	Clostridium hystolyticum	Approx. 37
	Clostridium nigrificans	Approx. 55

ALTERNATIVES TO TIN CANS
There are many technical, but few commercial, rivals to tin cans for general protein food handling whilst precooking is the favourite method of preservation. New processing techniques and changes in market patterns could encourage alternatives, as could further rises in the price of tin metal. The alternatives to be appreciated are glass, plastics and aluminium thick foil.

Glass is in general too heavy to be economic for distribution and the sensitivity to thermal shock makes it a slow material in processing. However, the clarity of glass is an advantage in marketing but this applies only to decorative foods and most protein foods are not decorative, therefore the main development of glass containers is likely to be in conjunction with the marketing of fruit.

Plastic sterilisable flexible pouches exclude microbes but not oxygen, although recent laminates have sufficient barrier performance to give contained food a reasonable life. The pouches were explored during the 1960s but were neglected by food manufacturers until tin prices increased, although recent rises in plastics prices have removed the initial price advantages of pouches. Most laminates are three-component in structure—one layer for strength, one for oxygen exclusion and one to act as a sealing layer by welding. The heat-sealing layer can be adjusted in strength to become a peeling bond, allowing opening of packages by simple pulling apart. A common laminate is polyester or nylon for strength, PVdC for the gas barrier and polyethylene or ionomer for the heat-sealing. Filling speeds of 40/min are common and the indicated market is at such medium-filling rates—half-way between hand-filling of jars and automated rapid-filling of cans.

Thick aluminium rivals plastics and it has superior barrier performance, being an absolute barrier with undamaged foil. As a rule, the foil is coated both sides with one coating acting as a heat-sealing layer, sealing being possible through the food. In effect, aluminium foil can be used for packages which are filled completely and will then exclude all contamination, which can be taken as superior to the possibilities of plastics or cans. Sealing by cold-folding or crimping is also possible with aluminium and there is no practical limitation to filling speeds.

The subject of rivals to cans is well-documented and need not be repeated in this book, but the main consideration in choice is cost relative to performance and filling conditions, and any package is a rival to tin cans for short-term storage.

Part 2

Animal Proteins

Chapter 10

Meat

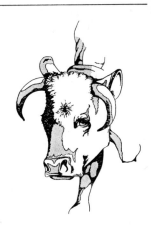

PRODUCTION EFFICIENCY

Recorded annual meat-output in the world is of the order of 100 million tons with an associated output of 10 million tons of dairy protein. On a basis of 20% dry protein for meat, total world land animal protein including eggs and offal is towards 35 million tons dry weight or 10 kg *per capita*/year, to which can be added perhaps another 5 kg of fish. As a source of edible protein, meat by conventional rearing is not efficient, using about three diet calories to gain one growth calorie. The inefficiency is however justified because the diet calories used can be, and should be, of a form unsuitable for direct consumption. Hence, local supplies of meat depend mainly on availability of feed unfit for humans, of which grass is probably the most important. Rearing animals can be regarded as a system of converting poor-quality food products into first-class protein with a balanced amino-acid pattern in which myogen, myosin, globulin and stroma proteins are particularly valuable. There is also a less-valuable fraction, for example gelatin, which lacks tryptophane and is more valuable as a binding agent than as a food. The conversion system uses two classes of animals:

Ruminants—which have digestive systems capable of dealing with high levels of roughage and low levels of nutrition in feed, and have rumens which allow internal production of microbial protein from a range of substances including urea.

Scavengers—which have no distinctive advantages in their digestive systems but will accept food rejected by humans and can therefore be used to convert reject and waste. They also glean food from places where harvesting for human diet would be impossible.

The animal population is therefore divided into those species which are herded over pasture to consume high quantities of vegetation, and those species mainly confined and fed richer food. The division is indistinct mainly because modern farming methods involve the feeding of high-quality protein-rich substances to animals designed for low-quality feed, and restrict the movement of animals which interferes with the energy-conversion factors in digestion.

The ratio of energy-input to protein-output is difficult to define and calculate. Cornell University studied the subject and produced a list including probable human effort, supplied fuels, etc. in the input, all of which vary according to the location and organisation of production. Broadly, meat requires up to fifty times more input per weight of protein produced than do other common protein sources, although free-ranged herds requiring no more than supervision and slaughter need much lower energy-inputs than rearing under intensive conditions, and protein from horticulture obviously demands more input than that from large-area mechanised farming of arable crops. The ratio therefore depends on how much input can be gained from nature and how much has to be supplied by the farmer. It is important to appreciate this when evaluating industrial sources of protein, in which almost all the energy-input after the initial supply of plant and equipment comes from self-regenerating microbial activity.

Man uses only a very small fraction of available animals, having developed agriculture during a period of excess supply in which he could select his animals according to demands for food or the ability of animals to provide carrying or dragging strength. It has now become essential to widen the selection to include any animal species which can provide food. For reasons of preference and prejudice it is difficult to introduce many new animals into the meat market for direct consumption, but it is not difficult to include them in manufacturing and possibly in the extraction of purified protein for compounding. Nor is it difficult to use unfamiliar animals for animal feed as replacement for the conventional fishmeals. With regard to the direct consumption of meat, a number of trends and attitudes have to be respected. There is prejudice against animal fat as a potential cause of heart failure and there is a growing need to standardise meat as far as possible for the sake of easy handling and undemanding cooking. There is also now more acceptance of processed and compound meat and wider appreciation of foods which have been previously cooked, subsequently frozen and require the minimum of culinary effort to become attractive meals. Therefore the growth area in the meat market is in the production of compounds, mainly because compounding reduces the proportion of waste per beast and it allows the supplier to use sophisticated methods of handling. In theory, this should produce a much lower retail price for the meat but in practice there is no significant price reduction for the consumer. Compounding can be either wet or dry, the wet compounding using a wide range of additives and the dry compounding using mainly cereals or soya. In the United States dry meat compounding accounts for about 15 000 tons of soya/year, which is not high and does not represent the full market for meat–soya combinations.

PRE-PACKAGING

The handling of meat has not changed much since man first killed reared beasts for distribution amongst his neighbours. The proportion of beast not sold as meat is roughly 30%, of which half is lost during rough division and the other half in trimming for retail sale and cooking. The trimming proportion varies according to the fat and bones acceptable by the customer but a fair comment is that only one-third of live weight arrives at the table as muscle meat.

Some 20% of the total loss is inevitable by the extraction of skin and other inedible fractions, although these components have value other than in direct cooking. Roughly 10% of total loss is from drying out, contamination and rancidification of fat. The two-thirds of the beast which is eaten as meat can be roughly divided into half for the table and half for processing including manufactured products for the table.

Moving abattoirs to the beasts, instead of siting them near population concentrations, could save about 5% of carcase weight. Early division, even if only into primal cuts, could save up to 8% loss of weight during hanging. On the other hand, airtight sealing of cuts in bags at an early stage could result in false conditioning with consequent loss of value and possible loss of weight by rejection. It is essential that the correct amino-acid pattern develops in conditioning to tenderise the meat, and that oxymyoglobin development is kept below 60% or there will be a dull colour.

Cutting the carcase whilst hot is said to be almost impossible, which makes it difficult to control the cooling of carcases by division into evenly-sized blocks. The ideal system would be to cut into primal joints at the time of slaughter, followed by controlled chilling and freezing. The alternative under examination is to reduce the carcase to 1–2 °C at a rate which does not produce cold-shortening, then cut and store at the low temperature but not frozen, with the oxygen removed to prevent fat and blood oxidation. This is said to be economic at 30 000 tons per year or more but it is suspected that the economic level could be much less. There is justification for combining primary cutting with trimming and then sealing cuts in oxygen-starved atmospheres, although this system needs a sophisticated distribution network in which consumers will accept pre-packaged, pre-cut and pre-valued meat.

In the United States about 90% of retailed meat is pre-packaged but most countries pre-package less than 10%. The main difference between USA and other markets is that the Americans waste less meat up to retailing but more after the meat reaches the table. Up to 50% of USA meat reaching retail distribution is now vacuum packed, which is probably nearing saturation point insofar that even in the USA there is a significant fraction of the population requiring direct vision of meat before purchase and claiming the right to select joints or cuts relative to observed value.

Meat is mainly selected by impulse according to its colour, whether seen directly or through clear film. The important reaction is oxidation of myoglobin to oxymyoglobin, converting the ferrous iron content to ferric iron sufficient to give the shade of red which consumers associate with good meat. Vacuum packaging or the use of an inert gas deprives the meat of oxygen, slows down the production of oxymyoglobin but allows the production of metamyoglobin, which dulls the colour and causes the meat to become 'dead' in appearance. It is also possible by oxygen starvation to produce false biodeterioration in which unusual microbes become active, giving a green colour which converts the natural red to a muddy brown.

In effect, the supplier can cut his weight-loss by pre-packaging as soon after slaughter as is possible but he can incur sales-loss if the pre-packaging depreciates the meat. Pre-packaging is being forced on suppliers by the need of self-service stores to have a form of meat which can be handled under their conditions, which includes the disturbing fact that almost two-thirds of retailed meat is bought on the last two days of the week. Hence, if the packaging system cannot give satisfactory life to fresh (chilled) meat it needs to be organised on a weekly-batch programme, which is not economic. Suppliers therefore encourage self-service outlets to concentrate on frozen pre-packaged meat which can be supplied ex-store on a regular basis.

United States distribution is not typical but the organisation in the United Kingdom resembles that in most developed countries. In the United Kingdom, 70% of beef consumed is near 900 000 tons passing through wholesalers. Farmers sell 40% direct to wholesalers and 60% through auctions. The wholesalers supply 45% to public abattoirs and 55% to private abattoirs. The resultant dead meat combines through wholesale dealers, who supply 65% to meat markets and 35% to consumers direct. Retailers get 95% of the final meat. Hence, the bulk of meat passes from farm to auction to beast wholesaler to abattoir to meat wholesaler to retailer to consumer. Throughout this long journey the bone and other waste is carried at high cost (£4/ton has been quoted but it could be higher) and has no longer an outlet in retail sale since the population became reasonably affluent. More serious perhaps, there is multiple addition of profits along the chain and the final retail price does not relate to producer prices. In the United States at least a quarter of meat is vacuum packed at the time of slaughter, or at least as soon as the carcase has cooled and conditioned. This is possible because 90% of the meat is sold through self-service outlets whereas in the United Kingdom and similar markets the sale through self-service is probably 15–20% only.

Losses in retail distribution include dehydration in open display but the main loss is rejection after contamination or decay. Contamination is inevitable in open display and most traditional butchers use the contaminated meat for low-price or free issue to pet-owners. Most of the contamination is visible and, in fact, is likely to cause harm but is obviously a cause for rejection.

Decay in organised open display should be minimal if the retailer knows his market and can organise his supplies accordingly. The common problem is that retailers cannot obtain skilled labour which can relate cutting to the market pattern and it is becoming imperative for retailers to sell pre-cut meat to a stated pattern of cuts which is unlikely to coincide with the cuts from a delivered carcase. If he accepts the meat in carcase form he is left with unwanted cuts which will develop decay if not used. During periods of inflation the unwanted cuts are likely to be those with high prices and the retailer is faced with the need to use top-quality meat for mince or sausage which he must sell at low prices. Retailers cannot afford to have meat in stock or on display with signs of decay or discoloration.

Decay of pre-packaged meat in retailing arises mainly from the need to advertise the quality of the colour by using warm lighting. This lighting is rich in infra-red, which is absorbed to increase the temperature of the rich red meat, the influence being more when the meat is trapped inside clear film. One point to appreciate is that the film may be selected for its ability to transmit the red colour of the meat, which means that it will also transmit the infra-red light. The United Kingdom Meat Research Institute found a temperature difference of up to 12 °C between the exposed and unexposed parts of a display cabinet or, to be more specific, found temperatures of 12 °C in cabinets supposed to hold the meat at 0 °C. A difference of 10 °C could quarter the shelf life of the meat and it can be presumed that some meat remained in the warm display when the store closed overnight.

MAMMALS AS A SOURCE OF PROTEIN

In his development of a meat supply, man has concentrated on mammals, mainly because they conveniently feed their own young and provide incidental milk for humans, and also provide very useful hair, which can be flayed from the beast as a tough, waterproof, warming layer. Mammals have warm blood and inherent thermostatic control which allows the animals to thrive in extremes of temperature and has contributed to their domination in most environments. The arctic fox, for example, can maintain its body heat in temperatures down to −80 °C. Whereas the echidna is able to vary its body temperature between a range of 22–36 °C. Other mammals are able to drop their body temperature to slightly above freezing during hibernation. However, for most mammals there is a constant blood temperature and a constant outflow of vitality regardless of the atmospheric temperature. This is achieved by their ability to adjust their body temperature by internal heat production or surface heat loss by evaporation. This constant body temperature has allowed the development of delicate reactions within the body, notably brain reactions which result in superior logic and memory. The ability of beasts to learn and obey was used by early man when he used his potential meat for temporary labouring duties, further encouraging the selection of mammals.

Mammals are not a large class numerically. There are probably three-quarters of a million species of insects as compared with only 50 000 species of vertebrates. Of the vertebrates, some 20 000 are fish, 8600 are birds, 6000 are reptiles and 1500 are amphibians. Mammals number 5000 species, divided into three subclasses. There are egg-laying mammals, mammals which carry their young in pouches and mammals which carry and feed their young inside the mother body. All provide excellent protein. The 5000 species of mammals fall into eighteen orders whose members are remarkably diverse in design and habits. For example man is closely related to the shrew but the otter is a very distant relation of the beaver. Populations vary in pattern too much for any estimate to have purpose but rodents dominate in all examined territories. Carnivores must obviously number less than their victims and numbers of animals per area increase as the animals become smaller. Rodents have been and are important in the diet of hunting and scavenging man. They account for between one-third and one-half of living mammals, have a high rate of reproduction and should therefore be studied in detail as potential in the meat manufacturing business. The largest rodent is the capybara which is up to 1 m in length. At present rodents provide food for the Carnivora order of mammals, including cats and dogs.

Of more interest are the hoofed mammals, which are divided into two orders according to the design of their feet. Those with an odd number of toes are Perissodactyla and those with an even number of toes are Artiodactyla. Hoofed mammals with odd toes include horses, tapirs and rhinoceroses. Horses are of value to man partly for the meat and milk they provide but more for the sustained strength arising from the individual protein composition. Hoofed mammals with even numbers of toes include almost all domestic animals in all world societies. The even number of toes is seen as a cleft in the feet of so-called cloven-hoofed animals, the subject of much religious and social complication. Almost all projects of domestication of animals have been based on land area, this emphasis on land-based animals dating from the time when beasts were needed for their labour. Intensive rearing has used several layers of animals per area, but there has been no commercialisation of the mammals which have forsaken life on solid ground.

Mammals vary in their feed requirements to the extent that a cat will die if it can find only grass to eat. They also vary in feeding ability, the giraffe being unable to survive on ground-level vegetation only, and the rabbit being unable to survive if it has to reach higher than its up-lifted teeth. (Mammals have four kinds of teeth, variously modified to suit the diet and social conditions.) Few mammals are completely specialised in their diet and they can, in times of need, survive on strange foods, but exceptions include some tropical bats which die if denied the nectar from night-blooming flowers and moustached white-nosed monkeys which must have the fruit of elaeis palm. The majority of mammals are vegetarian but do not always select tender green shoots and leaves, as is shown by the Egyptian gerbil and the American pocket mouse which can exist on seeds with moisture contents below 10%. Bark is a standard item of diet for the moose, for beavers in winter and for porcupines. Obviously, therefore, there is no need, with selection of the animal, for feeding to be restricted to oilseeds or grain or other common equivalent.

Ruminants, however, are specialised in that they feed exclusively on foliage. They have four stomach chambers, food being chewed briefly before being passed down to the rumen. In the rumen there is a bacteria population which prepares the food for the next stage in the reticulum, which returns the pulped foliage to the mouth for second-stage chewing before passage to the final chambers for digestion. Since the feed is low in quality the animal needs large quantities and larger animals, such as the elephant, which needs up to 150 kg per day, spend their entire lives grazing and chewing. There is potential in farming carnivores so that unattractive rapidly-breeding smaller animals can be converted into reasonably-sized masses of meat. The problem with carnivores is that they are unsociable and need space for development. However, the farming of marine mammals, using coarse fish as feed, is attractive, seals needing about 5 kg/day. Most of the interest in rearing un-familiar animals is in those which display flexible eating habits and can be provided with a varied diet according to local gluts, e.g. deer, rabbits and rodents in general which will eat meat as well as vegetables. The most outstanding omnivore is the rat, which includes other rats in its range of diet, and few other animals offer the same potential as a source of protein by intensive rearing.

Effective breeding relies on the frequency of sexual activity, which varies amongst mammals. In cold climates the activity is timed to allow reproduction during the warmer months of the year. In tropical climates the date is less important and animals disregard the time of the year. Mating is, as a general rule, promiscuous but there are exceptions, e.g. foxes and wolves form long-term pairs and are faithful. The record for promiscuity is claimed by a rodent, the jird, which has been observed to mate 224 times in two hours with little regard for the identity of the partners. Gestation periods vary from eight days for a marsupial cat to twenty-one months for an elephant. The number of young per occasion also varies from one to twelve in nature, and weaning periods are as low as three weeks for mice.

The potential value of unfamiliar mammals in protein production is influenced by the social organisations. Most mammals will herd but need a yet undetermined distance from other animals if health and temper are to be maintained.

Studies of animal sources of protein have included investigation into the dik-dik antelope. This can survive arid deserts without drinking any water for long periods. In general, large animals lose body heat by sweating and small animals pant out the heat in their respiration. Both control mechanisms rely on evaporation. Some small antelopes pant very little and allow their body temperatures to rise during hot periods. Their dung is dry and their urine is highly concentrated. The dik-dik is the most effective heat-controller amongst the common desert animals, even superior to the camel. It has only about 200 sweat glands to the square centimetre, compared with 1500 for cattle. If the body loss of water reaches danger level the dik-dik cuts its evaporation rate down to 50%, saving a possible 100 g of water per day. The kidneys are capable of producing double-strength urine. Furthermore, when the dehydrated dik-dik finds water its colon is capable of absorbing water at a very fast rate.

There is some possibility of farming dik-dik. The animal cannot survive on fully-dried grass or feed, but can thrive if left to graze at dusk, when many of the desert vegetation is absorbing moisture from the fall in air temperature.

The common ancestor of cattle was a fearsome beast which was probably tamed or confined in the early periods of development as a subject for religious sacrifice, particularly since the horns resembled a crescent moon. It is probable that the beasts were made to drag vehicles on their last journeys, more to prevent escape than to carry loads, and it was inevitable that the dragging ability should be applied to less devotional duties.

The beast was the aurochs (*Bos primigenius*), black and 2 m high with long horns. The last specimen died in Poland in A.D. 1627 after the breed had been diversified. By 2500 B.C. there were hump-backed versions of the type now being revived as an animal fit for survival in difficult terrain. Early Egyptians had a hornless strain and a piebald strain, both of which have led to some useful breeds. By the time of the Roman Empire, there was common cattle breeding and by the nine-tenth century A.D. there were special milk cows. There were also special beef cows and a few dual-purpose cows.

Cattle fed on open pasture and given free movement are likely to produce tough beef. Male beef is in general superior to female beef. Bulls are anti-social animals and are castrated to cool their tempers, then being known as steers. Steers are fed with a view to producing marbled meat, which has strings of fat between the muscle fibres. Steers can look forward to a life of about eighteen months before slaughter.

REPTILES AS A SOURCE OF PROTEIN

There are 6000 species of reptiles in four main groups; lizards (3000 species), snakes (2700 species), turtles (200 species), crocodiles (23 species) and a single tuatara which has a group of its own. The interest-ing group is the turtles, which are known as excellent food and are the only reptiles favoured by the majority of people. Other reptiles, when consumed, are mainly the subjects of witches' brews or other occult diet. As far as most societies are concerned, reptiles—other than turtles, which evidently had better gods during the development of mythology —are evil.

Turtles range in weight from a few grammes to half a ton and are characterised by the shell, which restricts body movement and thereby makes it necessary for the turtle to have a unique system of breathing. With some variation, breeding starts at three years old and turtles may live to be one hundred years old if they escape pollution or capture. They appear to be classified according to the technique used to hide the head in the shell, including:

Cryptodira—folding the neck into an S shape
Pleurodira—laying the head and neck sideways under the shell

There is also the broad division of turtles into sea-going types and land-based types, with a very untidy understanding of which is related to which. The shell of a turtle has the backbone fused to its under-surface. The shoulder and hip bones are where the rib cage should be whilst the ribs are flat and strengthened as supports for the structure. It is claimed that turtles can live for a year without eating and can lay fertile eggs four years after mating.

Lizards and snakes are the most flourishing reptiles at present. Snakes probably developed from lizards, the only essential difference being that lizards can close their eyes whilst snakes have to offer a perpetual stare, which may account for much of the dislike of snakes amongst humans. The broad difference, if not the scientific one, is that lizards have legs whilst snakes do not. In lizards, sizes range from 5 cm to 3 m although many lizards can drop off their tails to confuse their enemies. Snakes may be up to 10 m in length and crocodiles which are said to start breeding at eight years, are, on average, 7 m in length.

Most of the reptiles which evolved were subsequently lost during the period of the great dying some 70 million years ago. Crocodiles appear to have survived because they are superbly adapted to be carnivores. Turtles also have sufficient flexibility of diet and ability to starve for long periods, to fit into new environments. The remaining reptiles can be classified according to their equipment for eating into:

1. Those designed for eating vegetation.
2. Those designed for taking whole animals into their digestive confinement.
3. Those provided with equipment for special diet such as eggs.

However, it is not uncommon for a reptile to change its diet. For example, although most young reptiles start as insect-eaters, the iguana later develops into a fruit-eater, and the green sea turtle which starts life with no clear preference in its diet develops into a strict vegetarian. Most adult reptiles have a strong preference in diet, which may be insects but can be any vegetable or animal food group. The ultimate in preference amongst reptiles is shown by the dasypeltis, which eats only eggs taken whole. Many of the snakes, which are carnivores, rely on poisons which are mixed proteins and enzymes, either haemotoxic or neurotoxic. Vipers have haemotoxic venom, which kills by heavy bleeding and tissue destruction, whereas the cobra family use neurotoxins, which paralyse the victim. Snakes eat living meat, which is a further reason why they are not popular amongst humans.

In organised farming, reptiles are animals to be understood more as pests than as potential meat, although turtles would justify planned rearing. The danger is that turtle eggs would be taken in sufficient number for turtles to become extinct. To gain more turtle meat the need is not for intensive expensive rearing but is for protection of the eggs in their natural locations. Sea turtles live at sea but nest on shore, making long journeys in which they use advanced techniques of navigation. Whether they could be domesticated to any extent is doubtful but if the eggs could be protected the eventual adults would add considerably to protein supplies in some famine areas. A mature sea turtle will lay two to five clutches of 100 eggs each every year, which may take up to three months to hatch into reduced-scale turtles. Normal protection of the eggs is by burial but predators often recognise the trails and find the eggs, therefore it could be an advantage for turtle eggs to be given deliberate protection in nurseries for subsequent release of the young to grow into meat.

Most primitive people living near turtle breeding grounds eat both the animal and the eggs. In parts of South America turtle meat is more common than domesticated animal meat and in the Amazon region there is a vast range of turtle recipes. Japan and China also have turtle dishes, and sea turtles have long been appreciated as fresh meat on long journeys across the Pacific and Indian oceans. Turtles also have an interesting history in the development of the United States, where they were emergency food for Indians and pioneers before cattle reached the remoter areas. Early in the twentieth century, terrapin turtles sold in the United States for up to 10 dollars each but gopher turtles were less expensive and provided equal culinary enjoyment. The most important turtle for meat is the green sea turtle, which is eaten in most tropical regions where it can be caught. In the South West Pacific area it has been a major source of meat and revenue for many years, and it is doubted if the Caribbean would have developed so rapidly had there not been a plentiful supply of turtles for ships to collect for fresh meat.

Turtle soup is a luxury dish using the cartilage in the lower shell. A 150 kg turtle can offer about 2.5 kg of the cartilage, known as calipee, and there is some risk that turtles will be killed for the cartilage with the rest of the flesh thrown away. Japan has its own version of turtle soup, using cultured turtles. The mixture is turtle, saki and seaweed. As a further point of interest in this respect, iguana also make excellent soup, based on female iguana, coconut oil, chile pepper and garlic. The iguana soup tastes excellent with red beans or rice. There is considerable doubt that the traditional real turtle soup based on only a fraction of the turtle is superior to the soup made from whole turtle or whole iguana. In terms of world protein supplies it is vital, however, to discourage the destruction of complete turtles for the sake of the highly-priced morsel, particularly since the cartilage is the least valuable part in terms of protein. It is also necessary to discourage the killing of turtles for the eggs before they are laid, and to further discourage the taking of eggs if this is likely to reduce the numbers of adult turtles.

Because of the number of associated religious and social prejudices, reptile meat is unlikely to become a major contribution to world protein supplies. For example, the third incarnation of Vishnu was as a turtle; when Siva lost his temper with the snake Vasuki and bit off its head, his throat turned blue from the poison; the Nagas and their wives, the Naginas, were half-snakes half-humans and were not popular. On the other hand, between incarnations Vishnu sleeps in the coils of a cobra, which is why Hindus are kind to cobras and are not likely to accept snake meat. Crocodiles also have religious associations. Herodotus mentioned, worshipped and petted crocodiles in Egypt, and it is still possible to find holy crocodiles in Asia being fed fresh goat meat. Conversely, vipers have been cooked and eaten in Europe as commonly accepted medicines.

There is also an inexplicable connection between snakes and milk in mythology worldwide. From Siberia through Europe to the Americas it is common for a saucer of milk to be provided for a visiting snake. In parts of Africa, where snakes are probably carrying the souls of relatives, it is common to provide milk for the house snakes. Several countries carry the rumour that snakes drink milk directly from the udders of cows, although it is doubted if any cow would stand still to be milked by a snake, quite apart from the fact that snakes cannot, and do not, drink milk. They eat live meat.

Projects for meat production from reptiles are therefore better left with turtles but snakes are of interest in protein technology as sources of medical protein, the curative powers of boiled snakes having some foundation in fact. Venom is a known origin of many potential curative drugs and surgical aids.

MEAT DEMAND

Demand for meat is controlled by many variables and is perhaps best studied in terms of proportional meat content in diet, which varies about a norm dictated by the social condition and psychological structure of the consumer. This norm can vary from nil for some religious orders and strict vegetarians to almost 100% for a few hunting tribes. Most consuming individuals have some fixed ideas about the eating of meat. Some regard meat consumption as barbaric whilst some will eat meat providing they do not see it in its original bloody condition. Others regard meat as essential in diet and extremists insist that meals must include a fair proportion of fresh meat dripping with blood at the time of cooking.

With such a mixture of attitudes it is almost impossible to set demand down in statistics but there have been many estimates made for marketing and production planning. A cross-reference shows that West Europeans consume a daily 85 g of protein of which 60% is of animal origin. In Eastern Europe the protein intake is nearer 100 g of which one-third is of animal origin. North American protein intake is about 95 g with two-thirds from animals, and roughly the same applies in Australia and New Zealand. In Africa, although it is incorrect to generalise on African consumers, daily protein intake is 50 g with about a quarter of this as animal protein. Much the same applies to most of Asia but the Asian picture is confused by the high proportion of vegetarians. In South America there is considerable variation, intakes ranging from 50–100 g and proportions derived from animals varying from 25–60%.

Averages rarely indicate true situations and they need to be appreciated alongside statements of the distribution of wealth within an area or society. In this respect, there is a vast difference between the demand, which is dictated by requirements and attitudes, and the market, which is dictated by attitudes and spending power. The common factor is attitudes, meat being an emotive subject included in religious legislation and related to the killer instinct in man. Most of the attitudes originate in the early development of man as a social animal.

During his nomadic period, man found it convenient for his food reserves to have legs and to act as vehicles during its life. Kept animals were selected if they could tolerate an erratic, or high-volume low-nutrition diet, according to whether the wandering was rapid or casual, through jungle or pasture or sparsely-vegetated desert or perpetual ice. The first requirement was that the animal should be able to carry or drag loads, roughly at the walking speed of man, and should be sufficiently docile or stupid not to attack the keepers. Later, the ability to provide milk was welcomed and there was preference for fast breeders which could provide a regular supply of fresh young meat.

When man settled on farms, priority in crops was divided between delightful foods for humans and storage foods for the animals which were still kept partly for their labour and partly for their meat. When agriculture became more specialised there developed a new system of rearing in which land held more than its fair complement of livestock and feeding was supported by bought stored feed. Intensive rearing is simply one stage further, with the animal lifted out of its natural environment and fed only on bought nutrition. The world has at present all systems of rearing, from mixed agriculture according to the original policy, through open-range grazing with or without added bought feed, to complete intensification in which the animal is confined and is fed only from bought nutritional mixtures.*

During the period when animals provided both pulling power and meat, it was necessary for societies to regulate slaughter by the introduction of religious laws relating to diet. It was also essential to discourage the slaughter of neighbour's animals by association of killing and cooking and subsequent eating with ceremony. The created impression was that anyone killing or eating without due public ceremony would suffer a dire fate in this life and the next. This preserved stocks, or ran them down to economic levels when required, and also reduced the probability of conflict between neighbours.

So-called civilised society may find it hard to accept but most of present-day prejudices or preferences with regard to meat can be traced to primitive religious instructions. Although it is now widely realised that meat is not unique as a source of protein, the present market for meat is higher than it need be because meat has become associated with certain ceremonies, and the ceremonies are part of cultures which bind societies together. A social group needs a specific culture, which needs ceremonies, which originated to control meat consumption and still require meat as a focus of attention. Also, a very large proportion of the world's population understand that the eating of flesh introduces some spiritual component into the human body from the animal and that this spiritual component has value, but frequently only if eating is with due ceremony. These ceremonial aspects of dining have been commercialised and to some extent organised to assist marketing. The concept of a main meal comprising meat plus two vegetables has been developed, and there is a developed relationship of foods to drinks. Demand for meat is thereby influenced by its association with other foods and the relative fidelity of consumers to developed ceremonies and to traditional mixtures in or out of such ceremonies. Most of these

---

* Inevitably, this practice of controlling diet to achieve maximum rates of growth has led to interference with body activity—mainly the addition of chemicals to prevent sickness and to accelerate growth but also to modify the composition of the final meat. In effect, man has accepted responsibility for the body chemistry of the animal but it is strongly doubted if he yet has the education to know exactly what he is doing. Fortunately, body chemistries are self-regulating to a degree and there has not yet been the widespread damage to humans which could develop from interference with animal chemistry and structure.

traditional mixtures are local and are encouraged by local convention, not the interaction of flavours or balance of components. Much of meat marketing concerns the provision of the correct type of meat to coincide with seasonal prices and availabilities of associated vegetables, and the provision of the correct type of meat for ceremonies and traditional occasions. Almost all fresh meat and much of preserved meat is consumed with some measure of ceremony and convention, from the roasting of whole animals in public to the inevitable provision of bacon for breakfast by English landladies.

Consideration of the protein content of meat is rare in personal consumption but it is found in institutional catering and in discussion relative to feeding the starving millions. There is some confusion in quotations of protein content, mainly because it is rare for statistics to state if the content refers to original meat, trimmed meat or meat served as a meal. The proportion of food which is digested protein, and therefore of value to the body, is almost never quoted.

For the record, and with the understanding that protein contents vary considerably and can be partly ineffective under the influences of bad cooking and poor digestion, the protein contents of common meats at the time of cooking are roughly:

	Percentage dry protein
Bacon	25
Gammon	31
Corned beef	22
Boiled beef	30
Roast beef	24
Fried steak	20
Grilled steak	25
Brain	12
Boiled chicken	26 or 16 including bones
Roast duck	23 or 12 including bones
Roast goose	28 or 16 including bones
Boiled ham	20
Chopped canned pork	16
Heart	21
Kidney	27
Canned luncheon meat	11
Grilled mutton chop	24 or 14 including bone
Boiled mutton	25
Roast mutton	25
Stewed mutton	18
Roast partridge	35 or 21 including bones
Roast pheasant	31

	Percentage dry protein
Roast pork leg	25
Roast pork loin	22
Stewed rabbit	27
Fried UK-type sausage	13
Blood sausage	5
Sweetbreads	23
Tongue	19
Roast turkey	30 or 18 including bones
Veal	30
Roast venison	34

How much of this protein is absorbed depends on what happens to the juices from cooking, how much the cook leaves in the dish and the consumer leaves on the plate, and then on the ability of the digestive system to absorb. It will be noticed that the retail prices of meats bear very little relationship to the protein content, beef being particularly overpriced.

Price–demand relationship

Although the meat fraction may contribute only one-fifth to one-third of the total food value of a meal it can account for up to 95% of the total cost, ignoring heating and incidental overheads. In times of inflation, therefore, meat is an inevitable target for economy but such economy is inhibited by the conventional requirement for meat in a meal. The consequent reaction to inflation is a change of the character of the meal, away from recipes which by convention need meat as specified, and towards recipes which use alternative protein sources, notably cheese and eggs. Within the pattern of convention relating to meat dishes, inflation brings alteration of the menu rather than effort to use a cheaper meat cut against instructions in the recipe. Broadly, inflation brings change in eating habits more than change in the composition of listed recipes.

The average housewife may not be familiar with protein contents and amino-acid patterns but she is aware that low-priced cuts of meat are likely to contain high proportions of fat, bone and connective tissue. If, therefore, she is faced with the necessity to reduce expenditure on meat she will aim for the highest quality of cut within her revised economic limits, and will also aim for the highest possible edible bulk in cuts. In the circumstance, flavour and toughness are minor considerations, it being presumed that a revised cooking programme will overcome any such problems. The emphasis switches, therefore, from meat for roasting, grilling and frying, to meat for boiling or stewing or otherwise wet-cooking with a high proportion of associated vegetables.

This trend was evident in the 1970–1972 inflation period but there was also increased demand for processed meat to replace fresh meat rejected because the retail price had risen too quickly. Subsequently, the domestic demand for middle-quality meat brought inflation to the manufacturers of meat products, and meat products also increased in retail price. Consequently, more demand was passed on to middle-quality fractions, particularly since much of the meat was being bought for home freezers. Buying for home freezers in effect put purchase six months ahead of consumption and produced an extra demand (in the United Kingdom probably an extra 5% on demand when meat first showed significant price increases).

MEAT VARIABILITY

The consumer welcomes variability by species in that there is a choice of beef, pig meat, sheep meat, poultry, etc. and she welcomes variability by cut insofar as it provides a range of suitabilities for different dishes and a range of prices. Although suppliers appreciate the market demand for many types and grades of meat there is some serious effort to standardise meat to the higher levels, and to introduce changes in flavour which disturb the species–meat classification. It is possible to produce mutton tasting of pork and it is only a matter of time before the flavour need not indicate the beast.

Growth patterns differ amongst beasts and produce differing textures and constructions. Within a species it is practical to adjust composition and rate of growth by breed selection and within any given breed it is possible to control meat quality by feeding, growth conditions and the condition of the beast at the time of slaughter. The final dead muscle therefore depends for its composition on the growth history, sex, stress level at the time of slaughter and age. The muscle can then be conditioned to become meat which is suitable for the distribution pattern, i.e. manufacturing meat, prime cuts for domestic freezers, retail cuts or slices for pre-packed self-service, institutional catering, etc.

Bone structures are fairly common within a breed but fat content and distribution are an economic consideration in trimming. It is now established that fat is not needed to bring out the flavour of muscle and it is also widely thought that animal fat is conducive to heart trouble.

Hence, there is a rejection of fat by consumers and suppliers need to reduce the fat proportion of beasts. This can be done partly by breeding, as in the derivation of low-fat pork, or by organisation of feeding and conditions of rearing to give the maximum conversion of feed to protein. Consumers, because they are having to pay more for meat, are also seeking tenderness and flavour beyond that familiar in most meat cuts, and are demanding new standards of fat and water retention by the tissues. Water retention is particularly important for supermarket display, the loss of fluid producing unsightly stains and wet patches inside clear packages.

Meat and fat
Meat sells mainly by its image of excellent nutrition which is a joy to eat. The image of excellent nutrition is less effective since a fair proportion of the population have learned about second-class proteins becoming first-class by mixing, and particularly since animal fat became associated with heart failure. For example, butter has rapidly lost its image of superiority amongst table fats and is now regarded mainly as no more than an alternative to margarine, possibly with a better flavour but probably conducive to heart failure. The relationship of animal fat to heart failure is still obscure. Toughness of meat increases with age of the animal and is due in this respect to cross-linkages in the collagen and elastic protein. Such cross-linking comes from oxidation of the side chain in lysine amino acid and it can be inhibited by copper deficiency and by the introduction of specific enzymes. It is possible that it can be controlled in growing animals but there are doubts that anything can be done with old meat, including old human meat. The elastin protein is a major component in artery walls and is somehow responsible for fat build-up resulting in heart failure in humans and presumably in cattle. It is now thought that elastin protein contains hydrophobic centres associated with water-pockets, kept apart by polar amino acids, and that this structure is likely to attract fats and fatty breakdown products. There is concern that the manipulation of growing meat, including the addition of extra enzymes, might contribute to fat accumulation in consumers.

To some extent the demand for animal fat alongside meat was upheld by the tradition that meat must be cooked with its own fat to bring out flavour, but there is now evidence that meat needs no fat to bring out the flavour and, in general, there is no reason why any consumer should buy fat with the meat. Obviously, the meat industry regrets the lost market when fat is rejected. Therefore there are now developments of meat containing vegetable fat instead of animal fat, so that it can be sold as meat with fat which is unlikely to cause heart failure but which can add flavour in the cooking. The process is remarkably simple and opens up possibilities of many changes to the composition of meats.

Ruminants break down supplied protein and vegetable fats by bacteria in the rumens to produce their own versions of the proteins and fats, which are then saturated fats. If the supplied vegetable fat is protected on its way through the rumen it becomes absorbed into tissue as vegetable, or unsaturated, fat. This protection can be achieved by treating the protein with formaldehyde (in the same way that casein protein is made into insoluble plastics casein) and then using the treated protein as a barrier layer around the fat globules. The commercial system sprays casein with formalin and fat to produce a fatty dried protein concentrate similar to dried milk. The resultant product passes through the rumen into the abomasum where the stomach acid breaks down the treated protein to release the vegetable fat for direct absorption. Such modified dairy protein has been used in feeding trials which show reduced cholesterol levels in five out of six subjects. Modified meat is produced only two days after introducing the special feed and after eight weeks of such feeding the meat can reach 30% unsaturation in its fat. Vegetable oils used are mainly sunflower and safflower and this is of interest to arable farmers, particularly in Australia, where up to 20 000 tons of vegetable seed could be needed for 10% of beef to consist of unsaturated fats. The estimate is that about 10% of potential beef eaters are likely to suffer from excess saturated fats and would pay extra for the special beef. The market is, however, much wider since it has been shown practical to produce pork-flavoured meat from grass-fed sheep given a special diet for two months before slaughter, which are cheaper to produce than grain-fed pigs. Since most essences can be carried by fats it is obvious that in due course meat can be made to adopt any required flavour, including intensification of its own flavour for relatively flavourless cuts. Work on these lines has been done by the University of Dublin, which has produced lambs in which the unsaturated fat content was boosted five times. Twenty-four lambs were weaned two days after birth and fed on the casein–vegetable oil product until they reached a body weight of 8 kg. The flock was then divided into groups of six, each group to be fed on a special replacement diet including linoleic acid. (Linoleic acid is a common unsaturated fatty acid in linseed, cottonseed and many other vegetables and is regarded as essential in the diet of ruminants, deficiency causing the animal to fail in the production of body fat.) Growth rate was 300 g/day to a weight of 36 kg, after which eating trials showed the meat to be identical in flavour to that of normal lambs. As a further indication of the probable scope of chemical manipulation of body fats, an egg with unsaturated fat has been developed, but this evidently failed to produce a chicken containing vegetable fat.

Simulated meat

Simulated meat is a direct outcome of the implied social need to include meat in a ceremonial meal, associated with fear of animal fat and widespread psychological antagonisms against slaughter. From the commercial point of view, simulated meat is vegetable protein presented to consumers in the form they demand, which is similar to genuine meat but without the animal fat and divorced from the act of slaughter. It can be first-class or second-class protein but the pattern of amino acids is not important to the types of consumers who buy other foods providing any amino acids which are missing.

Soya and *Vicia faba* beans are common sources of the vegetable protein. The United Kingdom version by Courtaulds is based on *Vicia faba* and is made to have flavours of chicken or beef, being supplied frozen ready for heating to table temperatures. The comparison is:

	Protein (g/ounce)	Fat (g/ounce)	Carbohydrate (g/ounce)
Beef (raw)	4.8	4.5	0.0
Chicken (raw)	5.1	2.0	0.0
Kesp	6.2	5.9	0.03

Kesp (see p. 281) is textured on textile machinery to imitate the fibre of real meat. One advantage as far as housewives are concerned is the low shrinkage of Kesp, almost nil, against up to 30% shrinkage of real meat in cooking. During the initial marketing period, Kesp sold for 20–40 pence/lb 53–88 pence/kilo), which was roughly half the cost of real meat or chicken if bones were taken into account. The stated composition can be translated as 50% moisture, 22% protein, 21% fat and 3% minerals. The amino-acid pattern evidently follows that of soya and other beans. In terms of total economies, there is advantage in using vegetable protein for direct human consumption where 80% of available protein is likely to be absorbed. If the vegetable proteins were fed to cows there would be only a 15% conversion to milk or 9% conversion to beef.

Textured soy protein. Claimed analysis by Ralston Purina Company

	%	
Protein (N × 6.25)	93 (dry weight basis)	
Ash	0.9	
Moisture	63	
Fat	0.1	pH value 5.2

Amino-acid pattern	*g*/16 *g N*
Arginine	6.6
Histidine	2.4
Isoleucine	4.7
Leucine	7.8
Lysine	5.7
Methionine	1.2
Phenylalanine	5.4
Threonine	3.5
Tryptophane	1.1
Valine	4.8

Extruded soy protein. Claimed analysis by Ralston Purina Company

	%	
Protein (N × 6.25)	50 (dry weight basis)	
Ash	7	
Moisture	8.5	
Fat	1	
Fibre	3	pH value 6.8

Protein contents, genuine meat and imitations based on soya protein (%)

	Genuine meat	Imitation meat (analogue)
Seafood	16.5	70
Ham	17.5	60
Bacon	8.5	45
Beef	17.2	58
Chicken	18.5	70

	Protein content %	Price (cents/lb)	Production (million lb)	Applications
	Soya protein foods, USA, 1970			
Flour and grits	40/55	5.5–11.5	500/600	Bakery goods Dog food Sausages
Concentrates	60/70	18–25	35	Simulated meat Processed meat Baby food Health food
Isolates	90/97	35–45	25	Simulated meat Meat loaf Frankfurters
Textured extruded	50/55	28 plus	30	Simulated meat
spun	90 plus	50 plus		

NOTE: Textured extruded are made on a plastics-type extruder with high temperature and high pressure. Spun products are produced on textile equipment designed for rayon and nylon.

There is justified opinion that simulated meat will become a major item in the diet of affluent consumers. Affluence can be measured by the frequency of ceremonial meals, at which it is traditional to have meat or fish as a gastronomic focus. During periods of inflation there is conflict between the urge to save money by reducing meat purchases, and the urge to maintain status by retaining ceremonial meals. Simulated meat provides a low-cost focus for such ceremonial feeding. Under less pressure from inflation there is an urge to increase the frequency of ceremonial meals, in which case there is a need for a meat which demands comparatively little effort in its preparation. Mostly, this encourages cold meats but a very large proportion of the consuming public insist that only hot meals are fully beneficial. There are two fairly obvious market sectors for simulated meat in an affluent society:

1. For entertainment catering, particularly where pressure from inflation offers the entertainer the choice between a reduction of the frequency of entertainment or acceptance of imitation meat. In this sector, the convenience of handling is important but it could become more important that the simulated meat is without animal fat and is acceptable by all religious groups (strict vegetarianism is included as a religion).

2. For domestic catering in the very large number of families where meat is regarded as vital for health. It is probable, despite advice from Courtaulds and others, that simulated meat will be served to many families as real meat, notably in the so-called labouring classes.

However, it is doubted if there is much market for simulated meat outside affluent societies. There are developments which are intended to improve the quality of pulse proteins for human diet but there is no virtue in texturisation of such protein for impoverished societies.

Cured meats

One of the differences between cured meats and fresh meat is that the consumer looks for a different colour in buying. Fresh meat should be a familiar red or pink according to the animal or cut, whilst cured meat is associated with a delicate pink to brown. The colour is derived from the addition of nitrite and nitrate, although since nitrate breaks down to nitrite it is not essential to use nitrite in the original addition. The nitrite is converted to nitrosomyoglobin in the meat to give the pink colour. About 5 p.p.m. of nitrite will give sufficient pink for short-term storage but up to 20 p.p.m. may be needed for long-term storage. It would be possible to produce the desirable pink colour by dyes instead of nitrites but the inhibitive influence of nitrites is important in bacterial control. The nitrite also produces a distinctive flavour, which is why bacon and ham differ from common salt pork. Up to 100 p.p.m. may be needed to avoid botulism. Nitrite by itself does not protect against organic toxins but is one component in a complicated pattern of reaction in which some organisms cannot thrive.

In uncured meat the onset of putrefaction is obvious from the slime and odour of amino by-products, bringing instant rejection by the consumer. In cured meats the range of effective organisms is limited by the chemical environment and decay may not be obvious until after consumption. The most common toxic infection is caused by salmonella. It occurs more commonly in poultry than in hairy beasts and more often in pigs than in cattle. The degree of infection varies but is of the order of 1% of farm animals, up to 10% of animals brought for slaughter and higher in carcase meat. The main source of infection appears to be bought feeding stuffs but pellets are less likely to carry infection than loose grain or swill. Cross-infection between animals in transit is common and therefore it is important not to crowd animals for more than three days before slaughter. Cross-infection between carcases is also common and there is some evidence that infections are more active if the animals are subjected to stress before slaughter. There is also the opinion that sensitivity to infection is increased by high mercury and heavy metals levels in animals. In animals mercury links to protein receptors, 10% of it in the head and 5% of it in the blood. Toxic effects relate mainly to the central nervous system and encourage the development of bodily stress, leading to more sensitivity to infection.

Additives to feed
Feeds are formulated to encourage growth and, since they are limited in the number of components, they lack the richness of open-range diets. Additives are needed partly to encourage growth from a false diet but also to prevent sickness since natural preventatives are lacking. Exact formulation is difficult, because there is common ignorance of the true requirements of animal body chemistries and because most foodstuffs contain pollution, which is an unintended additive.

Mercury and heavy metals are known sources of contamination which influence the effective conversion of feed, and the mental condition of the animal. Most of the offending mercury appears to come from seed dressing passing into crops as organic mercury. Mercury is also scavenged by bacteria and then converted into soluble forms which can be absorbed by animal digestions. Most scavenging bacteria can concentrate the mercury compounds, notably from sea water, and this has resulted in excessive mercury in tuna from the USA and mussels from Japan. By the natural path of substances through consumers, such concentrated mercury reaches arable crops, mercury-rich rice already being evident in Japan. Mercury-based herbicides are known to be the origin of high mercury levels in grass, which may pass on the mercury through compost to horticultural crops or directly into animals through grazing. Lead is another commonly discussed contamination which passes through natural paths involving vegetation, consumers, sewage, and animals used to convert vegetation into flesh protein.

Farmers can do relatively little to control unintended additives but they need to be aware of the fact that any product used for feed is likely to contain some component which can interfere with growth of the animal. Farmers can control deliberate contamination but there is strong temptation to overload confined animals with hormones and antibiotics, on the basis that prevention of trouble is less expensive than rectification of damage. Common hormones used for this purpose are stilboestrol, hexoestrol, dienestrol, dianisyl hexane and a range of thyroid stimulants. However, there is a suspected link between cancer of the breast and oestrogens, and stilboestrol, amongst the oestrogens, is strongly attacked after evidence that it produces cysts in children and retards growth in unborn children. The main source in human diet appears to be chicken livers, probably because the hormones have proved particularly effective in intensive chicken rearing.

The probability of harmful hormone in meat after feed has been furnished with additives depends on legislation and the possibility of detection. At the time of writing, hormones in cattle feed is allowed in the United Kingdom and the USA but not in Australia after evidence that they produce malformed children. At least twenty countries ban the use of hormones but whether the law is obeyed is not known. The situation with poultry is complicated because antibiotics are said to be essential in economic battery-rearing. In the United Kingdom, sulpha-nitron and sulphaquinoxilene can be freely added but penicillin and tetracyclines need a veterinary prescription. Most countries have a thriving underground market in agricultural drugs and many birds are fed illegal doses or doses which may not be exactly as stated by the supplier. Therefore the quality of poultry meat in all countries using intensive rearing is suspect because the economics of rearing make it advisable to take precautions against infection and to stimulate growth. Also during the grain crisis of the early 1970s another problem of additives arose, as much feed grain changed hands a number of times and was likely to be not as stated on documents. Thus, in early 1972 in Iraq, farmers were supplied with seed grain dressed with ethyl mercury *p*-toluene, some of which was inevitably used as food. As a result 5500 farmers were admitted to hospital and several deaths were recorded. Since this event concerned humans it became known but there have also been many examples of misapplied grain causing damage to animals.

MEAT REFRIGERATION
Flavour and texture of meat are strongly affected by the rate of refrigeration, whether this is in chilling to about zero or freezing to the point where contained water becomes ice. In theory, the infections which occur during cutting and handling are best controlled by very rapid reduction of the meat temperature. EEC regulations from 1964 specify that carcases must be cooled to an internal temperature of below 7 °C

(3 °C for offal) after inspection and held at this temperature, air temperatures in handling operations being below 10 °C.

It is a fact that rapid cooling will inhibit bacteria and will reduce
evaporation and drip loss. The ideal refrigeration system quickly
produces a surface temperature very slightly above that needed for ice
formation in the meat. The problem then is to maintain the surface
temperature with a reasonable weight of warm flesh behind the surface,
as there is a danger of cold-shortening of the meat if heat extraction is
too rapid. Cold-shortening can produce tough meat if cooling is to below
10 °C within half a day of slaughter. New Zealand lamb was found to be
sensitive to cold-shortening and needed a pre-refrigeration period of 27
hours at 15 °C for certainty of tenderness. Beef has been found less
sensitive and may be conditioned at 8 °C, although some forms of beef
may tolerate the EEC specified early temperature reduction to 7 °C.
United Kingdom experience of lamb indicates that 6 hours' delay
before refrigeration should produce tender meat but most refrigeration
engineers within EEC support the use of early rapid refrigeration. The
support could well be because a long period is needed to remove heat
from a carcase and some delay is inevitable with economic heat-
extraction equipment.

In a typical chill-room it could take half a day for a filling of hot
meat to reach 5 °C on its surface, making it improbable that any meat
other than some lamb would exhibit cold-shortening. In fact, temperatures in chill-rooms are rarely measured and the EEC specification
would appear to be academic and not based on practical considerations.
After initial heat extraction, chill-rooms in practice run at various
temperatures up to 17 °C and are rarely found running at below 7 °C.
Nor is there evidence of offal being held at 3 °C.

Furthermore, it is common for chilled meat to be delivered in unrefrigerated vehicles for short-term storage without refrigeration in stores,
possibly for passage along an unrefrigerated cutting and packaging line,
then to be put on display. The appearance of the meat is improved by
warm lighting which, particularly through clear packaging film, encourages an increase of temperature. In effect, the meat passes through a
relatively uncontrolled history of heat input which makes a mockery of
the initial reduction to low temperature, although obviously any early
reduction of temperature is an advantage, as it helps to reduce the
danger of microbial putrefaction and lowers the probability of toxin
formation although it does not ensure purity in the final meat.

There is widespread ignorance of the actual heat history in refrigeration, not only in chilling but in deep freezing. Notably there is ignorance of the rate at which meat reaches the intended flesh temperature within the carcase or prime joint. As with chilling, there is significant difference between EEC regulations and practical possibilities, EEC calling for -17 °C for beef and -20 °C for pork. As a rule -10 °C has been found satisfactory but some meat is frozen to -30 °C with consequent economic loss from unrequired heat extraction. The very low -30 °C is claimed to be justified by the reduction of evaporation loss at very low temperatures. Tests have shown that storage loss at -10 °C is at least five times that at -30 °C but it can be doubted that the value of loss-reduction compensates for the extra cost of maintaining -30 °C. In this respect, it is less expensive to maintain a low temperature if the meat is concentrated in the space, by early boning and trimming and then compacting in solid units (filled boxes or film bags). On the other hand, if the meat is to be cut early and compacted it should be noted that sealed units build up a carbon dioxide atmosphere, which can be anticipated and encouraged by chilling with carbon dioxide, and will then give a shelf life of three months at about 0 °C. In this case, freezing may not be essential but it can help to delay the influence of the subsequent shipment and higher temperatures experienced in display.

Although the quality of meat depends on the pattern of heat extraction after slaughter, this needs to be related to the use of enzymes or other treatments. The thermal history starts with the initial cooling after slaughter. If this cooling is rapid there is reduced bacterial activity on the surface (less slime) and less danger of taint inside the meat. It is advisable for internal temperatures to reach 15.5 °C within 20 hours for beef, 10 °C within 15 hours for pork and, 7 °C within 12 hours for lamb. The rate of air flow and its temperature: humidity ratio across the surface needs study as an influence on slime formation and drying out. It can be appreciated that if different parts of a carcase show individual cooling rates there is justification for early division of the carcase into primary joints before the initial cooling, if only to accelerate heat removal. Cutting hot meat is, however, difficult and it is practical to wait for some cooling, but beef loses about 3% of its weight in this early cooling, pork loses about 2.5% and lamb loses about 7%. Rapid cooling can reduce this loss and there are claims of only 1% loss for beef and pork. The actual weight loss is probably less important than the time factor in waiting for the carcase to cool, particularly with many beasts to process in a crowded factory. Rapid cooling is also said to reduce drip by 50% and it is known to avoid watery meat in pork. On the other hand, rapid cooling can bring cold-shortening, i.e. contraction of muscle to about half its length and subsequent return to its original length.

The second stage in the thermal history concerns low temperature storage. It has been established that the longest life for meat comes from storage at slightly above the freezing point of blood, about -1 °C. Storage at 5 °C will cut the life by half and at 10 °C the life is cut by three-quarters. Humidity should be about 90% relative humidity and it would be critical if it could be maintained. High humidity encourages biological decay whilst low humidity encourages drying out. One problem is condensation after temperature changes in the air, a wet surface on the meat producing rapid decay.

Therefore, in the final analysis it is better to rely on common sense than to trust regulations. Experienced butchers know the quality of meat needed and the life required, and they also appreciate that chilled meat is likely to suffer an unchilled period in distribution, which needs to be considered in estimating the condition of the meat after chilling.

Deep-freezing

With regard to deep-freezing, this should not be done before rigor mortis has set in, as quick freezing before full rigor mortis damages the muscle, producing shrinkage and excessive drip. New Zealand lamb is held first at 13–18 °C for 24 hours, then reduced to 3 °C over a further 24 hours, and finally frozen. Long-term conditioning is common using one of the following cycles:

16 days at 0 °C
14 days at 2 °C
 8 days at 5 °C
 3 days at 10 °C

Recently, higher temperatures have been used, for example 37 °C for 5 hours. In using higher temperatures there is increased risk of bacterial decay since the carcase holds the high temperature beyond the specified period. On the other hand, the traditional periods of conditioning are too long and are suspected of being laid down for early cow meat, which needed a long period.

The freezing operation needs to be related to the bulk of meat involved. For example, a full carcase of beef may take several days and even a quarter may take 80 hours, whereas a carcase divided into primary joints may freeze within two days. It is important not to have a steep thermal gradient from the surface to the inner depths and it would appear to be unwise, and ineffective, to use an excessively low freezing temperature. The ideal appears to be a slow freeze at -10 °C to -20 °C. If a six months' life is needed the storage temperature for beef is -14 °C and for pork is -18 °C. Below -10 °C evaporation losses are not high but if the storage temperature is above -10 °C the evaporation losses can reach 10%. Therefore, the main problem appears to be that, using large masses of meat, rapid cooling can produce toughness by cold-shortening but very slow cooling can also produce toughness with off-flavour. Unrefrigerated carcase beef could take three days to cool to room temperature, by which time the onset of bone-taint is almost unavoidable. This is one reason why there has been development of primal jointing and freezing of relatively small masses. Freezing is now used for whole carcases, sides, quarters, meat without bone in cartons, and retail cuts. It is not remarkable that experience of refrigeration in one situation cannot effectively be applied in another. As said earlier, it is better to rely on common sense than to trust regulations, particularly regulations which specify heat extraction targets without stating the bulks of meat involved and the market to be served.

Domestic freezers can be regarded as extensions of commercial cold chains. In general, conventional refrigerators are being replaced by freezers including two-level freezers which act as conventional refrigerators and deep-freezers. Roughly three-quarters of domestic freezers have capacities over 250 l and over two-thirds have capacities over 150 l. About half of the low-temperature domestic storage equipment volume is of the deep-freeze type, which means a theoretical average temperature of -20 °C. During periods of inflation freezers are filled mainly with highly-priced products, notably meat, as domestic forward buying in anticipation of price rises. The contents of domestic freezers vary according to the owner and the season of the year but a rough breakdown is one-third flesh protein including processed meat and fish, one-third vegetables and possibly more for owners with gardens and one-third baked products including bread. Most domestic freezers also contain a little ice cream and other delights.

Freezer economics
The use of freezing as a preservation method for protein needs careful study. The equipment is likely to be the most expensive link in the long

chain between production and consumption, although the running cost should be low, of the order of 2% of the final product cost. In practice, operators of freezers accept relatively high running costs for the sake of certainty of function and ability to deal with the quantities involved. With higher accepted running costs it is possible to economise on initial capital cost, by using primitive freezers. Primitive freezers are common in the USA, where short-term estimation is common and low capital is favoured more than low running cost.

The main cost factor is the degree to which freezing avoids loss of product and allows more effective distribution. This can be given a finite value, as for example the avoidance of 5% loss at a market value of £500 per ton, or ability to sell an extra 5000 tons through home-freezer centres, or perhaps an extra 5% profit if the product is held in store until selling prices rise. When the benefit is identified, and given a cash value, it is then practical to decide the freezing rate needed. A slow freezing rate will produce ice crystals which grow, puncturing cell walls and leading to drip or improved tenderness according to the application. Fast freezing produces many small crystals of ice which do not grow but may prevent effective freezing within hidden depths of flesh or solid vegetable tissue.

A purchasing housewife will recognise the difference between a 20% drip and a 10% drip, but will not worry about 12% drip instead of 8% drip. Even at a very slow freezing rate the drip from meat is not important to the purchaser other than when observed as nasty slime in a clear plastics package. There is however an improvement in meat tenderness by reduction of the freezing time from about 3 hours to 20 mins, and an obvious economic advantage in quicker dealing with the product. As a general rule, there is no point in paying for an expensive rapid freezer if any improvement therefrom is not noticed by the consumer or does not bring some benefit in handling. It is also important to calculate the actual benefit from reduction of weight-loss by rapid freezing. Rapid freezing can, but need not, reduce a 7% weight-loss to below 1% weight-loss. Much depends on the product and the sophistication of the equipment, blast freezers showing weight-loss results between 3–7% for old designs but down to 1% for modern air-flow freezers.

The choice between freezer types is:

1. Super-fast freezers which put the product rapidly in contact with liquid nitrogen or carbon dioxide.

2. Fluidised-bed techniques which sit the product on a porous bed and pass refrigerant through from underneath.
3. Air blast tunnels, which are better entitled air flow tunnels because the air is with tightly controlled circulation.
4. Batch chambers, in which the cold air is circulated by convection and the rate of cooling is strongly influenced by the size and shape (and degree of packing) of the product.

Taking similar units of product, approximately 1 cm cubes, super-fast freezing might bring the temperature down to -20 °C in 1 min. A fluidised-bed freezer, which has to establish intimate contact between refrigerant and product, might take 6 mins but give a more even distribution of the cold. A blast or air-flow system might take anything from 1 hour to 1 day according to the efficiency of the circulation. Using liquid nitrogen or carbon dioxide gives an air temperature at the surface of the product of -60 °C for carbon dioxide and down to -150 °C for nitrogen (although -80 °C is more probable). A conventional air freezer offers temperatures of -20 to -30 °C. Using very cold refrigerant costs more money, of the order of 1 penny/lb for refrigerant and 1.5 lb of refrigerant/lb of product. The provision of facilities for less-cold refrigeration costs more money because it is slower and demands more space.

Thus, an air-flow equipment might cost £60 000 as accumulated costs, all in, regardless of whether it is used 1000 or 2000 hours/year. A rapid freezer might cost £10 000 as investment, and reach £60 000 accumulated costs after three years running at 1000 hours/year, or after only 1.5 years if run at 2000 hours/year. Broadly, both types of equipment show the same final cost after five years of running at 1000 hours/year but if 2000 hours/year are needed the cost of rapid freezing needs significant justification through improved quality or other benefit.

Inflation of product prices has made nonsense of much of the earlier calculations of freezer value. It is not uncommon for the initial capital cost of equipment to be rescued by one month of operation, and it is to be appreciated that higher selling prices allow more operating cost per weight of product.

Carbon dioxide
The use of carbon dioxide for chilling meat has been known for many years. Carbon dioxide can exist as solid, liquid or gas but the solid version, dry ice, has been the common form. It has been used for almost

half a century as blocks, broken blocks and recently as snow. Primitive practice is to hang blocks in nets within vehicles or stores and simply replace when exhausted. The use of carbon dioxide has diminished to some extent since the introduction of improved mechanical refrigeration and the development of liquid nitrogen. Even so, solid CO_2 is probably the most common refrigerant, particularly for erratic supplies and variable distances of shipment.

Carbon dioxide as gas has been used since the early 1930s for beef. The optimum concentration is about 10% CO_2 but up to 20% has been claimed as inert and bacteriostatic. Much of the development concerned beef from Australia and New Zealand to the United Kingdom, with increase of use up to about 1939 and then a decline. Liquid carbon dioxide developed for beef in the USA during the early 1950s. It can only exist as a liquid under pressure of 4 atmospheres and at temperatures below -56.6 °C, or at higher pressures with some slight increase of the temperature. When the liquid is discharged into lower pressure it forms a snow and cold gas, a much more efficient system of producing snow than grinding and blowing solid blocks of CO_2. When liquid CO_2 is blown over meat in a store or vehicle (or package) the snow provides a rapidly-cooling skin of refrigerant in direct contact with the meat and the gas provides an inert atmosphere, this being said to be more bacteriostatic than cold nitrogen.

The direct introduction of CO_2 snow to packages was pioneered in the early 1970s for chickens by W. and J. B. Eastwood and The Distillers Company Ltd. The system concerns dressed birds at about 10 °C in open cartons fed under a snow machine. It takes about 4 secs to apply from 0.5–1.5 lb of snow to a box of 8–10 chickens at about 30 lb weight. The weight of snow is adjusted to reduce the bird temperature to below zero within 1 hour. Liquid CO_2 is fed from a vessel holding at 300 p.s.i. and -18 °C. From this pressure:temperature ratio of the liquid it has been found that 90% of the cooling is from the snow. Claims favouring the use of snow are many and include:

1. Quick cooling of the bird, limiting dehydration and discolourisation.
2. Retention or even improvement of the natural bloom of chicken skin.
3. Inhibition of bacterial growth if the carbon dioxide gas can be sealed in.

Obviously during a period of inflation costs need to be dated. In late 1973 rough costing gave 2–4 pence/lb of bird, or about 10% increase to be passed on or compared against other refrigeration techniques. There has also been significant application of the snow system to other poultry, a few pre-packed cuts of meat and to processed meat, and one fairly recent development is to use a block of dry ice in the giblet pack in the chicken cavity. This is reported as reducing the temperature of the whole bird to zero within 4 hours and limits any cold-burn marks to the inside of the cavity.

Chapter 11

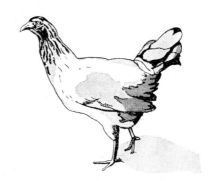

Birds and Poultry

Man has had a complicated relationship with birds since his origin. The ability to fly has been regarded as divine, birds being agents and messengers of sky-dwelling gods. The times and directions of flight have also had religious significance, and there is inexplicable divine inference in bird entrails. Navigational genius and extrasensory perception in birds has been used by man throughout the ages, from early watchdog geese to modern racing of pigeons, and most successful weather prophets rely on bird movements. In more practical terms, birds have been a vital source of protein in hunting and it has long been common to retain clipped birds as reserve food. In primitive nomadic societies, young birds and eggs were frequently the last suppers of the old and weak, who could no longer catch game or find suitable vegetation. More recently, the sensitivity of birds has been used for detection, as for example of methane gas in mines but also of slight sound waves. The sensitivity to pollution is of value under modern conditions and birds frequently indicate dangerous levels.

Birds can be seen in all parts of the world except the centre of Antarctica. They are relatives of reptiles, the earliest bird on record being archaeopteryx, which had feathers but was a poor flier. Its discovery as a fossil in Bavaria provided the first concrete evidence in support of Darwin. Over 2 million years ago there were probably more than 11 000 species of birds but most of the flightless or heavy birds have died out and we are left with probably 8600 species. There are calculations that the present range is less than 1% of all the species which have evolved, the grand total being over 1.5 million species. The largest living bird is the ostrich, which has the distinction of having only two toes, but there are records of larger birds. Notable are the elephant birds and the moas, which reached 4 m high and 300 kg in weight and survived into the eighteenth century. Rumours have it that elephant birds of up to half a ton in weight existed, which is possible since there are a few rescued eggs which hold up to 10.1 litres.

The species which remain from the turnover of 1.5 million total species since initial development have specialised to suit environments or, because birds can fly, to suit planned mixtures of environments visited according to a programme. An example of ultimate specialisation is the penguin, in which the wings have become flippers and the body has been designed for marine life in freezing temperatures. All but one of the fifteen species of penguin are to be found in the colder waters of the southern hemisphere. Specialisation may have been responsible for the high turnover of species amongst birds. At present, roughly 60% of species can be regarded as semi-specialist, insofar that they perch in conducive environments, far removed from the dangers which face birds specialised to diving, swimming, wading, clinging to storm-lashed cliffs or waddling through mud. Perching is the ultimate in safety precautions, particularly for small birds which can perch on very flimsy supports.

PROTEIN FROM BIRDS

It is evident that most existing bird species will suffer from increases in pollution and disruption of environments. With the constant increase in cost of land area it is also evident that there is more potential for organised protein production from birds than from mammals, since mammals occupy area whilst birds use vertical space, giving three-dimensional possibility to working. The orders which are available for exploitation are:

	Represented by
Sphenisciformes	Penguins
Struthioniformes	Ostriches
Gaviiformes	Divers
Pelicaniformes	Cormorants
Anseriformes	Geese and ducks
Ciconiiformes	Storks and flamingoes
Galliformes	Turkeys and various game birds
Gruiformes	Cranes
Columbiformes	Pigeons

	Represented by
Psittaciformes	Parrots
Strigiformes	Owls
Coraciiformes	Kingfishers
Passeriformes	Thrushes and most other birds which perch and sing

This is not a complete list, as it exempts the unsociable carnivores and birds which need long-distance flight in their conducive environments. Long-distance flight, apart from complicating the organisation of housing, demands a high proportion of wing relative to protein content and this would be less economic in protein production.

Most bird bones are hollow and many bones found in other vertebrates are missing from birds in the interests of low weight. The bones of, for example, a 1.5 kg frigate bird with a 2 m wing span may weigh as little as 100 g, which is less than the weight of the feathers. It is to be appreciated that if birds are to be used for intensive protein production the bones will travel with the bird but the feathers need to be removed before marketing, and they can be an economic problem.

There are two basic forms of flight. In one, the intention is to provide a short burst of powerful movement away from enemies. In the other, flight is geared to long-distance travel. Short-term flight is with quick-acting muscles and a limited supply of blood to the wing muscles, whilst long-term flight uses red muscle well furnished with oxygen-carrying blood. This muscle activity in flight produces body heat, which would kill if it had not an associated respiration system. In addition to a pair of lungs it is common to find at least nine air-sacs which provide extra oxygen and cooling. Since the extra ventilation makes the body sensitive to temperature changes there is advantage in feathers as insulation to contain body heat in cold climates, feathers being superior to fur in that they lay flat for easier air flow over the body. A common sparrow has probably 3500 feathers. Feathers on living birds are maintained by coatings of body fat from glands or by layers of dust derived from disintegrated feathers. There is continuous moulting from most birds but some ducks and other water birds shed flight feathers in seasons when they are consequently grounded. Penguins refeather by growing a new set which pushes the retiring feathers off the body.

All organisms are used by birds for food, from dead whales scavenged by gulls to the algae which is specialist diet for flamingoes. Young birds frequently consume their own weight per day but adults eat less. Grubeaters consume high proportions of water in their diet and may need a daily weight of feed of 40% of their body weights, whereas seed-eaters may need only 10% of their body weight. Seed-eating appears to be a late development as most vegetarian birds start off their families on insects. Pigeons are exceptional in that they start off their families on a milk secretion. One-fifth of all birds feed mainly on nectar. This involves hovering, which uses energy. It is calculated that if a human used energy at the rate used by humming birds he would have to lose 40 kg of perspiration per hour to keep cool. It is fairly obvious, therefore, that any protein project based on birds would need to inhibit wing action if conversion rates need to be economic.

THE FARMING OF WILD BIRDS

Wild birds are sensitive and fatality rates are high, it being extremely rare for a bird to survive into old age. In fact, one unknown in ornithology is how long specific birds might live if they discovered conducive environments without enemies. The total world population of birds is variously calculated between 10 000 million and 100 000 million, with a vague estimate that 60% are on dry land and 3% are on water, the rest being of no fixed abode. Densities vary from 1–40 birds/acre, not counting the birds using colonies for nesting. There are exceptions, notably the African weaver or Sudan finch, hated by farmers under various names which make the scientific name of Quelea important to remember. This bird seems to have no natural enemies which prove effective in control, and therefore exists in such vast numbers that estimates are impossible. Flocks darken the sky and are known to break branches from the weight of their perchings. They eat more grain in Africa than do the Africans living in the same central belt, and they could provide valuable protein if anyone could devise an efficient method of catching.

Wild birds increase and decline in number by cycles related to their food supply. Food gluts cause rapid reproduction of birds, which removes the glut and consequently produces starvation. Relatively little removal of the food supply can cause death to most birds, the energy from a full diet being essential for survival. If wild birds could be provided with a constant full diet the reproduction rates would be much higher than those in nature, and catching for food would not unduly deplete populations. Populations decline only if catching is excessive without the provision of extra food to encourage extra birds.

The farming of wild birds, other than in special circumstances, concerns species which live in colonies where extra food can be provided, eggs can be protected and adult birds can be harvested in number. Birds colonise for various reasons, of which the most important are protection against enemies and the availability of local food supplies. Some, such as guillemots, colonise because they can only mate in the midst of a noisy crowd. The largest bird colony is probably that of boobies and cormorants in Peru, some 10 million birds sharing the anchovy harvest with the fish meal industry of Peru, and producing rich guano fertiliser as a secondary export substance for Peru when the fish meal fails. It is probable that most birds could be encouraged to form colonies. Birds, other than birds of prey, are social animals and they have developed methods of communication. However, there are problems arising from proximity, almost all of which are related to mating habits, and densification of bird populations for protein farming could be severely limited by fighting cocks, although it is probable that birds reared in artificial colonies would not seek territorial areas for individuals. In natural conditions, birds who claim territories adjust the area of their individual claims to the population density. If food were to be provided it is probable that second generation birds would not seek individual rights, but they would fight in mating.

Clutches of eggs frequently equal or exceed the weight of the laying hen. A ruddy duck may, in fact, lay two or three times its body weight as a single clutch. Some birds lay a set number of eggs and refuse to lay more if any are removed. Other birds will lay new eggs to replace those taken away. This is the basis of domestic egg production, domestic fowls producing one egg per day to replace one egg taken away. There are two main groups of young birds, since relatively small eggs produce blind and naked chicks, and relatively large eggs produce lively clothed chicks which can run and peck without delay. Both consume a protein-rich diet and grow at rapid rates. Consumption is of the order of one body-weight of food per day and it is not unusual for a twenty- or twenty-five-fold increase in body weight to occur within weeks. Mortality is mainly in the first year and there can be allergic reactions during changes of diet as chicks grow to adults.

THE FARMING OF DOMESTIC BIRDS

Domestic fowls were probably kept 5000 years ago, the popular idea being that they were carried on polynesian boats as egg-laying sources of protein, to the potential Americas and the coasts of Africa and Asia. Through the ages there have developed at least 100 common breeds and many variations which are less common. Birds have been suitably fed and bred to become heavy with meat and capable of producing almost one egg per day through the year. Progress has been rapid during the twentieth century. Before 1900 it was unusual to find chicken farms with more than 500 birds, which would now be regarded as a reasonable number in a sample feeding trial before risking the main flock.

Poultry fit into mixed agriculture as scavengers capable of converting free-range food into attractive meat and as providers of eggs. They are by tradition the responsibility of the farmer's wife and are confined within farmyard limits, however the high conversion rate attracted factory farmers who developed systems of intensive rearing. Such systems produce rapid growth but ignore the egg output and result in meat which is widely regarded as inferior. There is growing rejection of battery-reared poultry meat, mainly following publicity of additives in feed, and farmers are seeking means of producing the flavour of open-range birds in battery-reared birds. The rejection is, however, unlikely to influence markets whilst red meat is expensive.

Per capita consumption of poultry varies considerably with season and the individual consumer. Without the influence of inflated retail prices for red meat a fair average in developed countries would be about 125 g of poultry meat in up to 500 g total flesh protein food per week. Most of this concerns relatively small birds but one aspect of inflation is effort by butchers to sell large birds as replacement for meat joints. Thus, turkeys of up to 8 kg have been promoted in Europe to replace the traditional Sunday meat joint. The position of poultry in the United Kingdom is of interest because, being a food importer, the United Kingdom offers a freedom of choice, and at the time of writing is not subjected to the impossible EEC regulations regarding inspection of birds before sale. The 1970 United Kingdom pattern avoids the main complications of inflation and is:

	Ounces *Per person per week* $(= 28.35\ g)$
Total red meat, of which	15.8
Beef/veal	7.7
Sheep meat	5.3
Pig meat	2.8

	Ounces *Per person per week* ($=28.35$ g)
Poultry	4.6
Bacon/ham	5.1
Sausages	3.7
Fish	5.5
Canned meats	3.37

Poultry are seen to be not overimportant in a market free from encouragement to consume poultry. The present high demand, occasioned by inflation, is deceptive. Since there is already objection to battery-reared birds there could be reduced demand if poultry prices increased towards the prices of red meat. The battery system of rearing is sensitive to cost changes, notably feed costs, labour costs and heating costs. In all respects the owner of a battery system is under pressure to increase retail prices and there is some probability that free-range birds will prove less expensive than battery-reared birds.

Other birds than the conventional chicken are also being examined, mainly seeking birds which do not suffer disease and can be reared without antibiotics. The target is a 'clean' bird which is acceptable outside the influence of inflation and which may sell at a higher price. Quail is of interest because it produces superior meat, matures within forty-five days, needs very little space and supplies eggs which have better nutritional value than hen eggs. The meat is of particular interest because it is low in cholesterol but high in vitamins, and the amino-acid pattern is said to be ideal for delicate digestive systems. Also the possible price range is said to be ideal for the rearer to make a profit.

Domesticated birds have been developed to be completely different from wild birds in their structure and requirements, and emphasis has been on chickens, which can thrive in simple circumstances. Most of the ducks, which are reared to perhaps only 10% of the numbers of reared chickens, originate from mallards, and in the United States there is emphasis on turkey, it being certain that there are now more turkeys in the Americas than existed when they were wild. Mexican wild turkey had been domesticated before Cortez arrived, Cortez taking it back to Europe in the 1500s. Noah was the first pigeon-fancier on record, and it is known that the Egyptians reared pigeons for food and communication long before chickens reached Africa. Pigeons originated from rock doves which became urbanised around temples, starting a trend which has resulted in most cities having pigeon populations. History also tells us that the Mediterranean area was rich in quail until local starving people found them excellent protein food. The children of Israel have been estimated to have killed 9 million birds within two days during one famine period. In more recent times, up to 1920 the Egyptians were exporting 3 million birds/year and more were killed for home consumption. Future history books may well record a similar drastic reduction of numbers of quelea in central Africa.

Only about 40% of birds can be eaten. The water content of bird meat varies considerably after cooking, from 20–75%. Raw chicken meat is about 23% protein and 2% fat, whereas boiled whole chicken has about 10% fat. Roast chicken has less fat, about 7.5%, but the protein is up to 30%. Roast duck can reach 24% fat with only 23% protein, and roast goose is likely to equal roast duck in fat content but with up to 28% protein. Roast grouse, to show the difference in game birds, is likely to be 30% protein and 5% fat. Other game birds, such as partridge, can exceed 35% protein but this is high amongst birds. Roast turkey is reasonably average with 30% protein and up to 8% fat. If bones are included in the original weight the protein contents and fat contents need to be reduced by about 30%. Wastage after cooking is high for poultry but if a fully-carved carcase is subsequently scavenged for its remaining flesh it is possible to increase the total protein derived from one bird by at least 25%.

MINERAL CONTENT OF BIRD MEATS

The mineral contents of bird meats are of interest. Being egg-layers, birds have less requirement for blood than mammals and the iron content is lower in the white meat. The minerals, presented in the conventional notation of mg/ounce, are:

	Na	K	Ca	Mg	Fe	P	S	Cl
Raw beef	19.6	95	1.5	6.9	1.22	78	57	20
Roast lean beef	20	101	1.8	7.1	1.5	81	80	21
Roast fatty beef	17.6	82	1.6	5.7	1.3	67	64	18.2
Raw chicken meat	13	115	1.7	8.2	0.2	70	76	17
Boiled chicken	28	108	3.0	7.5	0.6	77	83	17.6
Roast chicken	23	101	4.1	6.5	0.7	77	92	28.5
Roast duck	55.3	90	5.4	6.8	1.6	66	112	45
Roast goose	41	115	3.0	8.8	1.3	76	91	45
Roast grouse	27.3	132	8.5	11.6	2.1	96	97	38
Roast guinea fowl	39	122	5.5	8.2	2.6	83	103	51

	Na	K	Ca	Mg	Fe	P	S	Cl
Roast partridge	28.4	116	13	10	2.2	89	113	28
Roast pheasant	30	117	14	10	2.4	88	87	31
Roast pigeon	30	116	4.6	9.6	5.5	114	86	28
Roast turkey	37	104	11	8.0	1.1	91	66	35

Mineral compositions are to some extent a measure of the flavour of the meat. The game birds have attractive mineral compositions because they have changed little from their ancestors. The guineafowl is now much the same as that bred in Greece during the fourth century and the turkey is roughly similar to that enjoyed by the Amerindians and subsequently by Europeans after Turkish traders had bought it from the new Americans. Chickens have two main origins after their early domestication in the Pacific. The two development routes are from semi-tropical climates, producing lively small birds laying white eggs, and from colder climates, producing heavy peace-loving birds laying brown or cream-coloured eggs. In their development, both types of bird have also been developed as bantam versions, roughly half the size of their ancestors but laying relatively large eggs. All can be traced back to *Gallus gallus*, the original red jungle fowl which still scavenges in Asian forests. Most geese have descended from the greylag or Siberian swan goose. The most popular are Emden or Toulouse geese, which are excellent watchdogs before they become excellent meat. The mid-European geese are self-sufficient as scavengers in grass or over harvested fields, but are completely unsuited to factory farming. If geese and ducks were suitable for intensive rearing the mineral patterns would probably be similar to those of intensively-reared chicken.

Poultry are characterised by colour difference between the breast and leg. There are other differences, as illustrated by the vitamin pattern. Chicken leg shows much the same vitamin pattern as meat from mammals whilst the breast meat is much reduced in vitamin value. Broadly, the comparison is:

	Thiamine (*mg*)	*Riboflavine* (*mg*)	*Nicotinic acid* (*mg*)
Raw beef	0.07	0.20	5
Roast beef	0.05	0.22	5
Raw chicken breast	0.10	0.07	10
Raw chicken leg	0.10	0.25	5
Roast chicken breast	0.05	0.06	8

	Thiamine (mg)	Riboflavine (mg)	Nicotinic acid (mg)
Roast chicken leg	0.05	0.20	4
Raw turkey breast	0.06	0.08	11
Raw turkey leg	0.06	0.22	5
Roast turkey breast	0.04	0.06	8
Roast turkey leg	0.04	0.18	6

The vitamin pattern can be made to vary by alteration of the diet and it would not be difficult, if markets indicated the need, for poultry meat to be vitamin-enriched. If amino acids are expressed as proportions of total nitrogen, the pattern in poultry is similar to that in meat from mammals. The nitrogen contents of poultry meat and mammal meat are also similar.

Chapter 12

Dairy Protein

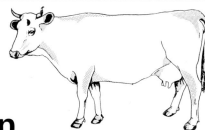

Milk is roughly one part solids in seven parts water. It is unstable and sensitive to biodeterioration, requiring consumption at the time of production. Mild heat treatment followed by low-temperature handling will give milk a life sufficient to allow local delivery, and UHT processing, which is short-period high-temperature heat treatment, gives a life satisfactory for wider distribution. There has been recent development of concentration techniques (reverse osmosis, ultrafiltration and ion exchange) which remove water from milk without spoiling the flavour. In effect, there is now no logic in developing markets for liquid drinking milk as produced or with mild heat treatment, since concentrates offer identical food value to consumers with much more convenience and economy in handling.

Other than heat treatment, the conventional preservation technique for milk is fermentation, introducing a little alcohol and acidity to inhibit evil organisms. Alternatively, the mixture may be divided into its components so that attacking organisms are given a restricted diet, or one effective component can be removed to discourage attack. Notably, water is removed to produce milk powder—preferably with reduced fat so that there is less fat oxidation. Under sensible processing conditions there is very little damage to the protein fraction, most of the deterioration problems coming from the fat and sugar. Compositions can be calculated from analysis of the two extremes of liquid milk and powder:

	Liquid milk	Skim milk	Whole milk powder	Skim milk powder
			(% composition)	
Fat	3.75	0.05	27.5	0.8
Lactose	4.85	4.95	38.2	52.3
Protein	3.30	3.40	26.0	36.0
Minerals	0.72	0.74	5.9	8.0
Water	87.5	90.0	2.0	3.0

The vitamin content is not particularly important in a mixed diet but is used as a marketing tool. Riboflavin and vitamin C are destroyed by sunlight and there is vitamin loss in heat treatment.

The casein exists as a colloid carrying the minerals and the fat as an emulsion with globules stabilised by a layer of protein and calcium phosphate. Common practice in concentration is to take the solids to 30% for whole milk and to 20–25% for skimmed milk. Skim milk can be taken to 35% solids by reverse osmosis and any milk can be taken to 50% solids by reverse osmosis followed by vat evaporation. Powder production starts from a concentrate at about 40% solids and can use spray or drum techniques. Drum dried powder has platelets of protein and lactose coated with fat. Reconstitution releases free fat and there is a cream line. Spray dried powder is granules of fat and protein coated with lactose, the particles being some three times the size of those of drum dried. Reconstitution is rapid because the sugar coating wets, but the final liquid lacks a cream line. Both types of powder contain air and are sensitive to oxidation if the air is not replaced by nitrogen or other inert gas. Bulk densities vary considerably according to the supplier, in the regions of:

	g/ml
Drum dried	0.3–0.5
Spray dried	0.4–0.9
Instant	0.2–0.4

Powder moisture content is 2–3%, at which level there should be a life of about one year, but less with high fat content and warm storage conditions. At 6% moisture content, which equates to 45% relative humidity, lactose crystals form and more water is released, causing caking and some degeneration.

Conventional liquid concentrates (so-called condensed and evaporated milk) thicken in storage at rates determined by the temperature, and need the cans turning over at intervals to prevent gel formation.

Subject to prevailing prices of alternatives, and applicable levies or subsidies, some milk is fed to animals. As far as returns can be trusted the proportions fed to stock are of the order of:

> France—21% of production
> Italy—17%
> Ireland—15%
> United Kingdom—2%

It can be calculated that about 40 million tons of world milk is fed to animals, not counting milk fed to animals at farm level without records. In 1970, in million gallons, the quantities of milk fed to stock included:

New Zealand	50
Canada	66
USA	170
Belgium	38
Denmark	43
West Germany	305
Holland	41
Finland	10
Eire	116
Sweden	22
Switzerland	110

The relationship of these consumptions, which are in effect representative of long routes to final protein, to other milk disposals should be appreciated. New Zealand puts 200 million gallons in applications other than butter and cheese and 50 million gallons of this is fed to animals. West Germany uses the stock feeding outlet for half the milk not needed for liquid, butter or cheese. Similar high proportions can be seen elsewhere for useful milk fed to stock. Much of the milk fed to stock is powder. Other uses for powder are infant foods, chocolate, ice cream, etc. with a general division of spray dried powder for human diet and drum dried powder for animals, although the division is not sharp. In the market for human consumption there is a rival in non-milk whiteners, which are mainly glucose and sodium caseinate.

Dried egg is a technical associate of milk powder, its composition being:

Shell 12.15%		White 57%		Yolk 30.85%	
Calcium carbonate	93.5%	Protein	10.6%	Protein	16.6%
Calcium phosphate	0.7%	Fat	0.0%	Fat	32.6%
Magnesium		Carbohydrate	0.9%	Carbohydrate	1.0%
carbonate	0.8%	Minerals	0.6%	Minerals	1.1%
Membrane protein	3.4%	Water	87.8%	Water	48.6%
Water	1.6%				

The liquid fraction of the egg comprises:

Protein	12.8%
Fat	11.8%
Carbohydrate	1.0%
Minerals	0.8%
Water	73.6%

Dried egg production started in China and has had a variable history, but technology is now fairly advanced. The liquid fraction is cooled to 4 °C and strained. Enzyme and hydrogen peroxide are added and the liquid is stirred for 12 hours to remove the sugar. The liquid is then pasteurised and sprayed into hot air. Removal of the glucose sugar is essential for a long storage life, most of the organic damage being traced to proteus or pseudomonas. Earlier, yeast fermentation was used to remove the glucose but it is now more common to use an enzyme extract from *Aspergillus niger*, the hydrogen peroxide being added to provide extra oxygen for the glucose to convert to gluconic acid.

Egg liquid is also sold for specialised markets, and there are blended egg mixtures of whole egg plus extra yolk. Developments include acidification of egg liquid for direct sale or for drying, sodium bicarbonate being added later if a long life is needed.

CHEESE
Every early society with milk to spare developed its own fermentation product as a liquid and subsequently as a drained solid. There has since been some regimentation of cheeses into common types but demand is strong for regional cheeses, despite the pressure to sell less natural hard cheese and to sell more processed cheese. Processed cheeses are manufactured from high-quality natural cheeses and are equal in nutritional value to natural cheeses, but are more suited to conditions of sale in self-service outlets and avoid the problem of packaging an active living substance. Confinement of natural cheese within barrier materials must

produce some change in the organic reactions and, since flavour and quality are functions of such reactions, most changes can be counted as damage. On the other hand, the making of cheese is a primitive process with danger of infection and it is practical to interfere with the organic reactions if only to make certain that they proceed as planned. For example, *Aspergillus flavus* can furnish toxin some 25 mm below the rind surface, and this, and other offensive contamination, can be prevented by dipping in wax or 0.1% sorbic acid, or by wrapping in some antifungal material. Nisin is one antibiotic which will inhibit spore development, and is a substance extracted from strains of streptococci similar to those used as cheese starters. Hence, it is regarded as safe and is used to about 2.5 p.p.m. to control clostridial development. Mites can also be a problem with cheese, penetrating some considerable depth and carrying infection. Since cheeses are results of organic reactions which continue to the point of consumption it is difficult to control quality by additives, some of which are whey proteins, which are the soluble proteins previously thrown away and are surplus dairy products. However, in the processing of cheese there is more freedom and unwelcome organic reactions can be stopped, the active life of the cheese being arrested at the time of processing.

Processed cheeses have two outstanding economic virtues when compared against natural cheeses. They can be manufactured with the addition of substances for which an outlet is required. Also, they can be produced in unit sizes and shapes ready for sale without waste in cutting and trimming. Processed cheese for slicing needs a low fat and moisture content down to 40%. For spreading more fat and moisture is possible but if the moisture exceeds 55% there must be addition of gums to emulsify the fat.

Natural cheese is manufactured by coagulation of the milk by enzymes and subsequent removal of the water fraction. The curd is then moulded and conditioned according to local traditions, reaching a point of perfection of flavour by a relatively slow final stage, at which point it should be eaten without further delay. For example, cheddar-type cheese is produced from milk heated to 66 °C for 15 secs to limit the microbe population, then supplied with a starter culture followed by rennet. The curd is cut to help drainage and given 2% salt. It is then pressed dry in moulds and conditioned at a ratio of 10 °C : 90% relative humidity for 3–9 months. Soft cheeses such as camembert are made with rennet but with a high moisture content, and very soft cheeses are made without rennet but with a high moisture content. Some cheeses are produced from milk with its original population of organisms, whilst some cheeses are from milk which has been heat treated. The finer flavour comes from the ripening, which varies and need not be at a constant temperature : humidity ratio for the whole conditioning period. Emmental, for example, has a secondary ripening period in which new families of organisms are encouraged to blow holes in the mass. Blue veins are also produced by secondary ripening periods. Each cheese is an individual and, if it is to be true to type, it must follow the original milk and process pattern. The following table is indicative of the variation, all values being approximations subjected to local variation :

	Ripening			Storage		
	°C	%RH	Period weeks	°C	%RH	Period weeks
Bel Paese	4.5	90	3–4	0	85–90	8–15
Cheddar						
slow	4	75	35–40			
normal	7–10	85	4–25			
rapid	12–16	85–90	8–10	0	70–75	50
Cheshire	12–15	85–90	8–10			
Edam	12–15	90	3–4	12–15	85	
Emmental						
1st	10–15	85	2			
2nd	16–18	90	4–5	10–12	80	
Gorgonzola						
1st	9–11	85–90	8–10			
2nd	5–7	90	4–5	0	80–85	12–30
Gruyere						
1st	10–15	85	2–3			
2nd	16–18	90	4–6	10–12	80–85	
Parmesan	16–18	80	48–60	0	70–75	50–100
Roquefort	5–10	95		0	80–85	4–15
St. Paulin	12–15	90	3–4	0	90	

Until recently it has been common for the whey to be discarded in cheese manufacture, or perhaps to be fed to local pigs. The whey contains the solubles in milk and it is probable that over 10 million tons of whey are discarded from world cheese manufacture, most of this is into waterways where it encourages false micro-organic growth on the sugar–protein content.

The lactose sugar in whey has application in upgrading cow milk for human consumption and in preservation by sugars with reduced sweetness. The protein has value in new cheese manufacture but it also has application in bakery products, beverages and general food compounding. Reverse osmosis and ultrafiltration can give a 15% protein liquid which is suitable for spray drying. Such a liquid is likely to contain 5% lactose, which is excessive, and there are developments of extracting the lactose for fermentation to more protein. On the other hand, cow milk has only 4.8% lactose whilst human milk has 7% and there is a large outlet for lactose in infant foods. The composition of the whey fed to concentration equipment is:

Protein	0.7%
Lactose	4.5%
Salts	0.6%
Acid	0.6%
Water	93.5%

Reverse osmosis can take the total solids to 33% with:

Protein	4%
Lactose	22%
Salts	2.5%
Acids	2.5%

Ultrafiltration can take the total solids to only 18% with:

Protein	12.5%
Lactose	4.5%

The choice of process depends on whether one needs a sugar-rich concentrate from osmosis or a protein-rich concentrate from filtration. Developments in many countries have resulted in very high protein concentrates, up to 80% protein with only 1% lactose and 1.5% fat. A typical outlet is in biscuits using:

Butter	36.7%
Flour	22%
Sugar	12.5%
Whey protein	22%

Such biscuits are excellent diet in famine areas and are an acceptable form of food for school feeding programmes, alongside reconstituted milk.

Broadly, about 80% of available proteins coagulate in cheese manufacture and the other 20% is lost as whey. Of the coagulated protein about 80% is casein and some of the more important proteins are lost. The soluble proteins can be rescued in part by reducing the pH value and heating, this form of rescue providing an additive for new cheese, the additive causing new curd to be harder. There are also processes for the extraction of edible casein directly from milk.

The protein content of cheese varies about the typical values of:

	Protein (%)	Fat (%)
Cream cheese	3.3	86.0
Camembert	22.8	23.2
Cheddar	25.4	34.5
Cheshire	25.8	30.6
Danish blue	23.0	29.2
Edam	24.4	22.9
Gorgonzola	25.4	31.1
Gouda	22.6	26.6
Gruyere	37.6	33.4
Mysost	10.8	28.7
Parmesan	35.1	29.7
Stilton	25.6	40.0
Wensleydale	29.3	30.7

The actual values depend on the stage of conditioning and on the location of the cut within the cheese. Mature Gouda, for example, can show 26.5% protein, which is 4% more than young Gouda. Processed cheese varies but should be in the region of 23% protein and 30% fat, more or less according to the additives. The following are useful comparisons:

	% protein	% fat
Condensed skim milk	10	0.3
Dried skim milk	34.5	0.3
Dried human milk	27	30
Liquid human milk	1.2–2.0	3.7–5.1(according to stage)
Fresh eggs	12	12.3
Dried eggs	43.4	43.3

The pattern of amino acids in cheeses varies with its processing, particularly since whey protein may or may not be included, and since the final composition depends on the conditioning. As might be expected, since humans and cows are both mammals, the pattern for cheese protein resembles that for human milk (but not colostrum, the first milk after childbirth).

	Amino acids in milk and cheese (per g nitrogen)		
	Milk or cheese from cows	*Human milk*	*Human colostrum*
Arginine	0.23	0.21	0.36
Cystine	0.04	0.12	0.16
Histidine	0.17	0.14	0.14
Isoleucine	0.39	0.35	0.27
Leucine	0.62	0.59	0.48
Lysine	0.49	0.39	0.39
Methionine	0.15	0.13	0.11
Phenylalanine	0.32	0.25	0.30
Threonine	0.29	0.28	0.41
Tryptophane	0.09	0.10	0.14
Tyrosine	0.35	0.30	0.34
Valine	0.44	0.39	0.42
Alanine	0.23	0.24	
Aspartic acid	0.51	0.58	
Glutamic acid	1.39	1.24	
Glycine	0.12	0.14	
Proline	0.61	0.54	
Serine	0.36	0.30	

As a point of interest, the amino-acid pattern for egg white is very similar to that for colostrum other than in its high isoleucine, leucine and methionine and its lower threonine and tyrosine.

SOURED MILKS

Souring has been a historic method of preserving milk, the induced acid acting as inhibition of growth to many organisms. Original soured milks were consumed as produced but there are now sophisticated versions in which the flavour of the acid is hidden under the sweetness of added sugar and strong fruit flavours. Bulgarians rightly claim that the title yoghurt can only be given to bulgaricus ferments of untreated milk, preferably sheep milk but with cow milk included when necessary. Most early societies have included in their diet some form of soured milk to be consumed without division into curds and whey. As a rule the souring has been by specific bacterial action with a local culture passed from batch to batch through generations, leading to local mutations. The substance known as yoghurt in modern society is likely to be low-fat (below 2%) with a protein content of the order of 5%, of which part may not be dairy protein or fat.

True yoghurt is fermented by *Lactobacillus bulgaricus*, the fermentation producing almost pure lactic acid. From about 1950, *Streptococcus thermophilus* has been added, the streptococcus removing oxygen to accelerate the production of lactic acid whilst the bacillus provides amino acids to encourage the streptococcus. The better yoghurt is from sheep milk (but there are yoghurts from goat milk), this being free from any risk of tubercle bacillus. Sheep milk is rich in fat and in vitamin B12. Common yoghurt from cow milk has a fat content of about 3.7% and is not to be confused with the marketed upgraded version at 5% protein and below 2% fat. Common cow yoghurt can contain up to 8.5% of non-fat solids. The protein porportion of these solids may be increased by addition of milk powder or whey solids, or may be decreased by the addition of fruit and sugar to the mixture. Flavouring additions can be up to 20% of final weight and roughly 90% of yoghurt in developed markets is flavoured.

There are many soured milks other than yoghurts. Kefir is a version rich in lactic acid and carbon dioxide. Scandinavian versions are fermented by *Streptococcus cremoris* and can contain up to 8% fat. There are also fermented whey drinks and cultured creams with up to 35% fat. Poland has milk or whey champagne and there is tea-flavoured soured milk in Japan. Types of yoghurt are now sold frozen and there are yoghurt puddings and cakes. Obviously, with such a compounding potential and intention it is pointless to detail protein contents or amino-acid balances.

WHEY PROTEIN

To some extent, interest in whey proteins came from attempts to reduce pollution of waters near to cheese-making. It grew with increases in price of milk powder, when it was realised that whey powder could not only replace milk powder in baking and compounding, but had advantages. Notably, the proteins in whey are the soluble types which blend into water-based mixtures and subsequenty bake to a rich shade of brown. In terms of diet the interesting whey proteins are lactoglobulin and lactalbumin. The vitamins are useful, the comparison against milk powder being:

	Skim milk powder (mg/lb)	Whey protein (mg/lb)
B12 (μg)	25	10
Thiamin	1.6	2.2
Riboflavin	9	10
Niacin	5.2	4
Pantothenic acid	15	20
Choline	650	900
Folic acid	0.3	0.44

The full breakdown of skim milk is:

	% in milk liquid
Lactose	5.05
Casein	2.67
Non-protein nitrogen	0.25
Ash	0.75
Fat	0.10
Whey proteins	0.70
Water to 100%	

The whey fraction is 93% water and 7% solids, of which:

	% in whey liquid
Lactose	4.9
Coagulable protein	0.5
Non-coagulable protein	0.4
Ash	0.6
Fat	0.3
Lactic acid	0.2

Both can be spray dried to give the following comparison:

	% in dried powder	
	Skim milk	Whey solids
Casein	30.0	0.0
Lactalbumin	6.0	13.0
Lactose	51	71
Fat	0.5	0.87
Ash	9.2	11.0
Moisture	4	4

Of the proteins the amino-acid patterns are:

	Skim milk (%)	Whey solids (%)
Arginine	1.13	0.32
Methionine	0.81	0.25
Lysine	2.89	1.07
Tryptophane	0.49	0.22
Histidine	0.88	0.20
Isoleucine	2.54	0.74
Leucine	3.74	1.14
Phenylalanine	1.59	0.36
Valine	2.47	0.73
Threonine	1.70	0.83

The low casein is a particular advantage for bakery applications. Casein masks flavour whereas whey products enhance flavour. The high lactose is also an advantage in baking, extra sugar being possible in a mix without extra sweetness. Lactose is not fermented by normal baking yeasts, which means that the sugar proceeds through to the final bake to give a rich brown colour. Other advantages of whey solids instead of milk powder in baking include less sticking of pans and a firmer crust.

Whey solids are also used in ice creams, mainly as a low-cost extender. The ability to bring out flavour is an advantage in flavoured ice creams. As a rule, whey solids can replace milk powder to 25% within existing legislation for ice cream but there are many frozen desserts which can take 100% replacement.

Chapter 13

Fish

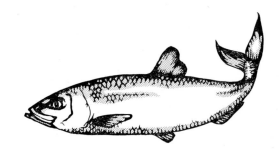

Fish, as a main source of protein food, developed only amongst populations living near seas, rivers and lakes and, since fish populations vary according to the waters, the developed selection of fish types varies considerably. Whilst meat on the hoof had a temporary function in transport and haulage, fish had no function other than the satisfaction of appetites. Also, whilst meat production involved the birth, growth and death of animals within compounds which also witnessed the life history of humans, fish bred and grew unobserved and without help. They were regarded as inexhaustible supplies provided by the good gods, to be taken as required and in quantities dictated only by the available catching labour and its skill, and by prevailing weather conditions. Hence, the religious significance of fish differs from that of meat. Fish are regarded as free gifts from the gods, who may be recruited to assist in the catching (as in the blessing of boats) and may be given a sacrificial commission from the catch, but are not unduly concerned with the fish after landing.

In more sophisticated terms, the cost of fish is mainly in the catching and subsequent handling. The cost of catching includes very high long-term investment in equipment, even in primitive communities where the equipment is only a boat and a net. Labour costs in catching are high partly because an advanced level of skill is needed but also because yields are variable and the labour is under-used for most of its time. The same applies to the very high labour cost in handling after landing, variability of landings causing inevitable idle periods. In contrast, the cost of meat is mainly in the breeding and growing, with comparatively little in the slaughter and distribution after killing.

Arising from the history of development, meat supplies are confined to a few species of animal and the meat passes from production to distribution in pure identified forms. Growing wild, fish catches contain the required fish at various stages of growth and also contain a variable collection of associated organisms. The catching of young fish and small unwelcome additions to the netload can be reduced by controlling the net size and the depth of fishing. It is, however, common to use fine nets and to disturb sea bottoms so that the catch is total, which reduces future yields and frequently spoils the seabed environment by bringing up settled pollution, disturbing marine plant life and revealing young fish to their hungry enemies. World catch is of the order of 70 million tons, of which about 40 million are not for direct human consumption. Loss levels are high from trimming and it could be doubted that most of the fish landed for human diet in fact reaches digestive systems.

There is now strong interest in the disintegration of fish tissue and the reconstruction into formed portions. This is an inevitable development from the cutting of boneless fingers and blocks from large fish. The advantages of reconstitution have been given as:

1. Economy and increased efficiency in transport and storage and freezing when the tissue is in flat-sided dimensioned small blocks.
2. Reduction of cutting waste since any fragment of tissue can be used regardless of its size or shape.
3. Ability to include unfamiliar fish which would not sell whole.
4. Ability to overcome variability of catches by the feeding of batches from many variable sources into a common disintegration plant.
5. Facility for the inclusion of other proteins such as whey protein or microbial protein, in effect producing an entirely new range of compounded protein foods.
6. Avoiding market fluctuations by absorbing temporary surplus catches of particular fish types, as for example absorbing sardines during their prolific seasons.
7. Avoiding the marketing problems of fatty fish by dilution with non-fatty tissue to the level of consumer requirement.

Since man is said to have originated from marine animals there is some justification for the claims that fish protein is the most suitable for human digestion. In fact, its suitability for sensitive digestions comes mainly from the ease with which its components can be reached after the tissue has opened from slight decay or from slight cooking. This is important in cases of protein deficiency, where the high potassium content of fish is an asset. The association of calcium with fish protein is also of benefit. Fish protein concentrates are being developed for feeding in famine areas as soon as problems of carried odour can be overcome. Odour-free products need expensive solvent extraction but there are developments of enzyme hydrolysis of the concentrate to give almost 100% pure excellent protein lacking only tryptophane, which can be introduced directly. There are also hopes of the development of compounds based on fish protein concentrate and groundnuts, the organisation of higher-value markets for oilseeds being important to many producing areas. In many coastal regions of developing countries there is a fruitful supply of fish but the types of fish are not suitable for export and the local distribution systems are unsatisfactory for the development of local consumption as fresh fish. Such regions are frequently within reach of oilseed production which is facing competition from soya and potential microbial proteins. It is therefore intended to promote the combination of fish and oilseed protein, partly to find application for the unused fish and partly to overcome problems of low world prices for oilseeds at the point of production.

In developed countries the trend is rapidly away from whole fish in retail sale. Handling whole wet fish is inconvenient and uneconomic, and was tolerated only whilst fish prices were sufficiently low for consumers to accept mess and slime in cooking. Currently the emphasis is on frozen cut fish, including that which is subsequently thawed and sold as fresh. The quality of this retailed fresh fish has declined mainly because a higher proportion of the catch is being supplied into the market. These changes in marketing are being forced by higher costs of catching which together with overfishing of grounds, a higher pollution rate which depletes stocks or drives them into distant waters, and a general increase in labour costs in handling has led to higher retail prices. It is obvious that these increased prices would have been inevitable even if inflated meat prices had not increased demand for fish. Unlike other sources of protein, fish can be costed according to the handling only, whereas other sources need consideration of feed cost, housing and supervision during growth.

At present world fishing fleets are designed for the familiar pattern of fish distribution in waters, but they need to be completely redesigned. In existing catching circumstances the fish start to digest themselves from the moment of death and the decay process is rapid and obvious in odour and flavour. Drip is heavy and there is pollution of vehicles, storehouses, display cabinets, shopping baskets, kitchen surfaces, cooking vessels, dustbins and disposal systems. Freezing has developed partly because it allows supplies to be married to demands but also because it confines odour and restricts drip up to the cooking stage. The market for unfrozen fish must therefore decline because social structures do not include provision for handling offensive substances if ways can be found to remove the offence before the substance comes into contact with people.

The meat industry is sufficiently well organised to reject only the fractions which are not suitable for digestion but the fractions rejected from fish are those which are not attractive to consumers and can be cut away without difficulty. Only very small fish are eaten in their entireties, bones and all, although it is not uncommon for the backbone to be removed from these by the ultimate consumer. Up to half the weight of large fish may be rejected in the production of fillets or steaks and there is a need for outlets for this primary waste in human diet.

Preserved fish are bought on a basis of value for money, value being calculated in terms of weight and flavour, responsibility for quality being placed on the supplier. Fresh fish is bought on a basis of freshness and texture, quality being associated with familiar appearance—clear eyes, white flesh, low slime and no ammoniacal smell. The percentage of edible matter reaching the stomach after purchase varies from about 50% for bought whole fish to 100% for fillets and boneless steaks, although not all this is protein and the relative protein content is changed by the method of cooking.

	Percentage of purchased fish eaten
Whole bass	47
Bloaters without head and guts	65
Whole bream	47
Skinned catfish	64
Cod steaks	66
Cod roe	95
Headless conger	60
Dabs without guts	90
Skinned dogfish without bones	90
Elver eels	100
Haddock middle cut	60
Hake middle cut	63

	Percentage of purchased fish eaten
Halibut middle cut	66
Herring without head and guts	77
Kippers	45
Sole without head and guts	62
Mackerel without head and guts	61
Canned pilchards	97
Plaice without head and guts	49
Pollack middle cut	68
Fresh salmon	73
Canned salmon	98
Skinned skate wings	95
Sardines	100

This list is sufficiently long to indicate the general situation. About 60% of whole fish without head and guts reaches the digestion. Obviously, this varies with the method of cooking and the character of the ultimate consumer but it does give an approximate proportion of product available for development of compounding techniques for undesirable fish fractions.

The fish bought for table use contains about 40% water, which equates to about 75% water in edible tissue without bones, skin and guts. This is higher than in meat but it is to be appreciated that meat has a higher proportional fat content. One reason why fish is superior to meat in hospital feeding is the lower fat content and higher water content, needing lighter cooking to give a more digestible meal. Because the cooking is light and rapid there is comparatively little variation of final protein content amongst fish dishes, most values being between 17 and 22%.

SOCIETY OF FISHES

Previously, fishes have been regarded as one of the five main classes of back-boned animals alongside amphibians, reptiles, birds and mammals. It is now realised that they comprise a very large and complex group with more members than all the other vertebrates put together. They have an earlier origin than land-based animals and, from the complexity of the environments they endure, may yet produce a new class of organisms capable of thriving in the new environments man is helping to manufacture. Whereas land-based organisms can tolerate only a comparatively limited range of environments, fishes thrive in a very wide range of conditions, and have adapted their structures, habits and societies accordingly. They live in lightless depths under very high pressures, in shore-line mixtures of pounding waves and sharp rocks, in highly-radiated hot tropical waters, in constantly-moving shallow waters and in highly polluted oxygen-starved dilute mud. Some fishes even live only part of their life under water, including examples which can hibernate in dried mud waiting for the rains to come and other examples which travel overland to find new homes.

Water covers about three-quarters of the surface of the earth and the various species have developed to suit the differing environments, some species dying out or adjusting and some species surviving unchanged for hundreds of millions of years to the present. There are fishes which can breathe air, fishes which can walk and fishes which can glide in air. There are live-bearers and egg-layers. There are round fishes, flat fishes, and fishes which can change their contours as needed. There are lone fishes and there are fishes which combine in huge schools. There are fishes which migrate according to a programme, fishes which constantly move and fishes which live their entire lives in one hole or weed-bed. There are at least 20 000 species known and many more yet to be discovered or recognised.

The only common factor to all fish is the incompressibility of water, which controls their shape, breathing, movement, feeding, reproduction and communication. Within this basic restriction, fishes have formed their identities and, having established an affinity to an environment, maintain this identity by remaining in the formative environment. Hence, bottom-feeders hug the depths and scavenge slowly as ruminants graze on land, weed-livers rarely venture into open water, reef-dwellers establish a base in rocks and operate by short-distance journeys, whilst lone hunters constantly roam the high seas preferably behind schools of food which moves relatively slowly. In effect, the formative environment has more influence on individual fishes than does the family group. For example, the characin family includes long thin members which are almost eel-like, barrel-shaped members, flatter versions and a few which have fins suitable for short-distance gliding out of the water. Piranha, which enjoy living flesh in their diet, are members of this family but there are also insect-eating and vegetarian members.

There is a hypothetical division into fresh-water and salt-water fishes. The body fluid of fresh-water fishes is salty compared with the environment and there is consequent absorption of water inwards through the skin. Hence, the fish does not drink but passes the absorbed water to the kidneys and urinates frequently. The body fluid of a salt-water fish is less salty than the environment and there is dehydration through the skin (in the same way that housewives use salt water for dehydrating vegetables for pickling). Hence, a salt-water fish drinks profusely, loses the excess salt through the digestive tract and through the gills and rarely urinates.

There are relatively few strict vegetarians amongst fishes, which makes it difficult for man to cultivate fishes by providing vegetation as he can for land-based animals. There is a theory that, since plants are efficient conversion agents of ultraviolet light, fishes can be reared alongside perpetual sowing of marine vegetation. However, under the best conditions, vegetation is only about 3% efficient in conversion and this would apply only to water surfaces, and then only if the surfaces were clean and unpolluted. There is, therefore, more potential in plankton, which is a mixture of plants (phytoplankton) and animals (zooplankton) and is a subsociety within the broader society of fishes and other marine life.

Plankton are microscopic, and therefore productive in terms of weight/time. In a reasonable location the yield is of the order of 1 ton/ acre, which is about the same as a poor hay crop but better than natural grazing on land. The total weight of the vegetable fraction of plankton produced in the world far exceeds the total weight of land-based vegetation, probably reaching half a million million tons per year. The vegetable fraction, phytoplankton, is diet for zooplankton and fishes eat both fractions. The fishes eating the plankton are surface-dwellers moving about in schools with about 4000 distinct species recorded. These are the netted fishes and include herring, mackerel, anchovy, etc. Other plankton-eaters include whales and oddities such as the Mississippi paddle-fish. Plankton-eaters swim along with mouth open straining the water and releasing it through the gills. They are the most abundant of salt-water fish and are food for larger and faster fish. In these predatory fishes the killer instinct is strong and the level of damage to schools far exceeds the diet needs of the hunters. Hunting patterns are sophisticated and include herding schools of small fish ready for the kill.

The other section of the society comprises a mixed selection of scavengers and bottom-feeders. These consume anything resting on the bottom and have digestive systems capable of picking out anything which could be considered as diet. Some fish are fairly selective in that they seek shellfish or vegetation, but most scavengers justify their description and take in anything passing. Mullet and a few others simply

suck in mud, extract any food value from it and then reject the remainder. There are also bottom-feeding carnivores which are not strictly
scavengers but seek worms and such. Scavengers have an obvious place
in any projects relating to fish-farming or manipulation of the fish society
for greater productivity.

Temperature

Although fish have no mechanical restrictions to movement they are
prevented from mixing completely into an averaged society. The main
inhibition to movement is temperature, since this exerts a controlling
influence on diet availability and on the oxygen content of water. Cod
and herring, for example, are cold-water fish which do not venture south
of the United Kingdom or Virginia. As water temperatures increase
towards the equator the range of fish species increases but the numbers
decrease. Hence, an African river may have a thousand species but few
fish to catch whereas an arctic fishing ground might yield a full net of
mainly two or three species.

The hottest water is around the Red Sea area at temperatures to 30 °C.
The coldest is that in polar regions where the salt content allows freezing
at two or three degress below zero. The temperature gradient varies its
pattern according to air temperatures above, but includes a threshold
transitional zone some distance down, below which the temperature
changes very little. Even in shallow water with ice on the surface it is
rare for the bottom temperature to fall below 4 °C.

Although fish are found in all temperatures they thrive best in the
waters at 6–20 °C. Most fishes can withstand temperature variations of
up to 8 °C when they are adult but slight temperature changes can kill
eggs and fry. It is therefore important whether eggs are laid in the upper
fluctuating regions or in the constant-temperature depths. As might be
expected, plankton patterns depend on prevailing temperatures and
plankton die if they drift out of familiar waters. The upper limit of
20 °C for energetic survival of fishes effectively divides the society of
fishes into tropical and temperate types. Between the lines of constant
20 °C temperature are the tropical fishes and from these lines to the
lines of constant 12 °C are the massive shoals of plankton-eating fishes
found mainly on the western coasts of continents. At the lines of constant 12 °C there is a change of population to the large fleshy fish of the
cod and herring type.

The temperature lines are not geographic, being deflected by currents
and the proximity of land masses. Frequently, the currents are vertical

and thereby misplace hot or cold water, and at the same time lift food from the sea-bed for the plankton and hence the fish. The lines can also move quickly without warning, as exampled by the recent famine of anchovy off Peru. A more dramatic event was in 1882, when gales swept cold water across the bottom of the Atlantic, killing 1500 million tile-fish and ruining the tile-fishing industry of New England. In the case of Peru, the north-flowing Humboldt current up the west coast of South America meets offshore winds, which in effect sweep off the warm surface water so that the rich cold water swells up to feed the anchovy. If the winds fail the hot water is not swept away and the plankton die. In turn, the fishes starve and the seabirds find no food. In extreme situations the damage may last several years and the Peruvian fish meal industry cannot meet orders.

Feeding

Marine life started in environments which were completely unlike present fresh or salt waters. When fish developed paired fins and jaws they occupied all waters and developed individual feeding habits. Hence the main difference between them is in the mouth construction and devices for making contact and then dealing with food. For example, sedentary fish grew to resemble vegetation and rocks or mud so that victims would come within reach. Those eating shellfish developed incisors and carni-vores developed needle-teeth. As an extreme example of development, the archer fish fires water at insect victims to bring them down to the water surface for prompt consumption. Marlins rush a school of fish at up to 30 km/hour, spear and maim as many as possible and then consume the dead and damaged victims at will. In contrast, garden eels anchor themselves to the sea bottom for almost their entire lives and simply wait for food to drift by. This flexibility in feeding habits is made possible by the fact that the environment has roughly the same density as the fish and there is no gravity to limit movement. Land animals are constructed, with heavy bones and supporting muscles, relative to the unidirectional force through their feet (or bellies if there are no feet), whereas fishes are constructed relative to a complete envelope of fluid, which can offer drift-pressures but which can be used as a wall to be pushed against for movement in any direction. The support from the water also allows unlimited growth.

In basic terms organisation of the digestive system is similar to that of land-based animals. However, because the water provides a constant temperature, fish are cold-blooded and therefore the digestive system is not complicated by needs to provide thermal energy, but this does mean that if a fish meets the wrong temperature it has to move or die. Hence, many temperate fish migrate and fresh-water fish vary their depth according to the season. Some fresh-water fish hibernate or stop feeding when the water temperature reaches unwelcome limits.

The circulatory system is a simple cycle from the heart to the gills, where blood is oxygenated, around the body and back to the heart. The heart has two chambers and is a direct pump, water being passed into the mouth and out of the gills. Gills are lined with blood vessels which can, in some species, accept oxygen from air, as for example with carp which can use an air bubble in contact with wet gills when the water becomes oxygen-starved. Lung-fishes have lungs similar to those of frogs and newts and many primitive fishes have air-bladders.

Visual recognition of food is made difficult for fishes by the low intensity of light. The eyes are accordingly designed for short-range maximum-sensitivity reaction—short-range because sight further than about 100 m is impossible in most waters. The lens is towards spherical, which gives short-sighted vision, but it can be pulled back for long sight. The lens is, of course, filled with a liquid of the same refractive index as the water, whereas in land-based animals there is a vast difference between the refractive index inside and outside the eye. Hence, a fish sees a monocular distorted picture and consequently tends to eat anything passing, constantly taking and then selecting or rejecting.

The ear in a fish is purely a balancing organ but fishes make signal noises which are obeyed by mates or schools. The gas bladder and range of small bones evidently transmit sufficient vibration for fish to recognise inter-fish signals, to avoid ship propellers or to dive for cover if footsteps disturb a river bank. The sense of smell in fishes is highly developed and is needed to offset the poor light and badly-designed eyes. In effect, smell replaces taste as far as diet is concerned. Having been stimulated by smell and having found the source of the smell, most fish simply gulp down the food directly into the stomach.

The sense of touch is also highly developed, is over all the body and is peculiarly sensitive to changes in pressure which are recognised in terms of magnitude and direction through lateral lines along the body side, where there are specialised sensory glands.

Evolution
There have been, as far as is known, five basic classes.

Agnatha—Jawless fishes, which obviously had no hope of survival in environments which needed jaws, and which are exampled now by only lampreys.

Placodermi—Armoured fishes, which also failed to meet the requirements of exacting environments, insofar that the armour prevented free movement and restricted locomotive muscle action.

Acanthodii—Spiny fishes, in which defensive armour was supported in combat by offensive spines.

Osteichthyes—Bony fishes from which developed the range of scaly fishes which now dominate fish society.

Chondrichthyes—Cartilaginous fishes.

The main division of the classes took place roughly 1 million years ago, when the cartilaginous fishes split into round-bodied, which are now the sharks, and flat-bodied, including rays and skates as we now know them. The scaled spiny fish developed along the many paths mentioned and the other classes died out or graduated into land animals, whose true fate will probably never be known.

Reproduction and survival

Since aquatic environments are well furnished with predators and the shifting currents move food and heat about, reproduction is to excess in the hope that sufficient will survive to maintain the species. The simple form of reproduction is by the female shedding eggs whilst the male sheds sperm, accidental contact bringing fertilisation. Egg sacs are hard roe and sperm sacs are soft roe. However, some fishes use internal fertilisation and it is not uncommon for fish to change sex, or indeed to be self-fertilising. Each species has an ideal temperature range for spawning. Herring, for example, spawn twice a year in spring and autumn but some nomadic fish spawn regardless of the time of year, when they are by chance in the correct temperature. In the tropics, spawning can be at any time but it can coincide with the hot months before and after monsoons.

Most fish have a favoured locality for their spawning. Cod choose water about 30 fathoms deep and nearby fishermen take advantage of the situation. A few well-documented fish return to the same geographic locality for spawning, notably the salmon. Eggs and fry are produced in vast number with the understanding that most of them will be eaten. Cod deposit about 5 million eggs/fish and there is a count of nearly 30 million eggs from a ling. If one egg/million survived there would be no

problem of feeding the starving millions, although there would be subsequent disaster as the fish died from overcrowding and polluted the
water by putrefaction.

The egg may have some device for attachment to other eggs or to
weed, or it may simply carry an adhesive so that when it sinks to the
bottom it sticks to stones. The embryo feeds on a yolk and then graduates to the eating of plankton. Growing fry may then drift for long
periods before seeking deeper water. Cod fry drift for over two months
and then, in mid-summer, move first to the bottom and then away into
deeper waters. In their fourth year, when they are slightly above half a
metre long, they are ready to spawn. Hence, if fishing is to continue as
an industry, it is vital to avoid fishing the 20 fathom waters in which
young fish are waiting to become spawning adults.

As might be expected, some fish do not overproduce on the basis of
high loss of eggs and fry. Notable exceptions are those which live in
rough water where a random cloud of eggs would be broken up and
thrown on shore and be subjected to violent changes of temperature.
These fish combine a few hundred eggs in bundles which are then care-
fully placed in holes which escape the movement of the water. Alternatively, the fish may bear the offspring alive. This is common amongst
lonely nomadic hunting fish, there being little hope of accidental contact
between eggs and spawn if both are dropped some considerable distance
apart in deep water. As a rule, mother fishes have no interest in their
offspring and will eat them alongside any other passing diet, but there
are exceptions such as the dogfish which may carry its young for ten
months, after the manner of land-based mammals. There are also fish
which provide protection for a limited period, including those which
endure temporary starvation whilst their mouths are used as caves for
the fry. One pipe-fish uses a system of development within the male, the
eggs being inserted by the female into the male for fertilisation and
eventual release as fry. Bitterling fish lay their eggs in shellfish and a
number of fishes lay their eggs out of water for hatching, throwing occasional water over them to prevent drying out. The grunion lays her eggs
at the high water mark on beaches, fry being washed back into the
water in the next series of high tides a few weeks later. Fresh-water fishes
frequently use nests with the male acting as watchdog and keeper, and
as a rule, male nest-watchers claim a territory and are therefore unsuitable for intensive farming.

The general opinion is that when a fish becomes adult its survival
depends entirely on the food situation, the proximity of the environment

to the ideal and the agility of the specimen when predators threaten. In fact, there are social systems which have been accepted and studied only recently. For example, many species co-habit without mutual conflict but with mutual benefit, either in the form of protection or in some service. One such partnership concerns cleaner-fish, a very wide range of fishes which eat micro-organisms from the skin of other fish. Surface infection is inevitable in most waters and many species would not survive if cleaner-fish did not exist. The relationships are specific and the fishes to be cleaned appear to seek out their cleaners. An extreme example is the damsel-fish cleaning stinging anemones, which sting to death any fish other than their own personal few damsel-fish, which in return know their own personal anemone and clean no other. Another partnership is the wrasse and barracuda, the wrasse cleaning out bacteria pockets from the mouth of the barracuda, which is a vicious fish towards all others.

Migration
Much of the observed movement of fish is simply the seeking of food or a more attractive temperature. There are, however, movements which are programmed and defy complete explanation. In particular, many fish use specific spawning grounds. For example, plaice eggs shed in the lower North Sea result in fry off the Dutch coast, and although the resultant adults wander around the various coasts they return to the original location for spawning. Cod also have a number of such favoured spawning grounds. Up to the early 1940s it was thought that migration programmes were fixed during formative evolution, but in 1941, the Santee-Cooper dam in the United States penned bass which had a migration programme involving return to the sea, and the bass now use the fresh-water lake instead of sea, reaching up local rivers to spawn with sufficient success to generate a thriving local fishing industry. Therefore, it is now appreciated that perhaps migrations can be adjusted or diverted to provide easier and richer catches.

POLLUTION
There are many reported occasions when pollution of waters produces death of fish. Cyanide in the Garonne river in France killed 22 tons of fish. There have been several similar incidents along the Seine and off-shore from the Cote d'Azur. There is strong opinion that the Mediterranean area could become sterile within one generation, there being very little tidal action and insufficient depth of water for fish to find refuge.

Probably more serious than the dramatic deaths, which are obvious and emotive, fish populations suffer disease and deficiencies in polluted waters, progressively reducing in number as they die younger and breed less. Furthermore, many of the diseases are likely to be passed on to consumers of fish, as are parasites in fish made weak by sickness. For example, the fluke *Nanophyetus salmincola* thrives in fish and mammals. The transfer of micro-organisms from fish to land-based animals is common, including Salmonella and Shigella as common infections but also to include a wide range of organisms yet to be identified. *Vibrio parahaemolyticus* is a familiar cause of enteritis amongst fish-eaters. Other evidence of the influence of pollution on fish includes:

Haemorrhagic septicaemia (bleeding blood-poisoning) from transmitted virus or bacteria.
Sock-eye in salmon and trout, probably by a virus in eaten eggs.
Ulcers in many fish but notably in salmon and trout.
Cold water disease, in which the young fry die before leaving the yolk.
Gill bacterial infections, of which there are many.
Kidney bacterial infections.
Bibriosis.
Pseudomonad septicaemia.
Forunculosis.
Fin rot, which is a generic term used to cover many complaints.

One problem of infestation, infection and the building up of foreign chemicals in tissue is that troubles are spread by predators eating the fish or their offspring. It is not practical to confine the problem in an area for effective treatment, or to prevent contamination of fish through the agency of, for example, bird droppings.

It is difficult to establish how much pollution will influence total availabilities of fish protein. Since 1948 the world catch has been multiplied by three to nearly 70 million tons if fresh-water fish is included. The Pacific contributes about half the commercial catch, with roughly 24 million tons out of the Atlantic and only about 3 million tons from the Indian Ocean. It is probable that the Indian Ocean could contribute 15–20 million tons and this is the area least likely to suffer pollution. There is a possibility of 5 million tons of anchovy from the Pacific coasts of North America. The thread herring is not fully exploited and there are untapped reserves of sardines off West Africa. It is possible that the combined oceans could furnish 100 million tons of fish per year but it is also possible that half of the catch would have passed through polluted waters. It seems inevitable that processing will be needed, partly to include fish species not now regarded as delightful but also to compensate for contamination. Some of the contamination may be within the limits of extracting processes but that which resists extraction or neutralisation will have to be reduced in concentration by bulk disintegration and blending.

FISH CATCHING

Techniques
If fish can be reached by mechanical devices or chemicals they can be caught. There are many systems, varied according to the condition of the water. Chemical systems, such as the use of derris, are silent and unobtrusive and of considerable value in the extraction of fish from forbidden waters but are not a major contributory factor in protein production. Mechanical devices are mainly either sharp points or nets.* The use of sharp points reduces the total yield but selects the fish by size and therefore encourages a continued supply. The use of nets increases total yield and, although young fish may not be landed because the net size is adjusted they may be considerably damaged and abraded which could result in easier development of disease. The gills of young fish passing through nets are notably sensitive.

There are four essential techniques of using nets. One is to stretch the net across water which is moving too rapidly for fish to retract when movement is inhibited by entanglement in the mesh. Relative damage to smaller fish is slight because they are simply extruded through the mesh by the back pressure. The second system is to drive fish schools before a long net until they exhaust their strength and fall back into the mesh. This technique is applicable to fish which move in schools and it removes complete fractions of such schools at the depth and width netted. Damage to young fish is high since, if they are forced through the net they are twisted in passing through the mesh and are under pressure from the

* Recently there have been disturbing developments in suction methods of catching. These use herding devices, such as artificial hunting cries of dolphin or electric shock waves, to drive schools along a set path. A ship then meets the school and dips a vacuum pipe. All the members of the school within reach of the resultant water flow are sucked into the ship to be extracted by filtration. This obviously catches all stages of fish development and causes damage to young fish even if they are returned to the water. More serious, perhaps, the fringes of the water stream will collect young fish whilst adult fish may have the strength to escape. The proportion of young taken must, therefore, be higher than the proportion of young in the school.

rest of the catch. The third system uses the herding of a thin population of fish by enclosing a large area and slowly reducing the netted area until the catcher has a solid mass of fish. In general, small fish swim out of the net through the mesh without damage, being stressed neither by water pressure nor compressed fish. By the time the thin population has concentrated to the point where it could suffer damage the smaller fish have escaped unharmed to grow ready for the next occasion. The fourth and final technique is to stretch a long net across a run of fish and leave it for a long time, preferably overnight. The fish become entangled in the mesh and can be picked off when the net is drawn in. Smaller fish suffer little damage but there is considerable damage to the fish caught and it has reduced value after being held for hours after death in warm water without the removal of the self-digesting guts. The danger of overfishing comes not from the taking of too many fish for eating, but from the taking of fish too young to have reproduced and from the damage to similar young when they have to force an escape from nets, particularly if the nets approach the young fish from behind and they have to turn to escape.

Netting is productive if applied to slow-moving schools of plankton eaters, particularly since such schools can be traced using sophisticated equipment. The schools seek the plankton and by inference the best net fishing is where the plankton thrives. There are 326 million cubic miles of water on earth and 97% of this is salted. This water holds about four-fifths of the total protein in the world but it is not evenly distributed. Ocean covers nearly three-quarters of the earth's surface and absorbs 70% of solar radiation. Up to 3% of the radiation is used by the vegetable fraction of plankton in depths down to 25 fathoms, producing a probable 80% of all plankton growth on the earth. The lowest level of production is in mid-ocean, which accounts for 90% of the area. Reasonable production is found within the 100-fathom line, accounting for 7.5% of the area. The highest production is along west coasts in subtropical waters, notably where up-swells bring cold water and nutrients up to meet sun-drenched surfaces. The total up-swelling areas are probably less than 0.1% of total ocean area but they supply half of the world's fish.

One estimate is that demand for fish will force an increase in the world catch from its present 60 million tons to 100 million tons and even 200 million tons by 1985. Without radical changes in the pattern of ocean currents this can only lead to overfishing and particularly over-extraction of young fish before they have time to reproduce. Most estimates of future supply indicate a reduction of catches in familiar fishing grounds, partly from less regeneration as more small fish are taken but also from the influences of pollution. Pollution is expected to cause migration of sensitive fish into deeper water for breeding, where conditions are less conducive to hatching. The composition of water inside the 100-fathom line is expected to change by pollution and it is anticipated that the interface of seawater and air will become too contaminated for the correct pattern of plankton growth, since toxic micro-organic growth is known to change the oxygen intake and the spectrum of light penetrating the upper layers. It is therefore anticipated that inshore fishing will progressively decline and that deep-water fishing will have to seek more distant grounds. The most economic fishing technique in the future is forecast as that using a mother processing ship with smaller catching boats, as exampled by the 43 000 tons factory ship *Vostock* with fourteen supporting smaller vessels.

The use of a large factory ship brings the problem of landing infrequent large bulks at ports which would be almost idle between landings. There is an obvious limit to the number of ports which can handle such bulks and few developing countries would be able to establish an associated distribution system. In fact, the processing at sea would have to be geared to prompt reshipment as exports when the mother ship reached port. There is also a limit to the number of large factory ships which could operate since they would have to seek only the large-volume runs of fish, which are seasonal and would presumably be fished by all the factory ships together. It could become essential to relate selected fishing grounds to approved factory ships and to severely restrict fishing in breeding grounds.

Alternatively, organic waste from land could be used to enrich waters in the shelf areas as a primitive effort to farm fish in their own territory, using the factory ships to take out the fish-food and bring back the grown fish. It might also be proved practical to control slightly the water temperatures, particularly to cool waters which do not have a cross-wind to wipe off the hot surface from cold rich seawater. The Institut für Verfahrenstechnik has devised a technique of diverting the upwards flow of cold enriched waters through tubes of 10 m diameter and connected lengths of 200 m, each length having a pump. Whether the energy input of such a technique would be justified by returns is doubted and there could be more potential in schemes to use air bubbles to lift the cold rich water to the surface, particularly since air-injection would encourage plankton growth in hot water.

The need for restrictions

Most of these plans to avoid a famine of fish require international co-operation and high capital investment. However, by tradition, fishing industries are parochial with a high proportion of small organisations which have not shown inclination to cooperate with each other, with national governments or with international authorities. It is therefore difficult to imagine how fish output can show long-term increase if present fishing organisations and techniques are preserved. The so-called 'Cod War' between Iceland and the United Kingdom was indicative of the problem.

United Kingdom deep-water fishermen land about 300 000 tons/year of which one-half to two-thirds originate off Iceland. Norwegian waters provide about 13.5%, Bear Island region about 10% and the Barents Sea about 17.5%. Iceland expressed a need to have a fifty-mile limit within which catching could be limited to domestic boats which could be trusted not to take too many small fish, and with a set limit of catch for foreign boats—mainly British and German. The fifty-mile limit was declared in September 1972 and in December the United Kingdom trawlers were given entry but with restrictions. The waters were divided into six zones to be fished in rotation with one zone open to United Kingdom trawlers at any one time. Also, the United Kingdom trawlers were limited to those 180 ft long and there were adjustable limits to numbers of boats and total catch. The United Kingdom trawlers inevitably complained that they had the worst areas and that rotation fishing was unproductive. They claimed that the organisation would reduce United Kingdom catches by 70%, and that it would have been satisfactory simply to limit total catch to 75% of the 1971 weight. Iceland replied that 1971 had been a good year and they would use proportional limitation if the United Kingdom agreed to an average year. Iceland then complicated the issue by presenting different schemes to the United Kingdom and West Germany, whilst the United Kingdom complicated the issue by passing it to the International Court of Justice. There is no doubt that the United Kingdom trawlers have increased their take from Icelandic waters. Nor is there any doubt that Iceland needs to preserve its stock, since she is 80% dependent on fish and has no other significant economic asset. By 1975, Iceland should have at least forty new trawlers and will therefore need a build-up of stocks during 1973–1974. This situation is related to the anchovy catch off Peru, where shift of the current or failure of the winds has resulted in failure, and reduced catches are needed in 1973–1974 for stocks to recover. In fact, the same situation is likely to develop in all deep-sea grounds since overfishing will reduce breeding and stocks will fail to recover because the grounds will not be left fallow.

The situation in shallow water differs from that in deep water. Deep-water fishing is capital-intensive, even for a small operator, and yield is roughly proportional to investment. Inshore fishing is highly fragmented and largely uncontrolled, and is labour-intensive with yield roughly proportional to the skill of the labour. Most of inshore dispute concerns the allocation of areas, it being understood that fishermen will protect their own stocks if outsiders are excluded, but will take all they can if there is complete freedom of access to all comers. It is accepted that any statement of rights which is based on distance will be unfair, and to some extent ignored, but it is difficult to define rights in any other way without long-term discussion. Free fishing in all inshore waters would destroy the grounds within five years, and the destruction could be beyond recovery because the ecological balances would no longer exist.

This potential destruction of inshore ecosystems gives rise to more concern than the excessive removal of small fish. If local small fishermen are forced out of business there will be introduction of replacement industry, which will accelerate marine pollution, including the development of industrial haze (which influences the phytoplankton pattern) and a change in the composition of effluent into the sea (sewage is said to be relatively harmless to fry but industrial chemicals can be highly destructive).

As far as Europe is concerned there is unavoidable dispute about inshore fishing rights. In 1964, the United Kingdom introduced a firm twelve-mile limit and banned exhaustive equipment such as 50 mm nets and chain-trawls. A 50 mm net not only takes fish too small but also wipes the slime from smaller fish and thereby opens the skin to infection. A chain-trawl drags the bottom and disturbs all livestock up into the net, taking all but the very small fish and even these are mainly damaged beyond recovery. However, after the 1964 restrictions, United Kingdom catches inshore increased whilst catches out of Dieppe and Ostend, where similar control was not applied, progressively reduced, despite the fact that many of the eggs laid in British waters grew to fish in Dutch and Belgian waters.

FISH SPOILAGE
The first consideration in marketing fish is to control loss, decay and

damage so that a high proportion of the catch can be sold at maximum retail prices. Control is by deceleration of the decay mechanisms, mainly by reduction of the temperature and by the prevention of damage from abrasion and crushing. At normal temperatures the lipid component (the substances containing fatty acids) oxidises and an unpleasant odour is produced. This odour is sufficiently powerful to prevent consumption of the fish before it can produce serious toxins. The oxygen can be excluded by canning and the oxidation process can be modified by smoking, salting or drying, processes which also limit the range of effective micro-organisms which might produce toxins. The advantage of control by reduction of the temperature is that the frozen fish can later be thawed and, as fillets, can be sold as fresh fish. Chilled fish, which is fish in ice for reasonably rapid distribution, is also sold as fresh fish. However, temperature reduction does not provide full control of decay, a temperature of below -30 °C being necessary for all processes to be declared inactive.

In fresh and chilled fish the problem is bacterial and enzymic spoilage, whereas in frozen fish the problem is denaturing of the tissue, when contained water becomes ice, and the development of rancidity. Both market areas have the basic problem of fat oxidation, which can be delayed by wrapping in barrier packaging. Exclusion of the air can give chilled fish an extra few days of life but care is needed not to introduce a false biodeterioration pattern. The bacterial activity in an oxygen-starved mass differs from that in a normal tissue and there could be danger from the prevention of the fat oxidation which acts as a warning of decay in ventilated fish.

The difficulty in wrapping to exclude air is that the wrapping also retains drip. This drip looks unsightly and it could encourage *Clostridium welchii* and *Clostridium botulinum*. Both these occur on fish and produce toxins, although the toxin production is slight previous to the production of taint and odour from fat oxidation. Below 4 °C it is not likely that toxins will be produced and it is more probable that they will develop after purchase of the fish and careless storage by the housewife. Drip can be reduced by treatment of the fish with polyphosphates (5% sodium polyphosphate and 5% sodium phosphate). All fish starts its decay and spoilage history from the damage sustained in the nets, in being brought inboard and then in processing on the boat.

Fish is unique amongst protein foods in that it is still mainly a wild uncultivated crop and the harvest is uncertain in terms of quantity, quality and the pattern of species involved. It is also individual in that most of the catch is in locations which prevent early delivery to the consumers, making it inevitable that decay will occur. The variability of catch makes it impractical to introduce sophisticated processing methods at the time of catching, but the rapid decay makes it essential to introduce at least some preventative techniques.

When white fish are landed on board they are gutted and, in the majority of boats, are then stowed in ice. This reduces the temperature and thereby slows deteriorative processes. It also allows crushing and abrasion which liberates enzymes, these enzymes increasing the biochemical activity. Common practice is to reduce crushing by stacking on shelves to about half a metre height, adding more shelves and fish to the hold height. Damage levels in shelved storage are high and there is increasing use of fish boxes at about $770 \times 440 \times 200$ mm, made from plastics. Fatty fish are difficult to gut on board and spoilage rates are high. Rapid mixing of fish and ice in boxes is claimed to give the ungutted fish a life of up to five days. More recently, mainly for herring, there has been use of insulated containers holding about 1.3 tons of fish mixed on board with half a ton of sea water and half a ton of ice. Nitrogen gas is blown into the container from its base to encourage mixing and therefore rapid cooling. The fish will then remain fresh for about two days, after which it needs more ice to last another two days. One outstanding advantage in using containers of this type is the ease of handling on return to port.

With present fishing methods a boat can stay at sea for up to two weeks for white fish or up to five days for fatty fish. The sea-time can be extended by using freezing at sea, freezing between plates to slabs roughly $1000 \times 500 \times 10$ mm. Such blocks are difficult to handle and if the catch includes fatty fish there is a danger of oxidation. Decay can be reduced by spraying the blocks with water to give a layer of ice but a better method is to freeze the fish in bags of water, completely enclosing the fish in ice and thereby delaying decay even in fatty fish. Herring frozen without added water are calculated to consume about thirteen times more oxygen than herring frozen with added water, the with-water shelf life at $-10\ ^\circ$C being equivalent to the without-water shelf life at $-23\ ^\circ$C.* Early bags were polyethylene film but they slipped in handling and most bags are now coated paper or film in paper.

The fish trade claims that the market divides sharply into two sectors

* The uptake of oxygen varies with the shape and size of the units of fish. Cutting a herring into fork-size cubes could increase the uptake four times that of the original herring, reducing an anticipated life of one week to less than two days.

of fresh fish as landed and fish pre-cut and pre-packaged as fingers or steaks trimmed square. Fish as landed needs effective display and most consumers can recognise quality. Fortunately, display lighting can be cold but there is still significant decay in the selling of whole fish. There is consequent emphasis on pre-processed fish, sold through cold chambers and frequently sold in collated semi-bulk for home freezers. Packaging for retail sale is made difficult by the rapid rate of decay, particularly if the fish is held in a sealed package for some time so that it develops visible drip and obvious odour. In selling fish from the slab the odour and drip is to some extent lost but pre-packaged wet fish cannot lose its drip or odour, or be subjected to a wash-down when decay becomes obvious. It may be in better condition than that exposed in open sale but it will look worse because the fish exposed can be given a periodic wash or be turned to allow drip to escape. Opinion is divided on packaging materials between high-barrier laminates and low-barrier films. High-barrier laminates contain odour, making the package suitable for mixed display, but the containment results in poor appearance of unfrozen fish and a distinct odour when the package is opened. Low-barrier film allows passage of water vapour and thereby prevents fogging inside the package and gives a better appearance for unfrozen fish, even if the higher rate of release of odour through the package wall makes such a package unsuitable for mixed display. Broadly, packaging is only fully practical for frozen fish, which does not have problems of odour and dehydration in short-term storage and display. Frozen fatty fish need a high-barrier package to restrict oxygen which degrades the fats.

There have been many interesting efforts to reduce damage from dehydration. One approach has been to dip the fish in water before freezing, producing a thin skin of ice with the hope that dehydration will take water from the ice and not from the fish. It has been found difficult to obtain full coverage by the ice layer on spiny fish and on fatty fish. Better coverage is found using starch or alginate in the water before dipping but results with ice layers have not been encouraging, and plastics films which contain water and exclude oxygen seem to be the best solution.

Fish need only about 0.05% oxygen to fat for rancidity to occur. Since it is uneconomic to use very high vacuum in packaging, or to use completely pure gas-flushing, even if an absolute barrier were used for packaging there would be some oxidation of fat. In an atmosphere deprived of oxygen the fish might reduce its hydroperoxide development to about 10% of that of exposed fish. In theory, this gives a shelf life some ten times longer but there are other factors concerned in shelf life. In practical terms, enclosure in an oxygen-starved atmosphere with a reasonable barrier package should double the shelf life.

FISH MEAL

Fish meal is not to be confused with fish paste. Fish paste can be regarded as an anticipatory product, opening the market for a very wide range of reconstituted fish products for human consumption. It has about two-thirds water content, which is about the same as most headless gutless fish, probably about 15% protein content against about 20% for the original fish and possibly 10% fat and 7% carbohydrate which were not in the original fish. Within the limits of definition of a variable product, fish paste has the calorific value of fried fish and is rich in minerals but has lost some of the protein content in processing.

Fish meal, on the other hand, is the solid fraction of fish after the oil has been pressed out. Swarming small fish, too numerous to be absorbed by fresh-fish markets after catching, are caught as raw material for factories set up to press out the oil. Efforts to relate a fish-meal development to the supply of fresh fish have not proved satisfactory. Fresh fish for sale into the retail market is variable in supply and is expensive to trim. Fish-meal production needs a high-volume raw material which needs no attention between the catching and the pressing. It also needs a high-volume market to justify the capital expenditure on plant. A small factory producing paste from fresh-fish discard could be economic but a fish-meal factory needs to handle large volumes of raw materials which can be trusted to arrive.

The Peruvian industry has 105 factories at the time of writing but recent history may encourage the closure of some. In 1971 there was a rich run of anchovy and orders were booked for the 1972 catch. In 1972, the total catch fell to 895 000 tons, which was only 45% of the 1971 total. At the end of 1972, Peru had outstanding orders for 400 000 tons of meal at an agreed price of $165/ton. In effect, this meant that 2.5 million tons of the 1973 catch would be required for meal selling by contract at 1972 prices. Meanwhile, a shortage of soya had inflated world prices for fish meal by about 50% and it was important to establish new contracts at the new prices before new protein introductions in animal feed markets. If the waters were fully fished in 1973, using one-third of the catch to pay off the 1972 debts, there could be almost no catch in 1974. On the other hand, if the anchovy were left alone for a year there could be a 60% normal catch in 1974 and more in 1975.

In March 1973 there was a trial two-weeks catch of 1.2 million tons but this was in a narrow belt of cold water and was not fully indicative. Available anchovy were calculated at about 3.5 million tons instead of the normal 15 million tons and 115 boats were taken out of catching for fish meal and applied to catching for retailed fish.

The Peruvian failure accelerated developments of fish meal for human consumption, the theory being that if meal was to be in reduced quantity it needed to find higher prices by upgrading to qualities suitable for human diet. The Technical University of Norway has investigated the influence of drying on fish proteins, leading to a definition of a Q_{in} value, an integration of drying conditions and initial moisture contents. When this Q_{int} value has been related to drying capacity there is no doubt that fish meal will cease to be only a component in feed and will become a significant component in food for humans.

SHELLFISH

Original armoured fish may have evolved to back-boned scaly fish and shellfish and original shellfish may have evolved to armoured fish and subsequently to back-boned scaly fish. Or, they may all have evolved from some common ancestor which for reasons yet to be determined left no fossil traces. However produced, we are left with a broad division into organisms which hang flesh on the outside of a skeletal framework, and organisms which enclose their tissue in an outer protective hard layer. In general, the hanging of flesh on a skeleton has allowed mobility and the development of complex body members and functions, whilst the enclosure of flesh within a shell has resulted in limited movement and a simplified body organisation within the limited volume. It has also limited the size to which shellfish can grow because large sizes demand heavy unwieldy shells, only possible where there is the available raw material and no need for the organism to move. Any such massive shellfish which might have evolved were probably incapable of moving out of changed environments or were unable to manufacture sufficient shell thickness to exclude parasites. Shells which have survived use all the tricks of mechanical engineering. Surfaces are suitably curved to be strong and may carry corrugations or ribs. Stressed points have reinforcing thickness and flexible joints are operated by long-reach muscles capable of rapid contraction. Mating surfaces are exact in their contours and it is usual for the flexible joints, which are the locations most suitable for penetration, to also be footholds so that they are hidden from enemies.

Feeding is by filtration with a relatively inefficient system of rejection. Large solid particles of contamination are likely to be covered and included in the inner surface. Unreactive contamination is likely to be thrown out but reactive contamination becomes absorbed into the tissues and, because the shellfish body chemistry is unsophisticated, remains there with little influence on the shellfish. High concentrations of contamination can be built up in tissues from long-term absorption of traces, to become toxic for animals which eat the shellfish. Likewise, micro-organisms can become established and thrive without damage to the shellfish but with dire consequence for those using the shellfish as diet.

The lack of mobility and the apparent disregard for contaminated water cause shellfish to remain in polluted waters whereas fish move out to find cleaner feeding grounds. In fact, since shellfish are scavengers they may increase their multiplication rates in contaminated water which contains useful substances alongside contamination. Shellfish need two main components in an environment—a firm surface on which to sit and a plentiful supply of organic matter in the water for food. Hence they prefer shallow water or, better still, an area which is alternatively wet and dry or an area which is repeatedly stocked with waste from tide-washed shores. In effect, this puts the shellfish in reach of shoreline contamination and also in reach of shoreline animal predators. They are therefore frequent causes of poisoning of fish, seabirds, animals eating seabirds and humans eating shellfish. The full story of the many shoreline disasters has been well documented and need not be repeated, but it needs to be appreciated that not all the serious contamination leading to a toxicity chain comes from industry. It can come from natural events. Industrial pollution of shoreline water is effective because its location is within reach of the humans working in the industry concerned, but natural pollution is of less concern to man because it is likely to occur in a much larger area of water and is, in fact, more probable in deep water than in shelf-water or shorelines. There is much more release of chemicals from deep-water volcanic action than from washed-down land-based effluent, but most of the temporary disruptions of marine ecosystems are out of sight and mind of land-based societies.

Most humans suspect shellfish and they do not account for a high proportion of diet; many humans are allergic to certain shellfish groups, probably from the accumulated toxins and very few humans can tolerate a diet mainly comprising shellfish as the protein content is not outstanding. Typical protein contents are:

	% protein without shell
Cockles	11
Boiled crab	19
Boiled lobster	21
Boiled mussels	17
Raw oysters	10
Prawns	21
Shrimps	22
Scallop	20
Whelks	18
Winkles	16

In terms of bought value shellfish are inferior, the shell included in the purchase reducing the effective protein content to, for example, 4 in crab and 5 in boiled mussels. Even so, demand is maintained because shellfish are established in luxury cooking and have the reputation of providing flavours and minerals which cannot be obtained elsewhere.

It is only a matter of a short time before almost all natural grounds of shellfish accumulate too much toxin and the only hope for the market is in artificial environments or through farming techniques which can operate away from shoreline contamination. There has been some success with the growing of mussels on ropes which can be towed into clean water for growth and then towed back to civilisation for harvesting. There is also some rising interest in the culture of shellfish in relatively clean water around developing countries but there are problems of bacterial contamination.

Mussels grow rapidly on diatoms and deritus and they could become a major source of protein. Mussel farms in Holland produce up to 40 tons/acre and there are farms in Spain with a total output probably more than 150 000 tons/year. There is an estimate that in India there could be farming sufficient to feed 20 million people. Even if the 40 tons/acre yield is ignored as not practical for widespread development and 15 tons/acre is used in calculations, protein production rates from shellfish of the mussel type could be 50–100 times that from farmed land animals—and growing on ropes would allow production to be some distance from areas of consumption, the harvest being towed in as required.

If shellfish are related more to food processing than to direct consumption there is a vast range to develop on farms. (The Pacific oyster can grow to 300 mm length inside two and a half years, giving a growth rate at least twice that of the common oyster.) No one yet can give accurate estimates of yields and costs, partly because farmed shellfish will probably not be those familiar and partly because costs may involve water-cleaning equipment and processing of the food for the shellfish. Also, there are indications that the farming of shellfish may prove more economic if associated with the farming of other groups of organisms.

Shrimp farming has been inhibited by the lack of a suitable method of preserving algae for feed. Recently, algae have been cultured, centrifuged to concentrate and then frozen. Up to 98% survival is reported of shrimp larvae fed on the frozen algae alone and it seems that the frozen algae can last several months without depreciation.

WET FARMING

Man has concentrated all his farming effort on air-based environments between a level half a metre below ground level and a height he can reach into the sky. Water has been used as a carrier of chemicals and as a reacting component but not as a medium for growth, it being presumed that natural sources of protein growing in water would continue and multiply according to the experience that natural regeneration rates are inversely proportional to population densities. This experience can only apply if the environment is not damaged and present environments suffer the joint attack of over-extraction and damage to environments.

Encouragement of yield by confinement has been known for centuries, as for instance in the growth of fish in irrigation water and the establishment of barriers which prevent fish from migrating away from local catchment areas. Despite publicity, however, there has been comparatively little serious farming of aquatic life other than that for sporting fish. Farming is needed of both vegetable and animal proteins, and of mixed proteins derived from the comprehensive mixture of total life in water culture. The animal fraction, being rich in methionine but short of tryptophane, is notably important as an intended associate of oilseeds in diet, oilseeds having tryptophane but only half the desirable content of methionine.

The main problem in fish farming is variability of waters, making it difficult to transfer experience from one environment to another and making it essential to carry out expensive previous investigation and probable modification of the water involved. The variability can be exampled by study of mercury levels in fish, mercury being a common subject of investigation and analysis. In the United Kingdom, the mercury content of all foods is below 0.005 mg/kg although pig offal has shown 0.03 mg. Most fish falls within the range of 0.03–0.2 mg for regional fish and 0.01–0.04 mg for imported canned fish. The local variation is shown as:

	mg/kg mercury
Most inshore fish	0.2
Thames flat fish	0.8
Thames round fish	0.4
Shellfish	0.16 (but up to 0.32 from Irish waters)
Pike	0.47
Trout/salmon	0.17

In terms of mercury content, flounder has more than whiting and whiting has more than plaice. Of the mercury, 40–90% is methyl mercury, which is a danger. Mercury is used as an example because it has been investigated and can provide statistics. Suitability of water for fish farming depends, however, on the entire pattern of composition and the temperature, and the ability to retain oxygen. It also depends on the pattern of micro-organisms, notably the content of bacteria which can concentrate heavy metals. Probably more important in the pattern of micro-organisms is the ability of the population to carry out biodeterioration without damage to the gas balance in the water. Special attention is given to the exclusion or control of micro-organisms which can cause sickness in fish. The outer layer of a scaled fish is slime, which is living cells and is a natural barrier against infection. If this slime is removed by handling or overcrowding it is easy for infection to reach the scales, where it is retained and can thrive on the tissues beneath. Since fish farming relies on handling and overcrowding it is inevitable that slime layers will be damaged.

Most present fish-farm projects rely on complete enclosure and forced feeding. So far, there has been very little effort directed at open-range fish farming, concentration of required fish within reach by deposit of food or improvement of the temperature–oxygen situation. The emphasis on total enclosure has been mainly because there has been associated emphasis on sporting fish for stocking profitable enclosures. The record for final cost of a single fish, taking into account rearing cost and rental of the length of river bank, is over one thousand pounds sterling for one salmon. With such orders of value available for sporting fish it is not remarkable that fish farming for food has been neglected.

Cold climates favour expensive fish, such as trout fed on fish meal whilst warm climates favour the mass production of fish for food. The farming of finned fish in temperate climates relies on summer heat for growth to an average yield of 300 lb/acre. The summer season of April to October in Europe can be extended by warming the water with sewage which also provides food, and there have been yields around Munich of 500 lb/acre. Europe takes three years to grow a reasonable size of carp but Israel can grow the same quantity of carp protein inside two years. The African equivalent, Tilapia, takes only nine months to grow to 0.5 lb and is then suitable for eating. Tilapia are vegetarian, which is unusual amongst fishes, and could be introduced to feed on unwanted vegetable growth where industrial heat is lost into waters. It appear that Tilapia could fit into sewage schemes, body waste from animals leading to zooplankton which Tilapia include in their diet. In Rhodesia and Uganda, Tilapia are said to have yielded 5500 lb/acre with water temperatures from 55–75 °F, which is over ten times the productivity of carp in Europe.

In the United Kingdom there is a municipal fish farm using effluent of BOD 10 mg/l, passing through eight ponds at 1 m depth, arriving at the last pond as water fit for drinking. The pollution is removed by roach to a weight of about $\frac{1}{2}$ lb weight, at which they are presumably sold to fishing clubs for sport. However, roach taste of mud, are full of bones and are therefore not acceptable for human diet and are possibly unwelcome in animal feed. It might be preferable, if a food market is required for the adult fish, to farm minnows, which, at 3–4 in. length were the original luxury dish known as Thames Whitebait. At this point it is worth noting that the smallest back-boned animals are the Philippine gobies, fish which reach only about 1 cm in length and are then caught for baking as fish-cakes. There are probably 50 000 tiny gobies per kilogramme of fish-cake.

Fish farming for food in developed countries is not likely to develop to any significant extent, although farming for sport may. The economic problem is the shortage of fresh clean water and the associated high cost of energy in cleaning available waters. There is constantly-increasing pollution from agricultural chemicals, industry and sewage, and the cost of cleaning can only increase in future years. Fish farming for food in developing countries is likely to develop but it is to be appreciated that many such countries have undeveloped conventional fishing, which takes less development capital than fish farming by enclosure and forced feeding. There could be consequent emphasis on the farming of seawater fish by enclosure of bays and this has been done in Scotland, where there has been farming of Halibut. The cultured fish has a poor colour, which may prove to be not important as it has improved flavour induced by driving the fish around the tank before capture so that fear improves the quality of the flesh. In this farm there is improvement by elimination of slow-growing specimens and effort to keep individual growth rates similar amongst individuals in the school.

The farming of shellfish is comparatively simple but, as with finned fish, the problem is finding clean water. In the case of shellfish it is vital to find and maintain clean water because the shellfish may thrive in polluted water and even show increased yield, but will concentrate toxins and retain infections. Since shelf-waters are becoming more polluted the only potential for shellfish farming appears to be in waters which are sufficiently distant from concentrated humanity to be clean, but are sufficiently close to markets for transport costs to be minimised. An alternative is to concentrate on shellfish which will hang on ropes or nets or platforms which can be retained in clean water for growth and towed to the harvesting station. There is also some slight interest in multiple-layer farming with recirculating water passing through a purification system, the claim being that potential protein output per square metre of growth area is up to 100 times that of the conventional farming of land animals.

As will be seen in the fuller discussion of algae, there is outstanding potential for cultivated algae, for direct feeding to humans but also as a component in mixed farming. The ideal would appear to be settlement of sewage with the solids taken for land improvement, the liquid fraction being used as a nitrogen source for algae, using the algae to feed fish and the fish to be converted into fish-meal by a simple process for feeding to livestock without delay. This is only one of several closed-cycle farming systems under examination.

SALT AND DRIED FISH

The common preservation techniques for fish in industrial societies are canning and freezing. In primitive societies there is extensive preservation by salting and drying. The techniques are prehistoric and are therefore variable according to the locality, and may be associated with smoking.

Despite the advancement of canning and refrigeration the total weight of salt and dried fish has increased during the past decade.

After landing, and preferably before tropical suns develop their full heat, fish are beheaded and split along their lengths, the backbone being removed. The fillets are then laid in vats or on concrete floors, in layers of one fish depth with salt applied to each layer. The salt removes the excess liquid, which is currently lost but may prove to have value. After about two weeks the flesh is fully impregnated with salt, at which stage they are ready for drying. In fact, the wet stack of salt fish may be ignored for months other than occasional turning and repiling. Before hanging, they may need washing. In very cold dehydrating climates (Canada, Newfoundland, Iceland and Scandinavia) the drying may be in the open air but it is now more common to use forced heat. Drying rates are according to the quality of the fish and the sizes of the pieces. Skin retards drying and there can be a slow drying rate for thick chunks of fish which have a low salt content. Stale fish takes up salt at a faster rate than does fresh fish, and it is not by necessity an inferior product in the final analysis.

As far as mathematics can be applied, a thickness of 25 mm of flesh will take one day to gain 10% of salt whereas a thickness of 50 mm may take half a week or more. Uptake of salt is also influenced by the temperature, being quicker at higher temperatures. However, higher temperatures increase bacterial decay rates and it is advisable to wait for the slow uptake at low temperatures. At 20 °C it is easy to find serious bacterial decay but at 0 °C there is very little growth of the non-halophilic bacteria during the period until the salt content is sufficient to control non-halophilic bacteria.

The analysis of fish at the three stages is:

	Water %	Salt-free solids (mainly protein) %	Salt %
Cod as landed	82	18	0.2
Salted but wet	54	26	20
Salted/dried	23	49	28

As will be seen, the term dried is comparative. The main consideration in the realisation of quality in salt and dried fish is the type of salt. This can dictate the technique used, which can be 'hard' curing or 'medium' or 'light' curing. Typical conditions for hard curing are of the order of

26 °C and about 50% relative humidity with an air flow of 100–125 cm/sec for nearly two days. Lighter cures are with lower salt contents, as produced by soaking the fish in brine instead of dry salting. A typical analysis of brined fish might be 73% water (from the original 82%) and only 5% salt.

In terms of protein value, there is merit in using brining techniques rather than dry salting. Proteins are thought to be damaged by salt concentrations above 9%, but it needs to be appreciated that low salt contents can lead to deterioration early, which also damages the protein. On the other hand, brining techniques are of special value for oily fish, which need immersion during salting so that the fats do not become rancid.

The rate of curing and degree of necessary salting depends on the chemical composition and bacterial population of the salts. Typical salts are:

Salt compositions as percentages			
Chlorides of:			
	Sodium	Magnesium	Calcium
Solar salt	89.5–99.9	0.0–1.3	0.0–0.05
Evaporated brine	97.0–99.95	0.0–0.15	0.0–0.35
Rock salt	94.6–99.5	0.0–1.0	0.0–0.4
Sulphates of:			Water-insoluble
	Magnesium	Calcium	matter
Solar salt	0.0–1.1	0.0 –2.2	0.0 –0.75
Evaporated brine	0.0–0.5	0.0 –1.5	0.01–0.05
Rock salt	0.0–0.15	0.12–2.1	0.12–3.55

Significant as they may be, the inorganic components are less important than the micro-organic populations. Solar salt and evaporated brine carry bacteria which result in pinking of fish flesh. Rock salt is more likely to offer fungi. The bacterial counts are of the order of:

Bacteria numbers/g (*maximum numbers*)		
Grown on salt-free media		
at 20 °C	at 37 °C	Grown on 10% salt
Solar salt	300 000	1400	337 500
Evaporated brine	710	120	73
Rock salt	1100	64	53

The actual numbers are unimportant since salts vary according to their derivation and handling. Rock salts are natural deposits which are contaminated after mining and grinding. Solar salts are from the evaporation of seawater by sun heat and winds, becoming contaminated from the atmosphere, above the original contamination of the seawater. Evaporated brines come from the production of brine in salt mines, subsequent pumping out and evaporation with applied heat. Commercial salts vary from those with over 99% sodium chloride to very poor salts with 80% sodium chloride or less. Solar salts are disfavoured for their high insolubles content and high populations of micro-organisms which can thrive at low temperatures (and high proportions of halophilic bacteria). The maximum calcium and magnesium content of a salt should be below 0.3% and 0.6% respectively as high calcium and magnesium contents are likely to produce a bitter flavour in the protein.

Salt for curing also needs to be examined for grain size and scatter of grain sizes. A fine grain dissolves too rapidly and there is accelerated extraction of water from the surface. This coagulates the surface protein and further salt penetration is inhibited. The early coagulation also encourages the fish to stick together, so that they rupture in turning. It is safer to use oversized grains, which may delay the process but will not damage the tissue by coagulation.

It is also common to dry fish without previous salting. White fish can be simply beheaded and split before being tied in pairs to stocks (such dried fish are frequently known as stock-fish, a fortunate name since the common application is as stock for fish soups). In Scandinavia it is common to hang the fish in dehydrating cold winds but other climates need artificial drying. In general, dried unsalted fish from artificial drying is vastly inferior to that dried by dehydrating freezing winds. Drying may take several weeks to reduce the water content from the original 80–85% to 15%, but the final product can have a shelf-life of several years and was a stand-by food for long sea journeys. It is used for soups but soaking in mild alkali will reconstitute an individual fish protein food, as used in Scandinavia for Lutefisk. The potential for dried unsalted fish is less than that of salted dried fish.

Deterioration of dried fish is common, mainly after unsatisfactory storage. Halophilic bacteria do not develop if the salt content is maintained above 5%, but there are halotolerant bacteria which can thrive in salt up to 20%—in fact, some will refuse to thrive if salt is below 10%. Halotolerant bacteria need to be differentiated from halophilic bacteria, which need salt to thrive whilst the halotolerant cousins do not need salt but enjoy its presence. Most of the spoilage is so-called pink spoilage, blamed on halophils which are variously identified under the two main references of Halobacterium or Sarcina. These need sodium chloride above 10%, and have the infuriating habit of changing form—which is why they have several identities. They can grow at temperatures down to 5 °C and up to 80 °C but prefer about 42 °C, at a relative humidity of 70–85%. The significance of this relative humidity is that it is the low level accepted as that which inhibits micro-organic growth on stored products. Hence, it is inadvisable to store dried fish in the same place as dried grain. Either the fish will suffer deterioration or the grain will have to be superdried so that it does not transfer moisture to the fish.

The halotolerant bacteria need more moisture. The main enemy is *Staphylococcus aureus*, which can result in enteric discomfort in consumers. In passing, it should be mentioned that the halophils which produce the indicative pink colour are not likely to damage consumers, but the pink colour is unpopular and can indicate halotolerant bacteria as well as halophils. Higher moisture contents are mainly indicated by a brown colour, which arises from *Sporendonema epizoum* or *Sporendonema minutum*. These can grow in salt from 5–25%, from 10 °C to 37 °C at humidities above 65% relative humidity and at pH of 6.0–7.0. It is also possible for them to grow at lower pH values, down to pH 4.0. Sporendonema is a difficult enemy because it can thrive without salt as sodium chloride if there is a reasonable concentration of other chlorides, or even of carbohydrates or glycerol. The brown colour which is the usual indication of possible toxins is related to histidine and alanine, and possibly taurine. The actual colour is thought to be a metal complex using trace metals and copper to 0.4 p.p.m. or iron to 20 p.p.m. seem to result in brown colour.

This account of the organic problems associated with salt and dried fish is brief and incomplete. If the moisture content can be kept very low there are few problems. If relative humidities are allowed to reach 90% there is real trouble from the growth of Aspergillus and Penicillium. From 70% to 90% the microbial populations are limited as described above, but it would appear that humidities below 65% are essential for full security, which may not be economic under practical conditions of supply and distribution.

Part 3
Vegetable Proteins

Chapter 14

Cereals

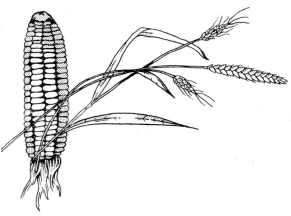

As a food group, cereals do not have high-protein contents and their amino-acid patterns are far from complete. They are, however, eaten in quantity in diet, providing a high total protein weight alongside a high total weight of carbohydrate. Protein contents vary with the species and the condition of the grain but are of the order of:

	% protein
Barley	7–8
Wheat	9–14
Oats	12
Rice	6
Rye	8

The protein content depreciates with milling and extraction, roughly:

	% protein at an extraction of—				
	100%	85%	80%	75%	70% of the whole grain
Wheat flour					
—low protein	8.9	8.6	8.2	8.0	7.9
—high protein	13.6	13.6	13.2	13.1	12.8
Rye	8.0	7.3		6.7	

Protein contents can be suspect, mainly because it is not uncommon for grain to be bought at, for example, 12% moisture content, to be left to absorb moisture, then be sold at 14% or even 16% moisture content. The amino-acid pattern is probably more significant, particularly with regard to the lysine content. On a basis of g/g nitrogen and accepting that three-quarters of the total phosphorus may be as phytic acid, the patterns are:

	Barley	*Wheat*	*Maize*	*Oats*	*Rice*	*Rye*	*Meat for comparison*
Arginine	0.31	0.27	0.31	0.41	0.53	0.31	0.41
Cystine	0.13	0.13	0.13	0.11	0.11	0.11	0.08
Histidine	0.12	0.13	0.15	0.12	0.14	0.13	0.20
Isoleucine	0.24	0.24	0.25	0.29	0.30	0.24	0.32
Leucine	0.43	0.40	0.75	0.44	0.51	0.38	0.49
Lysine	0.21	0.17	0.19	0.23	0.26	0.23	0.51
Methionine	0.09	0.10	0.13	0.09	0.13	0.10	0.15
Phenylalanine	0.31	0.29	0.31	0.31	0.29	0.29	0.26
Threonine	0.23	0.18	0.26	0.21	0.21	0.21	0.28
Tryptophane	0.09	0.08	0.05	0.08	0.09	0.08	0.08
Tyrosine	0.22	0.20	0.24	0.24	0.36	0.26	0.21
Valine	0.31	0.27	0.35	0.34	0.39	0.31	0.33
Alanine	0.28	0.21	0.62	0.32	0.35		0.39
Aspartic acid	0.37	0.31	0.77	0.26	0.28		0.57
Glutamic acid	1.28	1.73	0.96	1.15	0.67		0.96
Glycine	0.27	0.24	0.19	0.26	0.41		0.28
Proline	0.58	0.63	0.52	0.36	0.28		0.26
Serine	0.23	0.30	0.26	0.21	0.31		0.26

The low levels of lysine and tryptophane in maize are found in strains with a high zein : glutelin ratio. High-protein high-lysine maize has a low zein : glutelin ratio. There are hopes of using the high-lysine maize for chicken feed but maize-fed chickens have dark meat and yellow skins. To some consumers this means an old tough bird but in fact the meat is evidently more tasty and the cooked appearance is better than with white pale-skinned chickens. The high-lysine maize is said to have a lysine content of about 0.4 g/g N, which is superior to that of other cereals but short of that of meat. In terms of diet it replaces the mixture of corn-and-beans previously promoted for low-income consumers.

PRODUCTION
1972–1973 was a poor year for cereals, area having been cut back to

maintain prices and area-yields being below expectation. In the USA the maize harvest was delayed by bad weather and failure of monsoons reduced yields in Asia of rice. India, contrary to expectation, bought wheat and the USSR presented an unanticipated market for 30 million tons of mixed grain. By early 1973, European prices had inflated by 70% for wheat, 55% for maize, 65% for barley, 65% for rye, 80% for oats and 50% for sorghum, against early 1972 prices. Consequently, the 1973–1974 season started with reduced stocks and a late sowing of winter wheat in the face of poor weather. It was unfortunate that there was failure in all cereals, including rice to a situation where traditional rice exporters became importers. There would have been serious famine in rice areas if Japan had not stocks of old rice.

The main problem in production of cereals is that governments and trade organisations have attempted the matching of output to a calcu-lated weight which will bring maximum prices. Surplus production has been seen to be a cause of price depression, not a stimulation of product development. Such control has included payment for land left idle, which has proved to be inflationary since it represents an unprofitable and unproductive application of capital. The USA Department of Agriculture has forecast a rise of world wheat from a 1972–1973 level of 307 million tons to 331 million tons in 1973–1974, a fall in trade over the same year from 69–63 million tons but a rise in feed grain trading from 53–58 million tons. Of this, the USA can expect 1973–1974 wheat exports to be 26 million tons against 31.3 million tons in 1972–1973, feed grains being 35 million tons in 1973–1974 instead of 32 million tons in 1972–1973. On the other hand, the EEC predicts a massive surplus in 1980 of wheat, partly caused by development of other cereals which can be alternatives to wheat. It is forecast that the surplus wheat will replace oilcakes in feed, probably using denatured wheat.

All cereals can be expected to have a new pattern of production and marketing when new strains are developed. The ultimate target is a plant with very little height of straw, a short growing season with a narrow ripening period but very slow over-ripening, maximum response to fertiliser and a satisfactory pattern of amino acid in its protein fraction. The low height is important to allow production in areas which are subjected to high winds and driving rain. The short growing season is needed to produce ripe grain in short-summer countries. The reaction to fertiliser is to conform with opinion that synthetic feeding is the easiest method of increasing yield. The improved amino-acid pattern is to help feed starving millions where meat is rejected or is too expensive. There is some opinion that an ultimate cereal will offer a complete diet, using genetic manipulation and reproduction from cell culture.

The origin of maize is a wild plant with cobs less than 2 cm long, bearing about fifty seeds which were sufficiently light in weight to be spread by the wind. By the fifteenth century development of an improved strain had spread over most of the Americas. Columbus took a handful of seeds back to Isabella, who was not interested. By the nineteenth century the early Mahiz had developed into Maize and was a primary American crop. Yield was of the order of 20 bushels/acre until the findings of Mendel were applied to plant breeding. A pure inbred strain mated with another pure inbred strain produces a hybrid. Mating two such hybrids produces a double-cross. Such deliberate matings resulted in a yield of 60 bushels/acre. Today, 98% of the maize in the USA is from planned hybrid stock but, since 90% of it is for animal feed any depreciation of nutritional value is ignored for the sake of the higher weight of crop. In other countries, maize is important for human diet and the most dramatic outcome of planned mating is likely to be high-protein high-lysine maize—too good for animals but vital to under-nourished humans.

AREAS OF GROWTH

The effort to expand areas over which selected cereals can be grown is important in that it helps to avoid famine if one cereal fails. Thus, rice areas are accepting wheat as a crop, notably as a companion crop to sugar cane or in multiple-cropping and a typical multiple-crop is potato alternated with wheat.

At present, wheat production is mainly in the temperate land masses which have winter frosts. There are at least 1000 varieties with a vague division into hard and soft. Hard wheats are mainly for baking bread, soft for cakes and pastry, and one hard wheat, durum, is used for pastas and semolina. Other than a little cracked wheat, the main market is in flour milled according to market demands for percentages of extraction. The reject from refined flour is in fact the better part in diet if all com-ponents are considered and it is bought in a manufactured condition as a health aid by the same consumers who insist on white flour.

Rye production can be on soils and in climates which will not accept wheat. Production is mainly in wet temperate countries, where the high-energy composition of rye is appreciated in black bread. Oats can also be produced on poor soil but they need a calmer and drier climate than does rye. The conventional application is not in baked products but in porridge-type mixtures and as flakes. Barley can thrive in very cold, temperate and semi-tropical climates. European production is for brewing but it is grown for bread, porridge and pearl barley.

Maize production is mainly in climates which are too hot or dry for wheat. It is the most widely distributed cereal and is used, with local variations, for breads, porridges, flakes, additive to sweet or savoury dishes, or simply as stripped from the cob. The sister crops are millet and sorghums, which respond to primitive cultivation which might not produce good yields with maize. The grains are small and are used as flours for porridge, and for brewing when yields are high.

There are probably 3000 varieties of rice, which is a crop suited more to small-scale production than to estate farming. Production is mainly in Asia, where it has provided a foundation for social structures through the need in rice farming to use collective water control. Rice can be cultivated in most climates where water can be found and it yields the highest weight per area in return for the highest demand per area for labour.

The cereal market is influenced by alternative carbohydrate crops. Potatoes grow better in cool wet countries but are produced in every country, with at least 2000 common varieties. They are alternatives to rice in diet, being consumed mainly as a vegetable, but there is application to bread and pastry. The tropical version is the sweet potato. Cassava, which is also manioc, is easy to grow in hot climates but it has very little food value and is responsible for much malnutrition. Sweet cassava can be eaten raw or roasted but bitter cassava is toxic when fresh and is converted into flour and then cooked. The starch of cassava is converted into tapioca.

World output of cereals is indicated as:

	1972 million tons
Wheat	340
Rice	300
Maize	300
Barley	150

The total for all recorded cereals in 1972 was 1269 million tons, 60 million more than in 1970 but 40 million less than in 1971. Allowing for losses it is probable that the total dry weight protein in the 1972 cereal crop was 75 million tons.

Yield of cereals, various countries (100 kg/hectare approx.)			
	Wheat	*Barley*	*Oats*
Belgium	37.5	35.0	33.0
France	34.0	31.0	26.0
West Germany	37.0	33.0	31.0
Italy	22.5	16.0	14.5
Luxembourg	27.0	29.0	26.0
Holland	44.0	37.5	38.5
Denmark	44.0	39.0	37.5
Ireland	39.0	37.0	30.5
Norway	30.0	27.0	27.0
United Kingdom	40.0	36.0	32.5
United States	18.5	23.0	18.0

Chapter 15

Fresh Vegetables

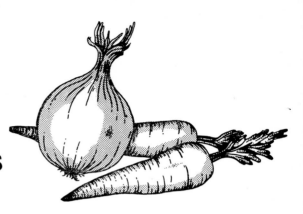

Vegetable proteins are mainly second-class, which means that they need mixing to offer a full pattern of amino acids in diet. This can be unfortunate where societies survive on a one-crop diet but it needs to be stressed that mixed vegetable protein is equal in value to flesh protein and it may be superior in its association with other components of diet (vitamins and minerals).

The broad division is into vegetation which is dehydrated for storage and vegetation which is grown to be eaten fresh, including that in which the freshness is extended in time by low-temperature preservation. This neat division is confused by a number of preservation techniques other than using low temperature or dehydration. Common preservation techniques include salting, sugaring, fermentation and heat treatment to kill biodeterioration agents before sealing in airtight packages. All preservation techniques are destructive but the destruction by low temperature is minimal and can be ignored. Destruction by dehydration can be considerable but is related more to vitamins than to the protein content. In very broad terms, preservation techniques do not reduce or damage the proteins to any significant extent but there are crops, notably pulses, for which care is needed in the application of a heating cycle for dehydration.

Sources of vegetable protein vary from very small agricultural holdings to vast areas devoted to single crops. As a rule, vegetables from vast-area single-crop production are inferior because quality has been sacrificed in favour of easy growth and maximum yield. Isolated crops are also inferior because emphasis on one vegetable disturbs ecosystems and there is selective biodeterioration with simplified cross-infection or cross-infestation. This has encouraged the use of chemicals for control in estate farming and, because some agriculturalists do not appreciate the difference between isolated culture and mixed cropping, in small agricultural holdings as well. There is evidence that arable farming must de-intensify and produce vegetation in a normal ecostructure of mixed plants and animals and micro-organisms. De-intensification is unpopular because it reduces yields, brings lower profit to farmers selling by weight, and damages the reputation of authorities seeking glory in output. The situation is now complicated by the development of high-protein and high-lysine cereals, which can offer required balanced nutrition but only with reduced yield.

In common diets, vegetables provide roughly half the protein. Most of this is from cereal, roots and pulses. The contribution of fresh vegetation is small, although the fresh vegetables are needed for the non-protein contributions. The relatively small intake of protein from fresh vegetables is partly due to the high water content of such vegetables and the fact that when cooked they are invariably boiled.

Statistics frequently ignore the contribution of gardens and local horticulture to food supplies, despite the fact that inflation encourages domestic production of vegetables and also raises the level of quality demanded by the consumer. The general rule in the vegetable market is that imported fresh vegetables sell on price whilst local fresh vegetables sell on quality. Both sources supply weight against payment and the economic factor in production is yield of acceptable quality, not nutritional value or protein content. Typical yields are:

	Tons/acre (divide by 2 for lb/sq. yd)
Broad beans	4
French beans	3
Runner beans	10
Haricot beans	0.75
Beet	12
Broccoli	8
Brussels sprouts	4
Cabbage	9
Cauliflower	6
Carrots	11

	Tons/acre (divide by 2 for lb/sq. yd)
Kale	10
Leeks	10
Onions	12
Parsnip	10
Peas	3
Potato	10
Savoy	15
Spinach	8
Swede	13
Turnips	13
Outdoor tomato	20
Indoor tomato	30

Protein components vary in content and in amino-acid patterns. The protein content as lifted is not important in any fresh vegetable due to be cooked, the following table showing how cooking can influence the arithmetic:

	Percentage protein	
	Cooked	Raw
Broad beans	4.0	
French beans	0.8	
Runner beans	0.8	1.1
Haricot beans	6.6	21.4 (as bought dried)
Beet	1.8	1.3
Broccoli	3.0	
Brussels sprouts	2.4	3.6
Cabbage	0.8	2.2
Cauliflower	1.5	3.4
Carrots	0.7	0.7
Leeks	1.8	1.9
Onions	0.6	0.9
Parsnip	1.3	1.7
Fresh peas	5.0	6.0
Dried peas	7.0	21.5
Potato	1.5	2.2
Savoy	1.3	3.3
Spinach	5.0	
Swede	0.9	1.1
Turnip	0.7	0.8
Tomato	1.0	0.9

The figures given in this table are suspect, partly because there is no constancy of quality in fresh vegetables but also because cooking can take many forms. Potato shows only 1.5% protein in its normal condition of boiled but it could read 2.8% roasted, 3.8% fried or 6% as potato crisps. The protein content is therefore influenced by the degree to which the method of cooking adds or takes water from the total weight and there is slight protein loss by incineration in dry heat cooking.

High-protein vegetables are being developed, mainly cereals and potato. The strains are individual hybrids which may yet show too much sensitivity to disease for estate farming, particularly since yields are not high. However, they could be of special interest to small agricultural holdings where high-protein crops are needed for domestic consumption, particularly where poverty dictates a diet comprising mainly the vegetation grown within reach, but it is doubted if the high-protein crops will be developed before the 1975–1976 season.

Among recent developments the International Potato Research Centre in Peru has produced tubers with 24% dry weight protein, three times that of a conventional potato. At the University of Nebraska, wheat has been produced which is more efficient at converting soil nitrogen into grain protein. At least a dozen USA seed companies now sell seed for high-lysine corn (maize) with the claim that the lysine content is double that of normal maize. It is interesting to reflect that the potato development starts from the original Andean potato, which has through the ages been bred to offer high-yield lower-protein replacements. The wheat concerned is Atlas 66 and 55 but other wheats are being bred into the programme. The maize programme started from realisation that the zein protein in maize is incomplete, lacking both lysine and tryptophane, whereas the glutelin protein is complete. Hence, high-glutelin maize was sought and crossed with high-yield maize. The result is said to be almost equivalent to milk in its amino-acid pattern. Rice contains the protein oryzenin which is equivalent to the glutelin in maize and could therefore also be the start of a programme for high-protein rice.

Bananas deserve special mention. Of fruit consumed fresh, they are the only ones which are non-seasonal. By volume, bananas are 76% water, 20% sugars, roughly 1% each of starch, fibre, minerals and protein. An average banana has the same calorific value as an average apple or orange but the low acidity makes it superior to other fruit for delicate digestions. Not widely appreciated, bananas are also ideal for drying and compounding. A powder mix of dried banana, milk powder and sugar is excellent diet. Plantains are the true cooking versions but their use is not international. A typical comparison might be:

	Apple	*Orange*	*Banana*
Percent waste	32.0	8.0	27
Protein percent	0.2	0.75	0.75
Fat percent	0.5	0.15	0.13
Carbohydrate percent	13.5	9.0	15.0

With regard to the comparative contents of minerals, bananas are rich in phosphorus, iron and potassium, but deficient in calcium. The combination of high mineral content and low acidity has reduced the incidence of protein deficiency in banana-eating districts. The processing of bananas has, however, been sadly neglected although the equipment needed is no more than a simple drier, crusher and drum mixer. Processing might have developed more if the banana did not have a convenient skin for holding and peeling. Bananas are second only to milk in terms of quantity eaten on a world scale as ready-to-eat food. They are the world's most popular fruit but, since much of the output is casual and unrecorded, output estimates are invariably inaccurate. The favoured estimate is 20–25 million tons with about 4 million tons passing into trade.

CASSAVA

At first sight, cassava deserves little mention in a book concerned with proteins. It is, however, one of the few crops which will thrive in most tropical regions, even if rains are unpredictable. Its contribution to diet, even to the carbohydrate fraction of diet, is limited by the cyanide toxicity. World output of cassava is probably 100 million tons. Yield is of the order of 9.5 tons/hectare, which is much lower than it could be on good soil. There are reports of cassava yields of more than 20 tons/hectare. In terms of energy content as an expression of carbohydrate food value, cassava offers 250 000 calories/hectare/day against only 175 000 for rice and 110 000 for wheat. Maize is the main rival with 200 000 calories/hectare/day but maize may be more expensive to produce. One calculation is that cassava can be grown to sell for fermentation at a field price of $6/ton.

Cassava starch contains less amylose than do the starches of maize or potato. Hence, it is a better starch for adhesives but could prove inferior in fermentation, although fermentation is relatively easy to encourage by adding sugars.

The toxicity is from a cyanogenic glycoside frequently known as mannihotoxin. This is toxic from the release of hydrogen cyanide in tissues after consumption. The toxicity levels and distribution vary according to the climate and farming techniques. Traditional cooking methods in South America and West Africa have overcome the problems, notably by boiling and by fermentation. Even so, there is some evidence in cassava districts of neurological damage, vitamin B12 absorption, and goitre. Goitre is one outlet for absorbed cyanide, the cyanide being converted to thiocyanate. It would seem logical to replace cassava as a common carbohydrate food, and to divert the cassava into fermentation processes, which evidently remove the cyanide, for the sake of microbial protein. The main production of cassava is:

	Million tons	Percentage of world production
Brazil	29.5	32.6
Indonesia	10.5	11.4
Zaire	10.0	10.9
Nigeria	7.3	7.9
India	5.2	5.6

The other third of world production is spread amongst about eighty other countries.

The production figures are far from accurate. Alternative statistics put the output of India at only 3 million tons, of Zaire at 7 million tons, of Indonesia at over 11 million tons. The true production may never be known but there are records of the patterns of application. India and Zaire consume about 95% of the crop with about 5% waste. Nigeria consumes about 80% with 20% waste. Brazil, on the other hand, consumes only about 35% and feeds nearly 40% to animals. Thailand consumes a little short of 40% and exports most of the rest.

Chapter 16

Oilseeds

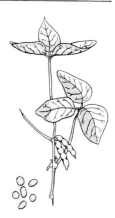

Oilseeds are grown for the vegetable oil and the residue of tissue which is protein-rich. World output in 1972, as far as records can show, was 119 million tons, 7 million more than in 1971 when the total was already 3 million tons more than in 1970. The probable protein contribution of oilseeds was 40 million tons, roughly half the contribution of cereals from about one-tenth of the original bulk, which is why oilseeds are valuable in animal feed. Outside the growing areas they are not popular for human diet other than in compounding, although the oils are popular as fats which do not carry a threat of heart failure.

The cakes are sensitive to micro-organic attack, notably from aspergillus with production of the toxin aflatoxin, which is known to kill poultry and is suspected of having a link with cancer in all animal groups. Sales of cake are inhibited by the common primitive handling which allows biodeterioration but there are hopes of improved handling, possibly with extrusion to pellets and airtight packaging of the hot product before it can become damp and infected. There is also effort to improve the flavour and ease of digestion of cakes so that they can be promoted for direct human consumption. The pattern of amino acids in the proteins is reasonably good but methionine is frequently needed for a full balance. The balance is sufficiently good for whole seeds or cakes to be used as meat substitutes to a limited extent, as butters, so-called steaks and recently texture as fibres for imitation meat.

About half the original bulk is left after full extraction of oil. Soya is the most favoured crop because it is conducive to estate farming, accounting for about one-third of production. Over two-thirds of soya is from the USA but only 2% of USA soya is used for direct human consumption. It is said that more soya might not be used in direct human diet because the raffionose and stachiose contents inhibit digestion, this being disputed in other sections of trades. It is also said that fish meal protein is more suited for development for human diet than is soya protein, fish meal lacking tryptophane which is claimed as easy to add whilst the methionine lacking from oilseeds could be an expensive addition. Fish meal appears to offer more potential than soya if it can be produced odour-free when there has been further development of enzyme hydrolysis, which evidently converts fish meal into a digestible first-class protein food requiring only the addition of flavour to be attractive for human diet.

With regard to developing countries and famine areas it is probable that there will be developments of mixtures of oilseeds with marine derivatives, as the oilseed is available from local agriculture but contains only half its needs of methionine, whereas marine derivatives, not only fish but all marine life, have excess methionine but need the surplus tryptophane in oilseeds. The fish meal or other marine derivative can supply mineral shortages in the oilseeds and can overcome any problems of phytic acid in the oilseeds. The balancing of compositions is not, however, the main consideration. Oilseeds and marine derivatives are low-cost local crops which can be developed in developing countries with general improvement of the economic and social situation. This is much simpler than relating a new meat or dairy industry to the oilseed supply or trying to improve the fishing industries by injecting heavy capital.

Methionine is water-soluble and is stable at boiling and evaporation temperatures. It can be extracted and added to oilseed foods to balance the amino acids. Synthetic or extracted methionine is widely used in cereal–oilseed feeds at a rate of about 0.5 kg/ton mostly for poultry feed. For pigs the required addition seems to be 1 kg/ton for lysine with some doubt if the methionine is also required.

The development of high-protein cereals is expected to have influence on oilseed demand. High-lysine maize can replace half the oilseed cake used in pig feed, the claims including a lysine content of 0.5% and a tryptophane content of 0.15% for the new maize, both of which are about double the concentrations in common maize. On the other hand, when protein contents are the main consideration as they frequently are in buying feed, low-fat soya contains more nitrogen than almost any competitor, 7.9% nitrogen which equates to 50% protein. It can be

practical to overfeed a deficient protein food for the sake of lower raw
and storage cost.

To ease calculations in compounding feeds it is common to use simple
percentages in statements of amino-acid patterns in oilseeds. American
sources claim the following:

	61.4% protein soya meal	Beef for comparison
Leucine	7.7	8.0
Isoleucine	5.1	6.0
Valine	5.4	5.5
Threonine	4.3	5.0
Methionine	1.6	3.2
Cystine	1.6	1.2
Lysine	6.9	10.0
Arginine	8.4	7.7
Histidine	2.6	3.3
Phenylalanine	5.0	5.0
Tryptophane	1.3	1.4

Comparison of soya protein against beef protein is not significant because
ruminants do not only rely on supplied protein but can manufacture their
own by bacterial activity in the rumen. One ton of urea supplied to the
bacteria can replace 5–6 tons of conventional feed, and can be used for
about a quarter of total protein requirements of the beast. Microbial
protein, however, tends to be lacking methionine, so the feeding of urea
instead of oilseed will not solve problems of methionine deficiency,
although it may well solve problems of lysine deficiency and thereby
become more significant as replacement for cereals. Even so, in 1966
in the USA, almost 200 000 tons of urea replaced 1.1 million tons of
44% soya, and there has been further development of feed-grade urea
in the USA.

With oilseeds under threat in the feed market from improved cereals
and from the feeding of non-protein nitrogen, some effort to find other
outlets is evident. In the United States, which as a major supplier can
indicate market directions, the non-feed application of soya in 1967
included:

Meat products—15 000 tons
Pet foods—60 000 tons
Beverages—5 000 tons

12·—WPR   *   *

This is remarkably low, a fact which can be related to legislation. There is no doubt that, given freedom of application the manufacturers would have used much more soya.

The Israel Institute of Technology have done much work on soya and related proteins. Subjects examined in detail include the use of protein concentrates in food compounds, effect of processing on soya protein, study of dextran sulphate and lipoprotein, soya protein as an aid in spray-drying bananas, bread from soya and the influence of storage on the lysine in soya. There are similar studies, though possibly not in such detail, in most countries, and it would seem that future products will be more sophisticated than the present feed.

Oilseed now accounts for about a quarter of compound feed, increasing in this application from 12 million tons in 1967 to 15.4 million tons in 1970. There could be a rapid increase in the proportion of oilseed used after the failure of Peruvian fish meal and the need for cereals for human diet. On the other hand, the soya failure coinciding with the fish meal failure encouraged grazing rather than feeding compound.

Oilseed residue for feeding animals is a relatively recent development. It developed during the 1960s and accelerated after 1967. From 1967 to 1971 the demand increased from 50 million to 60 million tons and is forecast to increase to 70 million tons by 1980. There are twelve major importing countries, all in Europe, and Japan imports whole seeds for crushing. Imports are entirely for feed with the proportion of oilseed in compound varying from 12 to 20% and with the type of oilseed varied according to the animal. Coconut cake is excellent for ruminants but has too much fibre for pigs and poultry. Groundnut cake can be suspect with regard to its population of fungi and cottonseed cake can be toxic to some delicate digestions. Soya dominates partly because it is more universal in application and appears to be less likely to carry toxic organic growth.

Production economics are slightly complicated by the joint production of oil and cake. It is probable, for instance, that there will be surplus oil through the 1970s because a heavy crop in Brazil and the USA was previously used to develop the feed market without attention to the oil. This early surplus started a continued lack of balance and it may yet prove necessary for a process to be devised for the fermentation of vegetable oil into protein. The world demand for beef and dairy protein has caused a glut of butter and future demands for oilseed cake can be expected to be for low-fat versions. Surplus butter will also inhibit the development of vegetable table fats, although it will not unduly influence demands for cooking oils in countries which prefer liquid oil to hard fats.

Soya has grown in importance partly because it has been backed by sophisticated marketing and partly because it is suitable for most animals. The United States has been able to supply regular deliveries of constant quality, but recent confusions after the USA crop failure at the time when Peruvian fish meal failed, and particularly the imposition of controls after deliveries were agreed, have reduced trust in the United States and have renewed interest in other oilseeds.

Groundnuts suffer from the problem of aflatoxin development in careless handling but they are favoured by the United Kingdom through the historic association with West Africa and East Africa. The same association encourages purchase of groundnut by France, whilst Germany favours palm and Scandinavia favours cottonseed. Rape seed is not popular because supplies vary and do not satisfy the demands of economic crushing plant, and rape is rich in glucosinolates which can be mild toxins. The final analysis in feeding animals is, however, input cost related to returns, and this is influenced firstly by the choice between grazing and supplying bought feed, then by the relative advantages of the various feed components including non-protein nitrogen, then selection of an oilseed cake if oilseeds are favoured.

West Europe is the market for oilseeds, with a 1971 consumption of almost 16 million tons of which almost 8 million tons were imported. The breakdown in 1970–1971 was:

| | Percentages of consumption | | 1971 imports |
	1970	1971	
Soya	56.0	59.7	47.3
Cottonseed	8.6	6.4	10.7
Groundnuts	8.1	6.6	10.3
Sunflower	4.4	3.4	4.6
Rape		6.1	1.2
Palm	2.2	?.2	1.6
Copra	4.3	5.1	5.1
Linseed	5.9	5.8	9.2
Others		4.7	4.7

The proportional increase of soya is to be noted but it is to be appreciated that future European attitudes to soya from the United States could inhibit further increase whilst negotiations relative to new associ-

ates of the EEC could encourage other oilseeds. The 1971 consumption
pattern in Europe was:

	Consumption (thousand tons)	Percentage imported
West Germany	4667	60
France	2090	61
Holland	1770	69
Italy	1467	23
Spain	1265	7
United Kingdom	1209	71
Denmark	999	60
Belgium	913	80

The export pattern is dominated by the United States, with 13 million
tons exported in 1970, the year which influenced feeding patterns in 1971,
and the EEC is the world's largest soya importer with 50% bought from
the United States. However, when the United States cut deliveries contrary to agreement it was inevitable that the EEC would seek alternative
supplies from Brazil. The cuts in deliveries also caused concern in Japan,
where over 90% of soya imports were from the United States (3.1 million
tons from the USA out of a total of 3.4 million tons imported).

OILSEED ISOLATES

In cereals the tissue is mainly endosperm with a small embryo. The seeds
store carbohydrate and the protein content is relatively low. In oilseeds,
the entire tissue is embryo with a thin layer of endosperm, and the
storage of energy is partly as oil and partly as protein. It is common to
crush the seeds to release the oil, selling the oil into the cooking-fat
market and using the crushed residue for animal feed. Qualities depend
inevitably on the original seed but also on the excellence or otherwise
of the crushing process. When needed, more of the oil can be extracted
by solvent and the protein fraction can be fractionated to meet specific
requirements. The broad commercial division in oilseeds is into cottonseed and the rest, cottonseed being an unfortunate commodity in that
it contains gossypol, an undesirable toxic pigment. Conversely, cottonseed is an attractive commodity in that it is a by-product of cotton fibre
production, and can therefore be shown to cost very little in production
(the alternative hypothesis is that cotton fibre production can be financed
by profits from seed, allowing cotton to compete against low-cost synthetic fibres). Most of the oilseeds are reasonably flexible in their climatic

requirements, and are sensitive to improvement by breeding. Hence, interest is in all geographic regions, particularly since the proteins obtained are only slightly second-class. The quality of protein can be expected to improve with development of protein isolation and subsequent division into specific mixtures. The comment below refers mainly to cottonseed, as the difficult representative, but the mentioned processes apply to other oilseeds. It is to be appreciated, however, that other oilseeds can be eaten and enjoyed in the original condition but cottonseed contains gossypol, which has to be removed before the protein is fed to animals without rumens.

The tissue of the original seed is a collation of packages, each of which holds a main constituent. The cells are in five zones of: nucleus, spherosomes, protein bodies including phytin globules, cytoplasm, and cell walls.

In cottonseed the protein bodies are about 5 microns in diameter, enclosing smaller bodies known as globoids and holding the phytin content. Around the protein bodies are layers of round particles which are lipid bodies, with diameters from one-third to three microns. The structure is punctuated by glands, diameters from 50–400 microns, containing networks of globules of gossypol. Gossypol is a reactive polyphenolic binaphthaldehyde which is mildly toxic to monogastric animals and also combines with lysine to reduce the effective lysine content of the seed tissue. The protein content includes about fifteen water-soluble proteins and a few water-insoluble proteins. The target in concentration and isolation is to eliminate unrequired cellulose and unwelcome gossypol, then to divide the protein fraction into groups as demanded by the applications. The normal intention is to manufacture three main products:

A high-protein product for human diet as cereal replacement

A lower-protein produce for animal feed

Undesirables, for which there is little application so far but there could be processing to microbial or algae protein.

The original cottonseed kernels contain:

	% *dry weight*
Protein	30 to 40
Oil	About 40
Ash	5
Fibre	2

Water-soluble proteins account for about one-third of the total protein and insoluble versions account for about two-thirds. A protein content of the order of 70% is accepted as the norm for oilseed protein concentrates. The gossypol glands account for 2–5% of the seed weight and the actual gossypol accounts for 0.8–2% of seed weight.

Polar solvents rupture gossypol glands. Boiling in water releases the gossypol to contaminate the protein fraction. The conventional solvent extraction used for oilseeds releases the gossypol into the oil. A typical solvent mixture is 39% acetone, 60% hexane and 1% water. It has been discovered, however, that the gossypol glands are tough and do not rupture with non-polar solvents. They can withstand fairly brutal treatment and be floated out in hexane or similar non-polar solvent. Obviously, extraction is easier and more effective if the gossypol is removed in neat little packages of reasonable size.

The simple process puts crushed seeds in hexane, waits for the non-protein particles to settle and then pours off the creamy mixture of hexane and protein bodies. Alternatively, crushed seeds can be mixed with a hydrocarbon mixture adjusted to a specific gravity of 1.378. Gossypol glands rise above this density and everything else sinks to the bottom. In the hexane-only technique the proteins are removed from everything else whilst in the mixed hydrocarbon technique the gossypol glands are removed from everything else. As might be expected, neither technique is exacting in its division.

An improvement is to pass the mixture of hexane and crushed seed through a cyclone, classification then being according to particle sizes, weights and shapes. Such a liquid cyclone process (LCP) can start with undefatted crushed seeds, which can save a process. The cleaned flour from LCP has the composition:

Moisture	3.2%
Lipids	1.2
Free gossypol	0.02
Total gossypol	0.065
Protein	66 (60 to 70)
Fibre	2.3
Ash	8.9

This flour is acceptable for human diet but is also suitable for air classification. The general target in air classification is five fractions showing a progressive reduction of protein content. A typical fractionation might be:

		Yield	% approx. Moisture	Protein	Fibre
Cottonseed					
Original flour		100.0	9.0	61.5	3.0
	Fraction 1.	36.0	8.5	70.5	2.0
	2.	17.0	8.5	68.0	2.0
	3.	13.5	8.0	58.5	3.0
	4.	7.0	7.5	56.0	3.0
	5.	26.0	7.0	48.0	4.0
Groundnuts					
Original flour		100.0	8.0	63.0	4.0
	Fraction 1.	37.5	7.5	76.0	2.0
	2.	24.5	7.5	67.5	3.5
	3.	26.5	7.5	48.5	6.5
	4.	6.0	8.0	44.5	7.0
	5.	5.5	7.5	45.5	6.5

In the cottonseed fractions the gossypol proportion increases through the grades, from about 0.3% in the first fraction to about 3.5% in no. 5. It is common with cottonseed to combine fractions 1 and 2 to give a high-protein flour at a nominal 70% dry weight protein, then to combine the other three fractions as a general feed additive. Similar recombination with groundnut flour extracts give a protein concentrate at a nominal 72% dry weight from nos. 1 and 2, a general feed additive from the rest.

Groundnuts are fairly common diet for humans as original seed or as processed products. One process of note is defatting, up to 70% of the oil being removed by pressing (2000 p.s.i. for nearly an hour) followed by boiling for 3 mins to expand the tissue and then drying and roasting. The final product has an attractive texture for eating which can be blamed on coalescence of protein bodies and the gelation of starch. Original groundnuts provide 100 calories per about 20 seeds but the defatted, boiled and roasted versions provide only half this energy and obesity potential. They also provide one-third more protein per weight of seed eaten.

The potential food value of oilseeds in aid programmes has not been ignored. CSM is a dry blend of gelatinised maize meal, roasted defatted soya meal, dried milk and soya oil. Cottonseed flour and groundnut concentrates are used in beverages. An edible cottonseed flour is being developed in India. Also in India, wheat flour is being improved by the addition of groundnut flour. There are many unpublicised uses of oilseed flours and concentrates, the protein content of diets being improved without public comment and without observed change in the texture and flavour of familiar foods.

Glandless cottonseed is under development and should be fairly common by 1980. It is doubted if a glandless version is justified since it is likely to be low in yield, and developments of gossypol extraction continue. The comparison of glandless and glanded cottonseed as flour is, roughly:

	Nitrogen	Moisture	Fibre	Total gossypol
Glandless (%)	9.5—10.5	9.9	2.7	
Glanded (%)	9.0	8.7	3.1	1.35

Future analysis will change this rough comparison. If a liquid cyclone process is applied to cottonseed which is dried down to 0.75% moisture, about two-thirds of the protein is obtained with a gossypol content of 0.3%, including 0.045% as free gossypol. About one-third of the protein is removed with the gossypol glands. Justification for a glandless cottonseed depends on outlets for high-gossypol protein fractions, the only major outlet being in feed for ruminants.

A factory processing 100 tons of seed per day could produce per day:

	Tons
High protein concentrate for human diet	18
High-gossypol animal feed for ruminants	13
Cottonseed oil	18
Hulls and other cellulose reject	38
Linters	10

Up to 90% of the gossypol is concentrated in the animal feed fraction, and it exists in glands which would rupture if exposed to polar solvents in efforts to fractionate. Obviously, a glandless cottonseed would provide a feed fraction suitable for a very wide range of animals. Glandless seed have been grown in the United States and Chad. There are developments in Egypt, Mexico and several South American countries.

The alternative to air classification is wet extraction. Air classification delivers a fraction which is rich in protein and sugars but low in cell wall reject. The quality of fractions from wet extraction depend on the applied chemicals and the precipitation acidity. Broadly, calcium chloride extraction results in a product which shows a low comparative content of protein and sugar but a high content of cell wall. Alcohol extraction provides a compromise between the compositions from air classification and those from calcium chloride extraction. Most current interest is in two-stage wet extraction, using water followed by alkali.

The water-soluble proteins account for about one-third of the total nitrogen. The protein bodies in cottonseed do not rupture in hot water at the high rates found with soya, groundnut or other common oilseed. Hence, a simple boiling technique is only partly effective, although almost total extraction can be by boiling at pH 10.0 followed by precipitation at pH 5.0. If the market indicates a need for a high-lysine high-methionine protein extraction, then a two-stage process is indicated. Started with defatted flour the stages are:

1. Take out the water-soluble proteins with water and precipitate at pH 4.0
2. Take out the alkali-soluble proteins with 0.015 N caustic soda and precipitate at pH 7.0.

Isolation of the protein fractions may not be necessary for the market available. From one-fifth to one-quarter of the flour content of baked products can be replaced by oilseed concentrate. In normal wheat bread, this increases the protein content to about 20% and provides an amino-acid balance from the mixture of cereal and oilseed. Up to 6% of isolate can be included in acid beverages, which may yet prove to be the major route of introduction of more protein to those who need it. Cottonseed isolate is inferior to soya isolate in meat products because the gelling characteristics are poor. On the other hand, cottonseed isolate may prove superior to soya in textured products such as imitation meat.

For the record, in anticipation of more area devoted to glandless cottonseed, the glandless flours comprise:

| | *% dry weight* | | |
	Acala	*Gregg 25-V*	*Watson G1-16*
Protein	65.9	63.6	58.8
Nitrogen	10.54	10.18	9.41
Lipid	1.2	1.2	1.3
Fibre	2.6	3.5	2.8
Ash	8.6	7.1	9.3
Sugars	5.1	3.2	6.0

The flour from normal glanded cottonseed, and the two main selective extracts, have the composition:

Cottonseed isolate compositions (%), USA Dept. of Agric opinion

| | Original flour | Isolate extracted with all proteins | Selected extract of | |
			Soluble proteins	Insoluble proteins
Nitrogen	10.73	15.58	13.08	17.24
Fibre	2.2	0.5	0.5	0.2
Lipid	0.9	1.1	3.0	0.2
Ash	7.8	3.4	14.1	1.0
Sugar	7.3	0.5	0.5	0.0
Amino-acid patterns (g/16 g N)				
Arginine	12.4	10.0	10.4	11.3
Alanine	3.7	3.6	3.2	3.5
Aspartic acid	9.1	9.0	6.7	8.4
Cystine	—	—	2.6	0.3
Glutamic acid	20.4	16.4	21.8	18.9
Glycine	4.1	3.5	3.2	3.7
Histidine	2.9	2.9	2.6	3.0
Isoleucine	3.4	3.4	2.6	3.1
Leucine	5.8	5.7	5.1	5.8
Lysine	4.4	3.4	6.0	3.0
Methionine	1.3	1.4	1.7	1.0
Proline	3.6	3.4	3.1	3.1
Phenylalanine	5.5	5.7	3.7	6.3
Serine	4.1	4.0	3.4	4.5
Theonine	3.0	2.9	2.9	2.7
Tyrosine	3.1	2.8	3.3	2.6
Valine	4.6	4.7	3.3	4.4

The relative proportions of lysine in the soluble fraction and insoluble fraction are important. For some deficient feed mixtures it could prove highly economic to isolate the high-lysine high-methionine fraction, which is the solubles, as a feed additive. The insoluble fraction, which originates in the storage proteins of the seed, has proved excellent as an additive in baking, increasing the bread protein content but not spoiling the bread texture or flavour. Since bread is a common item of diet in many protein-deficient districts, the ability to add isolate without changing the nature of the bread could be important.

Soy protein isolates. Range by Purina Protein Europe

Percentages							
Protein (N × 6.25)	90.0	90.0	95.0	93.0	91.0	95.0	95.0
Moisture	4.5	5.0	4.5	5.5	3.5	7.0	5.5
Ash	3.8	4.0	3.8	4.5	5.5	2.5	4.5
Fat	0.2	1.5	0.2	1.2	0.2	0.2	0.2
Fibre	0.01	0.5	0.01	—	0.01	0.2	0.2
pH values	6.7	6.7	6.7	6.7	3.3	4.5	6.5

Claimed amino-acid pattern (g/16g N)		
Isoleucine	4.6 *or* 4.7	
Leucine	8.4	7.8
Lysine	6.3	5.7
Methionine	1.1	1.2
Phenylalanine	5.4	5.4
Threonine	3.4	3.5
Tryptophane	1.3	1.1
Valine	4.8	4.8

Isolated soy protein. Claimed analysis by Grain Processing Corporation

	%	%
Protein (N × 6.25)	90.0 *or* 70.0	
Ash	4.1	4.1
Fibre	0.2	5.0
Moisture	3.9	3.9
Fat	0.5	0.5

Soluble protein 88%. pH value 6.8.

Amino-acid pattern	g/ 16g N		*Minerals*	p.p.m.	
Arginine	7.3 *or* 7.5		Calcium	1510 *or* 6200	
Histidine	2.9	2.4	Sodium	12 000	3900
Isoleucine	4.6	5.1	Potassium	10 000	3000
Leucine	8.1	8.4	Phosphorus	8000	8100
Methionine	1.0	1.1	Magnesium	995	2600
Phenylalanine	5.5	5.6	Copper	17	11
Threonine	4.0	4.0	Iron	140	120
Tryptophane	0.9	0.9	Zinc	86	90
Valine	4.6	5.7	Mercury	0.1 less 0.05	
Cystine	0.9	0.9	Lead	0.2	0.3

Isolated defatted cottonseed flour. Analysis by Grain Processing Corporation

	%
Protein (N × 6.25)	65.0
Fat	1.0
Ash	9.0
Fibre	2.5

Protein solubility 99%. pH value 6.3 to 6.9

Amino-acid pattern	g/16 g N	Minerals	p.p.m.
Arginine	12.4	Sodium	300
Histidine	2.7	Potassium	21 000
Isoleucine	2.6	Phosphorus	17 900
Leucine	5.7	Calcium	530
Lysine	4.1	Magnesium	1050
Methionine	1.4	Copper	19
Phenylalanine	5.6	Iron	125
Threonine	3.1	Zinc	84
Tryptophane	1.2		
Valine	4.5		
Cystine	1.2		

The Japanese developed many soya fractions, exampled by DX-100 with a composition of:

	%
Moisture	6.0 to 10.0
Protein	19.0 to 22.0
Fat	0.5 to 1.0
Minerals	3.5 to 4.5
Fibre	9.0 to 15.0
Polysaccharide	47.5 to 60.0

The main outlets for DX-100 type of fraction are in calorie-reduced compounded foods, special high-protein diets, as a binder in compounds with extra protein from the binder, and in flour confectionary to improve crumb strength, particularly since bakers are having to use lower-cost weak flours during periods of inflation.

Soya fractions have arisen mainly from efforts to develop markets in Europe. Soya has been an essential part of diet in Eastern Asia for centuries, and probably accounts for 15% of the protein in Japanese diet. There is some doubt that soya as crushed will be accepted on a wide scale for human food, although the proteinates are likely to become fairly standard in compounding.

Soya beans are first cracked in rollers to remove the hull and to break up the tissue into grits. Oil is extracted using hexane or other solvent, the grits being soaked in solvent and the oil being carried with the solvent in subsequent distillation. The solvent is then evaporated off and the crude oil refined with removal of lecithin. The grits which remain are the source of the proteinate. The processing conditions are variable and the final proteinate is not standard. Common compositions are with total protein content from 54–70%, the NSI (measure of solubility of the protein) percentage being from 10–50%.

The defatted grits have probably about 55% protein and can be used to upgrade protein feeds. It is not difficult to concentrate the grits to about 70% protein, at which level the concentrate can be used for compounding into meat. The degree to which it is suitable for compounding into the water/fat/muscle mixture of meat depends on the solubility of the protein. Soluble protein acts as a link between the water and fat of meat, reducing cooking losses and shrinkage and also preventing fat loss from compounds such as luncheon meat.

As compounded, soluble proteins form complex molecules which include the available water and fat. When cooled, the proteins coagulate to lock the water and fat in a firm stable matrix. The fat, for example, in a sausage, needs such a lock to prevent fat loss in cooking. A similar locking of fat is needed in luncheon meat, it being fairly common to see a migrated fat layer in tinned luncheon meat without added soluble proteinate.

Any stage in processing is likely to reduce the proportion of soluble in the protein. The processing choice is, therefore, between a fairly lengthy low-heat cycle which results in a high proportion of soluble in the final product, or a rapid reasonably-hot process for inexpensive but insoluble protein. The type with solubles is for binding water/fat compounds whilst the type with less solubles is for other non-binding compounding or for direct consumption.

Particle sizes are varied, the larger particles being of value in general compounding. In general, larger particles give texture to meat products whilst the smaller particles are more rapid in binding and should, since they suffer more work in production, be with less solubles than larger particles. Particle size influences the quantity which can be added to a compound, the common proportion in meats being from 1.5–2.5%. It is common to add the proteinate with the water demanded by the recipe used for the compound, preferably by mixing the water with the proteinate and then adding the slurry to the compound. A typical sausage recipe might be:

	%
Lean pork	40
Fat pork	25
Cereal	10
Seasoning/flavours	3
Water 20	
Proteinate 2	
22 — — — 22 added as a final slurry	

Proteinates hold about their own weight of water. They can be used to rescue the gelatin fraction in meat compounding. If rinds are cooked with proteinate and water the proteinate gels to bind the gelatin, after which it can be chopped for addition into the meat mix.

Cottonseed can also be used for proteinates, the claim being that a loaf of bread made from cottonseed flour is equal in protein to 2.5 kg of beef, indicating a market for protein extract as a compounding additive with cereals. Cottonseed protein concentrate is already widely used alongside carbohydrates in soft drinks, pastries and ice cream. Development started in earnest when the Lubbock, Texas cottonseed flour mill opened and the United States Congress was provided with protein-packed cookies. The cookies had protein contents from 10–18%, using Lubbock concentrate at 65–70% protein. Lubbock also produces 95–100% protein concentrate for snack foods. In Israel, cottonseed protein was used for baby foods. The concentrate was at 60% protein, the baby food being first developed as a dry powder for mixing in water. It was then mixed with wheat flour and drum dried to a final protein content of 35% with 15% fat. Subsequent processing was with sugar (50% sugar added) and with water in a proportion of 10 parts solid to 1 part water. The nitrogen balance was inferior to that of milk but infants on trial feed appeared to thrive.

Chapter 17

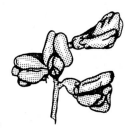
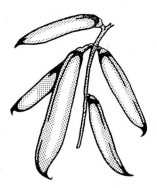

Pulses

Pulses are the edible seeds of the legume family, the term legume covering the entire vegetable crop, which may be grown for manure, animal feed, or for the seed which may be eaten with the pod. Pulses are basic foodstuffs, mainly for the protein content, but there can be deficiency problems in pulse areas if the vegetable protein is not supported by animal protein and many of the problems arise from difficulties in preparation of the pulses and their relatively difficult digestion.

The main pulses are peas, haricots, horse beans and lentils. All the seeds have an outer protective coat, the testa, which has little food value. Within the testa are two lobes, which are to become the first leaves, enclosing an embryo, and there is no extra food store, or endosperm, as found in cereals. All the food value is in the two cotyledons. It is fairly common to split pulses, which removes the worthless testa and also accelerates cooking so that food values are maintained. Pulses can be ground into flours, which do not keep well but are superior for cooking and can be compounded.

The moisture content which inhibits mould growth is below 14 or 15%, which is a little higher than for cereals. The composition varies with the growing conditions but is roughly:

Moisture content (%) of dried pulses at about 10 mg/100 g

	Protein	Fat	Carbo-hydrate	Fibre
Peas	25	1.0	57	4.5
Kidney beans	24	1.7	57	4.0
Lima beans	20	1.5	58	5.0
Broad beans	25	1.5	57	4.5
Lentils	24	1.0	59	4.0

The *Vivia faba* bean used for simulated meat is the broad bean as listed. There are many other peas and beans which could be listed but the table shows that all the pulses are roughly similar in composition if measured as dry seeds. The above values are for a typical moisture content of about 10 mg/100 g of dry tissue. Lima beans may reach 12 mg and broad beans may have only 9 mg, but 10 mg is a fair average.

The vitamin content of pulses is roughly similar to that of cereals. They are useful sources of iron and calcium but both minerals vary according to the soil. The protein content is offset by a high phytic acid content. Cereals are mainly deficient in lysine whilst pulses are mainly lacking cystine and methionine, therefore, a balanced diet involves mixtures of cereals and pulses, notably rice–bean dishes.

There is some danger of toxins in pulses if regular large quantities are consumed. There is understood to be one African society which has developed communal allergy to broad beans, although this could be due to overconsumption of beans without added cereal as deficiency can frequently be mistaken for allergy. However, the broad bean, or *Vicia faba*, evidently can retain its toxin whilst other pulses lose their toxins in cooking and certain societies in eastern Mediterranean regions are sensitive to broad beans, to the extent of giving the allergy an identity of 'favism'.

Dried pulses are durable but there is widespread loss in storage from biodeterioration, some of which is carried by the seeds from the fields. Preharvest infestation by bruchids is responsible for this storage loss. Bruchids are inside the seeds and continue their development after harvesting, emerging in due course through windows in the testa. Storage losses by infestation are individual in character, as other stored seeds suffer from external attack, but since pulses have a very tough testa which inhibits such attack they suffer internal attack. Since bruchids are inside the seeds they are impossible to reach with pesticides until they break their escape windows. The hole left in the window is then a target for fungal attack and the uptake of moisture.

If pulses are overdried, down to 12% for beans or 11% for peas, the protective testa becomes brittle and cracks. There is also some unknown reaction in the overdried tissue which makes the mixture impossible to soften in subsequent soaking and cooking. It is important to maintain humidities within very tight limits, high humidity producing mould growth and low humidity producing mechanical damage and poor cooking quality.

Chapter 18

Dehydrated Vegetables in Feed

Dehydration of vegetation varies in degree according to its intended function and the money available in production. Many countries have part of the year in which there is sufficient solar heat and dry air for drying by exposure. If vegetable tissue can be dried down to an equivalent of 70% relative humidity, micro-organisms cannot find sufficient moisture to be active and some insects are less effective as destructive consumers. The equivalent moisture content varies with the tissue but is mainly of the order of 10–12%. Where climates are unkind and do not offer dry heat it is necessary to use forced drying, but this is made difficult by the relatively low world prices for bulk commodities sold into a competitive market.

Food processing and the feeding of livestock compete for supplies of dehydrated vegetables. The price in the processing market is limited by the danger that overpricing will encourage rejection in favour of some other food group, as for example a decline of bakery products when they become too expensive. The price in animal feeding is limited by the availability of grazing and silage as an alternative. In food processing, substances are evaluated in terms of initial purchase price and convenience of processing. In the feeding of animals the intention is to convert vegetable protein rapidly into flesh protein and the protein content of the initial vegetable matter is important.

The growth area is in compound feeds. There is world-wide increase of consumption of animal products and, associated with this, an increase in demand for cake to satisfy demands of intensive rearing, although

1970–1973 price inflation has brought renewed interest in grazing and the feed industry is aware that there are developments of alternative proteins at low prices. From 1967–1970 the world consumption of compound feed increased from 49–60 million tons and the oilcake fraction of this increased from 12.1–15.4 million tons. Cake in compounds appears to be steady at about one-quarter of the total composition but it can be expected to increase its proportion if fish meal is not provided to replace that lost from Peru. It can also be expected that new protein sources such as algae and microbes will replace the fish meal and soya of feed mixtures more than the grain and oilseeds such as groundnuts and cottonseed.

The relationship of technology to economics in feed is complicated. There are illogical situations such as the feeding of dried milk to animals because it exists as surplus after excess butter has been manufactured, despite the fact that dried milk is urgently needed for feeding unfortunate humans and is too valuable to be used as simple replacement for soya and fish meal. Likewise, despite the need for grain in human feeding it is common for wheat to be denatured and used for animal feed, although a very high proportion of waste from human diet is ignored as a source of energy and protein for animals. A significant complication has been the deliberate restriction of crop output with the mistaken understanding that surplus will reduce prices and famine will bring more profit to the producers. During the early 1970s it has been shown that there is not a direct relationship between supplies and prices, mainly because speculation removes further stocks in times of famine and the consequent price is not the acceptable maximum for the market, but is inflated to the point where users seek urgent alternatives. To maintain market stability and profit to the producers there must be relatively slow changes of price so that intermediate users have time to pass on increases, and can buy forward at fixed prices which will allow sensible factory operation. It has now been realised that yield restriction is fully destructive and that prices are dictated more by ultimate consumers than by first-buyers. If there is surplus, there is associated effort in the market to find new uses and thereby increase demand. If there is famine the users seek alternatives and, as a rule, find new economy and satisfaction with consequent rejection of their original raw materials regardless of the quantity of future supplies.

Even if it could or would, an animal being reared is not allowed to have preference or prejudice relative to its diet. The composition is dictated by the farmer according to experience, availability and prices.

In this, he is influenced by political pressures in the form of regulations, added costs related to specific actions or materials, and a confusing medley of financial benefits. There is consequent variation in habits amongst farmers, as can be illustrated with regard to compound used in feed in Holland and France—countries with roughly the same order of affluence, much the same pattern of animal selection, and both within the jurisdiction of the EEC.

| | *Quantity of compound used per animal* (*kg*) | |
	Holland	France
Cows	907	94
Pigs	522	248
Poultry	36	25

According to simple economic theory there should be continued increase of the proportion of compound in feed because:

1. The demand for meat increases constantly.
2. The size of operation in animal rearing is likely to increase.
3. Inflation of land prices will encourage intensive rearing.
4. Grain will be needed more for human diet and its price will probably rise further.

Detailed study of this theory shows it to be suspect. The demand for meat could well fall rapidly if new sources of protein provide low-cost attractive alternatives to meat for the rising generation which is likely to depreciate the influence of tradition, preference and prejudice. The size of operation in animal rearing could well fall to take advantage of natural vegetation and avoid the inflated cost of supplied feed. Land prices could fall but it is more probable that there will be sharper differentiation between urban land and rural land, the urban land inflating in price at a much faster rate than that of rural land. Also, a fact which agriculture economists appear to ignore, there are vast areas in the world yet to be developed using agricultural methods other than those familiar to agricultural economists. With regard to grain and human diet, it is forecast that there will be surplus cereals by 1980. It cannot yet be stated if this will reduce the demand for compound in feed, or if it will be used for reserves after subjection to some preservative technique yet to be perfected, or if it will be part feedstock for protein culture through fermentation, or if it will be required as raw material for organic chemical industries seeking a natural alternative to oil.

Amino-acid patterns, cereals in feed, FAO opinion

mg/g Nitrogen	Barley	Maize	Millets			Oats	Brown rice	Sorghum	Wheat
			Bullrush	Foxtail	Ragi				
Isoleucine	224	230	256	475	275	237	238	245	204
Leucine	417	783	598	1044	594	453	514	832	417
Lysine	216	167	214	138	181	239	237	126	174
Methionine	104	120	154	175	194	113	145	87	94
Cystine	142	97	148	—	163	167	67	94	159
Phenylalanine	321	305	301	419	325	309	322	306	282
Tyrosine	194	239	203	—	225	209	218	167	187
Threonine	207	225	241	194	263	210	244	189	183
Tryptophane	—	44	122	61	—	—	—	—	—
Valine	315	303	345	431	413	321	344	313	276
Biological value	—	59.4	—	—	—	64.9	72.7	73.2	64.7
Protein utilisation	60.0	51.1	—	—	—	65.7	70.2	55.8	90.9

Amino-acid patterns, various feed components, FAO opinion

mg/g Nitrogen	Dried grass meal	Lucerne (Alfalfa) meal	Brewer's yeast	Blood meal	Meat meal	Fish meal	Dried skim milk	Poultry waste meal	Feather meal	Whale meal
Isoleucine	583	267	365	70	179	269	442	283	327	285
Leucine	837	496	500	782	374	452	568	510	560	450
Lysine	447	263	565	568	328	484	442	256	107	231
Methionine	131	84	100	93	89	171	134	130	19	313
Cystine	80	108	130	63	49	77	41	275	317	77
Phenylalanine	550	255	303	467	213	241	308	287	313	216
Tyrosine	194	112	259	227	140	193	134	189	154	207
Threonine	792	315	346	227	193	265	258	264	313	71
Tryptophane	55	95	—	319	55	60	6	66	8	87
Valine	661	306	459	539	278	318	268	430	540	294
Biological value	—	57.5	65.6	—	24.0	81.1	79.7	—	—	81.1
Protein utilisation	—	—	55.6	—	—	65.3	72.1	—	—	65.3

Amino-acid patterns, pulses and cakes in feed, FAO opinion

mg/g Nitrogen	Butter (Lima) beans	Cow peas	Dried coco-nut	Cotton seed cake	Ground nut kernels	Linseed cake	Palm kernels	Sesame seed	Soya bean cake	Sun-flower seed cake
Isoleucine	310	239	244	196	211	271	240	226	302	267
Leucine	509	440	419	363	400	382	421	419	489	399
Lysine	465	427	220	259	221	237	246	171	380	231
Methionine	78	73	120	89	72	122	164	176	89	154
Cystine	63	68	76	93	78	120	123	113	104	110
Phenylalanine	379	323	283	320	311	299	256	277	313	304
Tyrosine	202	163	167	184	244	170	182	195	237	162
Threonine	261	225	212	205	163	239	222	223	267	228
Tryptophane	63				65		63			
Valine	322	283	339	271	261	339	377	288	327	322
Biological value	54.8	56.8	69.0	67.2	54.5	70.8	—	62.0	72.8	69.6
Protein utilisation	47.8	45.1	55.0	52.7	42.7	55.6	—	53.4	61.4	68.3

It is standard in the feed market to evaluate components according to their protein content and amino-acid pattern. The synthesis of amino acids, and their extraction from rich sources, has disturbed this simple form of evaluation and has placed more emphasis on price as a factor in selection. Sunflower cake, for example, lacks lysine but can accept synthetic lysine to become a major consideration in feed formulation—very important to developing countries since sunflowers are easy to grow and have high yields. In effect, since the development of manufacture of amino acids for addition, and particularly since it has been found possible to manipulate amino-acid patterns in vegetable tissue, the amino-acid pattern has become less important than the total proportion of available protein in a substance.

Conventional feed components, Protein Content

N × 6.25% approx.

Cereals			
Barley	9.0	Groundnut cake	
Barley feed	13.0	—decorticated	45.4
Brewers grains	18.3	—undecorticated	30.3
Wheat	12.2	Groundnut meal	49.7
Wheat feeds	15.9	Kapok seed cake	26.9
Maize	9.9	Linseed cake	31.9
Maize germ meal	13.0	Mustard seed cake	
Flaked maize	9.8	—unextracted	18.0
Maize gluten	24.8	—extracted meal	22.8
Oats	10.4	Niger seed cake	32.4
Brown rice	8.3	Palm kernel cake	19.2
White rice	6.7	Palm kernel extracted meal	20.4
Rice bran	12.4	Rape seed extracted meal	36.8
Rice meal	12.9	Rape seed cake	35.3
Sorghum	10.8	Sesame seed cake	44.7
Millet, finger	6.0	Sesame extracted meal	46.4
Millet, bullrush	11.0	Shea nut cake	12.1
Millet, foxtail	12.1	Soya bean cake	44.9
T'ef (Teff)	8.5	Soya extracted meal	44.8
Buckwheat	10.3	Sunflower seed cake	
Findi	7.7	—decorticated	37.2
Job's tears	14.0	—undecorticated	18.5
Rye	11.6	Sunflower seed extracted meal	38.1
		Pulses	
Oilseeds		Pigeon peas	20.9
Castor bean	29.2	Chick peas	20.1
Coconut cake	21.2	Horse gram	22.0
Cottonseed cake		Hyacinth beans	22.8
—decorticated	41.1	Lathyrus peas	25.0
—undecorticated	28.0	Lentils	24.2

Conventional feed components, protein content—continued

Lupine	44.3	Stewed bone meal	7.5
Yellow lupin	41.8	Whole meat meal	60.0
Butter beans	19.7	Poultry by-product meal	55.4
Mung beans	23.9	Dried hatchery waste	45.7
Kidney beans	22.1	Feather meal	87.4
Peas	22.5	Dried whole milk	25.5
Velvet beans	24.0	Dried skim milk	32.8
Broad beans	23.4	Dried whey	12.6
Cow peas	23.4	White fish meal	61.0
Bambara groundnut	17.7	Menhaden fish meal	62.1
		Dried fish solubles	71.3

Roots

Cassava	2.8	*Various*	
Cassava flour	1.6	Dried beet pulp	8.8
Potato meal	9.7	Beet molasses	8.4
Sweet potato	4.9	—dried	8.9
Yam	7.1	Cane molasses	3.0
		Carob bean pods	4.7
		Carob bean seeds	16.7
Animal derivatives		Locust beans	26.0
Blood	81.0	Dried grass	15.0
Pure meat meal	72.2	Dried alfalfa (lucerne)	21.1
Meat and bone meal	50.3	Data stones	6.0
—solvent extracted	49.9	Trewers yeast	44.9
Cooked bone meal	26.0	Borula yeast	46.4

Main types of feed for intensive rearing

Poultry
1. Chick starter feed. Used for the first 6–8 weeks after hatching.
2. Grower feed used up to 16–18 weeks.
3. Breeder feed used for birds older than 16–18 weeks kept for egg production.
4. Broiler feed used for birds intended for meat. Starter feed is used to 5 weeks, followed by finisher feed for another 5 weeks, after which the bird is slaughtered.

Poultry feed needs low fibre, high protein and high minerals. Normal mixtures are based on 75–80% cereal plus 5–10% meat or fish meal plus 5–10% oilcake or extract. Up to 5% fat may be added for broilers. The protein content requirement decreases as the bird becomes older. Common materials used are maize, barley, sorghum and soya meal.

Pigs
1. Starter feed for use up to 2–3 weeks old.
2. Creep feeds from 3 weeks to fully weaned at 8 weeks.
3. Feeds for lactating sows and weaners.
4. Growing feed for use until the pig is 50–60 kg live weight.
5. Bacon feed.
6. Final fattening feeds.
7. Feed for pregnant sows.

Main types of feed for intensive rearing—continued

Feed for mature pigs may be concentrates above a basic ration of starchy roots. Feed components are similar to those for poultry but more fibre can be used. A typical creep feed might be 83% cereal plus 15% fish meal or dried milk. A fattening feed might be 95% cereal plus 3% grass meal.

Cattle
1. Feed for calves before they have functioning rumens.
2. Feed for adult cattle.

Feed for young cattle is similar to other creep or starter feed, low in fibre but high in protein. Feed for adults is intended to augment normal high-roughage feed. A typical feed for dairy cattle might be 45% cereals, 40% cake, 5% grass, 5% carobs. Feed supplied as extra to green roughage can be with reduced protein, probably by removing the dried grass and oilcake. Part of the oilcake might be replaced by urea.

Sheep
Feeds resemble those for cattle, the main division being into feed for lambs before rumen and feed for adults.

FEED PRICES

The period from mid-1972 to mid-1973 has economic significance, not only with regard to the inflation of feed prices but also with regard to the speed at which such inflation arrived in a situation which should not have caused inflation. The actual increases in cost to meat producers could have meant no more than reduced income and an inflow of temporary capital as bridging loans instead of permanent capital as investment. The rates of increase, however, disrupted planning in almost all sectors of world agriculture, producing completely new attitudes. Notably, many agricultural producers sought buyers for their land, invested the proceeds at perhaps three times the profit of working the land. Those remaining in agriculture looked for alternatives to bought feed, such as grazing, or converted to arable farming from livestock.

World output of cereals was:

Million tons	Wheat	Rice	Maize	Barley	Total
1971	353.8	309.1	305.6	151.5	1315.7
1972	347.4	295.2	302.9	152.4	1276.6
1973	364.3	317.5	313.2	157.6	1344.4

In effect, there was a 3% drop in availabilities in 1972, followed by a 5% rise in 1973. In theory, the temporary shortfall should have been overcome by taking from stocks and by temporary diversion of some markets, followed by a 1973 dramatic reduction in prices, rebuilding of stocks and rescue of the markets which were temporarily lost in 1972. In fact, there was speculative buying of grain and unwarranted hysteria which took world prices over the threshold of acceptability. In other words, much of the change in agriculture was permanent, not temporary as it should have been.

Typical price rises between the summer of 1972 and that of 1973 were:

	% rise
Argentina durum wheat	98
Canada No. 1 wheat	150
USA No. 2 wheat	150
Canadian rye	140
Canadian oats	100
Argentine maize	100

During the same period, soya beans increased in price by 95%, groundnuts by 90% and copra by 160%. Groundnut cake increased in price by 218% in the panic but later reduced to only 100%.

The pattern of conversion of bought feed to animal protein is too complex for generalisation but it can be calculated that doubled prices for feed relate to a 25% rise in the selling price of the final meat. Unfortunately for meat producers, the increase in feed prices coincided with consumer rejection of high retail prices and it is realised that a reduction (in real terms) of the price of meat is essential if the market is to be related to anticipated increases in meat output. Whether such an increase of meat output is possible is not certain, output having increased only from 107 million tons in 1971 to 109.5 million tons in 1973 despite the efforts of governments and international agencies. Also, higher feed costs are only one of many disturbing factors, there being inflation of costs of labour, land and energy. There is justified opinion that meat production will become restricted to output for local consumption using only local feed.

Furthermore, any country with organic waste needs to convert such waste to some useful product. There are routes to methane from organic waste, which could provide a platform for development of organic chemicals as oil supplies diminish, and routes to microbial or algae protein for animal feed. In 1971, cultured protein feed was roughly equal in price to oilseed or fish meal protein feed. By the end of 1972, cultured protein feed could be estimated at about half the price of the conventional feeds. It is probable that Scandinavia will produce all feed requirements from papermill waste, and that the north Americas will also replace agricultural or fishery feeds by cultured protein.

In effect, traditional feeds face progressive replacement at a rate at which plant can be approved and erected for alternatives. It is therefore inevitable that producers of traditional animal feed will seek alternative markets, as in the refinement of soya and fish meal for human consumption. They can also be expected to increase selling prices to acceptable limits for short-term markets—prices which are far higher than selling prices which would be needed if the market had hopes of being maintained.

non-legumes with nitrogen-fixing bacteria, partly to allow catch-cropping of feed crops on poor land.

As might be expected, increases of yield per plant bring consequent increase of sensitivity to disease and general weakness. In 1970, the United States lost one-sixth of the maize crop by Southern Corn Blight. In the eighteenth century potatoes were introduced into Ireland with a very narrow range of varieties. They yielded well in the excellent soil and climate whilst they were isolated from their normal pests. However, in the 1830s spores of *Phytophthora infestans* reached Ireland and the crop failed, with the result that 2 million Irish died, 2 million emigrated and 4 million were reduced to poverty. There is a danger that a similar event, but on a larger scale, could arise from over-emphasis on one crop and variety for the sake of weight of output. A similar event concerns Sri Lanka (Ceylon) which was the leading coffee producer in 1870 with a narrow range of trees which proved ultra-sensitive to coffee rust. Coffee was wiped out within a few years and the United Kingdom became a tea-drinking nation. Coffee rust has now reached Brazil but is being contained, probably because there is variation in the trees. In this respect it should be noted that Malling Research Station devised a new cloning system for coconuts, which are 4% excellent protein when fresh. Coconuts cannot be reproduced by grafting or layering, but need seed and a life-span of twenty years. The new cloning produces earlier yield with some certainty of output. It also makes all the trees in a plantation alike and sickness of one tree means sickness of all.

Chapter 20

Monoculture

A natural ecostructure comprises a very large number of plants, animals, micro-organisms, and temporary conditions of humidity, temperature, sunlight, air composition, etc. According to the temporary conditions there is encouraged survival to a selective degree for each organism involved. Consequently, there is survival of the fittest, which can be loosely defined as those organisms with a very wide range of tolerance so that they survive however the conditions change. Obviously, a steady state is never reached because environmental conditions show erratic variation and because, apart from interaction of organisms to conditions, there is interaction between the organisms. Hence, if a set of conditions is repeated it will probably find a balance of organisms different from that before.

The underground population breaks the soil and processes waste. The overground population performs its complicated sex life and circulates chemicals. Each organism has its selected diet and waste product, and its incidental influence on all other organisms within reach. However, man has interfered by the introduction of organisms which did not generate in the prevailing conditions and by the modification of the conditions, including removal of organisms which have no obvious contribution to the welfare of man and may be too efficient in preventing surplus of any organisms which do contribute. Problems have arisen because man has only partly changed the populations and conditions. He has not entirely reorganised creation but has simply reduced visible inhibitions and promoted visible growth mechanics. If one organism is encouraged by protection within an ecostructure there is consequent increase in other organisms which are associated. Conversely, elimination of an organism removes also those other organisms which are associated or forces the other organisms to develop new habits of diet and reproduction. Such changes would occur without interference from man but the human manipulation is drastic and is likely to result in severe disruption. The outcome may be negative, as in the failure of an organism by disease or destruction of its medium from chemical exhaustion, or it may be positive, as in the over-reproduction of selected weeds or pests when enemies are removed. The introduction of delicate hybrids for the sake of high individual yield is a particular source of trouble, such hybrids needing synthetic feeding and pest control.

Red rust of wheat was known to Roman farmers, who even had a god Robigus for it. It can mutate to meet change conditions, as exampled by the fact that Cambia and Cama wheats in the United Kingdom were regarded as rust-free until a new strain of rust claimed 25–30% of the harvest in 1972. In 1916, the United States lost 2 million bushels and Canada lost 1 million bushels of wheat to rust, the blame being firmly placed on intensive cultivation of a single sensitive wheat. The wheat failure brought effort to increase maize output, bringing in a hybrid maize which could give 25% more yield, this being improved in 1931 to become the T (for Texas) strain. Texas maize was promoted through the 1960s and by 1970 almost all USA farmers were growing maize with identical cytoplasm. Thus when Southern Corn Blight arrived it took one-sixth of the harvest.

Over 90% of southern USA rice is of only five varieties and the entire Californian rice crop is of only three. Roughly three-quarters of the potatoes grown in the USA are of one strain, as are 90% of the sugar beet and two-thirds of the sweet potato. Likewise there is genetic uniformity in the soya, groundnuts, pulses and green vegetables. The agriculture of the United States is therefore by no means secure against failure and the weakness is self-generated in the urge to increase yield.

In this respect, the United Nations have introduced a programme under the title of 'Green Revolution', based on the introduction of high-yield crops with a narrow genetic base. This is a recognised danger, particularly to world rice which already has a significant proportion of highly-bred strain in the plantings. More than half the population of the world depends on rice and following the loss of several thousand acres in 1969 in the Philippines there are genuine fears of a fungal disease called blast. There is a similar concern in animal husbandry relative to emphasis on narrow genetic bands. The fowl pest in the United Kingdom in 1971 has been blamed on narrowed genetics and there is opinion that foot-and-mouth disease in cattle would be better dealt with by allowing immunity to develop. The slaughter policy is also considered to confine infections and thereby prevent the fringe infection which could encourage natural immunity.

Chapter 21

Infestation

Damage from micro-organic attack can be reduced in vegetation by dehydration to a level equivalent to 70% relative humidity. Infestation requires sophisticated control and is responsible for significant loss of protein food. The earliest record of infestation was a flour beetle in Egypt in 2500 B.C. and a later infestation in the tomb of Tutankhamen by biscuit weevil, hump-backed spider weevil and tobacco weevil.

During the early days of agriculture there was unintended distribution of insect pests but infestation was largely ignored until the North American prairies were developed and there was a dramatic increase in the movement of grain. Control methods applied to growing crops and stored products evolved and have become a sub-industry, although the individual methods are open to criticism and the destruction of insects is not widely accepted as sensible or ethical. Notably, a very large number of social–religious groups prefer not to kill anything animal, although the same groups do not hesitate to kill humans in warfare and private conflict.

Technical support for killing contained insects is based on the concept that it is impossible to grow vegetation under revised conditions without associated revision of controlling mechanics for the carried pests. Technical objections are:

1. That synthetic control of one unwelcome organism has influence on all associated organisms, including those which eat the controlled pest, leading to disruption of ecosystems far removed from the point of control.

2. Control methods introduce a foreign stage in the natural chemical processing through growth, consumption and waste discharge. There can be the production of unknown toxins in falsified growth and there can be passage of fumigant or other applied chemical into digestive systems.

It is not therefore probable that infestation-control will become universal in agriculture and storage. It is probable, however, that control will increase but not using the methods which are familiar at present. Currently, insects are destroyed by mechanical devices or by exposure to toxins, almost all of which are also toxic to man. The favoured mechanical device is one which throws the product plus contained insects against a solid face, reducing the insect to invisible dust and, it is light-heartedly claimed, adding extra protein to the product. (However, disintegrated insects are edible but their contribution to useful protein is slight.)

There is also a wide selection of toxins used for killing insects and the list is likely to grow as insects suffer trace exposure which leads to immune strains. There can never be absolute chemical control and there is fear that the toxins used will become increasingly more violent with consequent increase of damage to man and his beasts. Most workers now regard chemical control as a temporary activity until radiation techniques and biological techniques are perfected. Most hope now seems to be on the introduction of insects which have high sexual activity rates but no ability to produce offspring.

The practical history of infestation control probably dates from the 1930s when moths in Australian dried fruit not only did damage but distressed warehousemen when opened boxes released clouds of moths. A pyrethrum–oil mixture proved effective but widespread control was not accepted pending legislation and a responsible code of practice, particularly since two children had died in 1933 when their home was fumigated against bugs. Widespread control of infestation dates from the 1950s, or possibly even the 1960s when more was known about the life cycles and habits of insects.

INSECTS AND THEIR REPRODUCTION RATES

There are at least 750 000 species of insect with more variation of structure than in any other class of animal. A few, such as collembola, have passed through the ages unchanged in visible structure but insects are adaptable and many are modern specialisations, such as diptera. The largest is probably the 25-cm long stick-insect and the smallest is probably the parasitic mymaridae at less than a quarter of a millimetre. They have been larger, fossils reaching 70 cm, and they will no doubt prove to have been or to be smaller. The pest insects are mainly 1–12 mm in length and are, in general, related to specific crop groups. Their crime in storage is not the quantity of food they steal but the damage inflicted with consequent easy entry of micro-organisms which can produce toxins. As with rodents the problem is not direct consumption by the pest but the associated physical damage and deposition of contamination.

Detailed division of the class Insecta is according to the specialised development, notably the wing structure or absence thereof. A full account is not necessary but it needs to be pointed out that each insect has its own life history and construction, making it difficult to devise a common method of control. The full life-cycle from the egg to the adult laying her first egg, can be as short as a few weeks for a common house-fly or up to seventeen years for a cicada. There is some justification for evaluating insects as sources of protein for poultry feed as *Sitophilus oryzae* has been shown to increase its total mass, under ideal conditions, at least 700 times within a period of sixteen weeks.

Insects feeding on growing vegetation are mainly univoltine, or producing only one new generation per year. Insects feeding on stored products and agricultural waste are mainly multivoltine, or producing two or more generations per year. This is not a sharp division, as indicated by the fact that *Ephestia elutella*, a warehouse moth, is multivoltine in warm southern United Kingdom storage but is univoltine when moved to the cold inhospitable warehouses of northern United Kingdom or Scotland. Ephestia moths cannot thrive without linoleic acid in their diet and similar special diet requirements can be found with most insect forms. Several have included yeasts which provide vitamin B to the hosts, giving extra support to the theory that disintegrated insects in grain products add to the value.

Although a full account of the divisions of insects is not of value in the present context, it is worth mentioning the orders:

Hemiptera are bugs and their mouths are designed for piercing and sucking. Mostly, they suck plant fluids but a few well-known examples suck blood from animals.

Diptera are flies, also designed for piercing and sucking, with at least 60 000 species selecting victims amongst all organisms including man.

Hymenoptera covers ants, bees, wasps and a few other groups. The mouth is designed for biting, licking or sucking, with considerable variation in the 100 000 species. They may provide biological control of infestation by parasitic action and their painful but rarely toxic injections have potential in medicine.

Lepidoptera contains at least 100 000 species but only a few are regarded as pests in food. They are the moths and butterflies feeding on selected diet including living vegetation, micro-organisms and animal fibres.

Coleoptera are beetles and they may live outside or inside vegetable tissue, numbering at least 200 000 species. Some are carnivores and the range of diet is sufficiently wide to include dung.

Acarina are mites, small other than when blood-suckers distend by over-feeding. They have very rapid rates of reproduction and are broadly divided into plant-eaters and meat-eaters. They are responsible for most of the itching diseases in animals and for some sinus complaints.

Reproduction rates of insects have been studied since the 1798 essay on population by Malthus, in which he outlined a geometric progression leading to starvation by overpopulation in a limited stock of food. The essay was used to justify wars as population control and has since been a foundation for economic theories, many of which have since been proved wrong. Given an equal balance of sexes, house-flies laying 120 eggs seven times/year would produce nearly 6 million flies/mating pair/year. If the population of wireworm in soils is higher than half a million/acre the potential reproduction makes it not sensible to plant wheat on the soil. Such types of calculation have a direct influence on food production and storage.

Studies of reproduction rates have also indicated that there could be more protein from the deliberate encouragement of infestation to the degree whereby the stored food was raw material for insect production. Notably, there is potential in caterpillar production, possibly with growth control so that no adults are produced beyond those needed for new eggs. On average, about 10% of eggs can be expected to be infertile and there are recognised micro-organic attacks on caterpillars which could remove 90% of hatched eggs. Broadly, with obvious wide variations, an initial stock of 1 million eggs subjected to the normal deterioration including bacterial attack would produce 3 million eggs as the next generation, or 30 million eggs if there is protection against bacteria. For some examples, such as the house-fly, the per-generation increase could be higher and the final total could be towards a 6 million times increase of feedstock weight. The breeding of eggs and grubs has so far been only for pet fish and fishermen but there is remarkable potential for schemes associated with fish-farming, poultry and pigs.

METHODS OF CONTROL

As mentioned, the crime of insects is not their theft of food but the associated damage which opens the food to microbial development. With this is associated damage by exothermic heat, damaged grain showing an increase of internal temperatures to the point of self-combustion but, before that, showing thermal displacement of moisture so that some regions of a bulk quickly develop microbial growth whilst other regions show dehydration with consequent damage to the tissues. Direct losses from eaten food relative to levels of infestation have been calculated but should be distrusted. One caterpillar of ephestia moth is thought to damage by consumption at least forty-five wheat embryos or about 4 g of tobacco leaf. The question could be asked if it is always sensible to protect a product with a few percent of second-class protein against the misfortune of insect attack, or to encourage insect growth with its generation of first-class protein to perhaps 25% of a harvest of grubs.

Chemical control dates mainly from the early 1940s when warfare reached Africa and Asia and there was a need for an insecticide to combat carriers of deadly diseases. DDT was produced and was thought to be the answer to all infestation problems. In fact, extensive use of DDT screened out the insensitive insects and removed the sensitive insects which had been their natural competitors. Consequently, the final result of DDT was replacement of a sensitive insect population by an insensitive population.

Common toxins used fall into the conventional classes of those eaten by the insect and those effective on contact by passing through the cuticle into the insect body. A more practical classification used is into fumigants, sprays and dusts. The chemical classification is according to the toxin used and this classification is safer for substances which can kill operators. The only recognised safe insecticide is pyrethrum, known since the middle of the last century and widely used under the name of Keatings powder. Other common materials are:

Organic phosphorus compounds—as represented by Malathion
Organic halogen compounds—of which can be listed:
    Dieldrin

DDT

BHC

Carbon tetrachloride

Ethylene dibromide

Ethylene dichloride

Methyl bromide

Sulphur derivatives—as represented by Carbon disulphide

To this can be added a few inorganic chemicals such as cyanides and phosphides. Arsenic derivatives have been used but residues on fruit produced sickness and it was not uncommon for arsenical insecticides to be used with criminal intent. The sulphur derivatives have historic interest and were mentioned by Homer, Eurycleia providing sulphur with which Odysseus fumigated the bedroom. More recently, hydrocyanic acid gas was used on wood and then on ships to prevent bubonic plague, to be joined in due course by methyl bromide as an alternative general fumigant. Solid insecticides are likely to be carried through to the point of consumption. Liquids and gas fumigants are absorbed by protein fractions in food, particularly if designed to penetrate the tough outer protein layer of insects and bromine carried through into diet is an accepted problem.

Physical control is by heat or refrigeration or mechanical destruction. It is common to destroy insects and eggs in flours by driving on to a revolving plate, but airtight storage is now recognised as efficient, as it was in ancient Egyptian grain pits. Modern use dates from the 1940s when Argentine lost markets in war-stricken Europe and had to store in airtight silos. Very recently, there has also been interest in radiation techniques, by gamma rays or accelerated electrons.

Biological control is by the use of predators and parasites. Most important are other insects—mostly beetles, flies and wasps, although microbial infections are gaining importance. There is also biological control by the introduction of sterile members into populations, and by the use of hormones, although the use of hormones is far from proven as safe for the eventual consumers of stored food.

As far as protein is concerned, a simple statement would be that control of infestation would vastly improve supplies, and would improve quality because insects in general appear to prefer a protein diet to that based on carbohydrate and fat.

Chapter 22

Green Leaf Protein

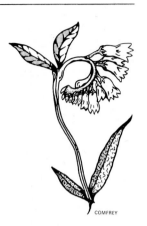

COMFREY

PLANT DEVELOPMENT

Two thousand million years ago there were organisms in the watery
primeval soup—algae—which had the accidental ability to employ solar
radiation in their chemistry. The near relatives were fungi, which lacked
the magic green pigment and had to use alternative body chemistry to
regenerate. The partnership between algae and fungi was established
and can still be recognised in lichens, in which algae absorb sun energy
and fungi provide mechanical protection and minerals.

Four hundred and twenty million years ago the first land plants left
their traces. Within the next 30 million years, which is very short in this
time scale, land plants became established almost everywhere they could
find water and heat. They were vascular plants, reproducing by spores
and thriving to become vast thick forests which are now our coal. From
this confused jungle came plants which bore seeds, as still represented
by conifers.

After another 150 million years there were plants which had flowers,
and insects arrived to carry out the functions of pollination and control
of micro-organic growth by direct consumption. It was inevitable that a
very large number of plant species should evolve and we now have
probably half a million species known if not fully listed. In fact, a full
library of plant species would be impossible although there are fairly
accurate lists of the 300 families. The long history of development can
be listed as:

Million years ago	Development	Group title	Resultant plant classes
2000 plus	Organised living things	Archaic bacteria	Chemobacteria Photobacteria Other bacteria
About 2000	Oxygen producing plants	Uralgae	Blue–green algae Red algae
600	Organised chloroplasts	Chlorophyta	Green algae Dinoflagellates Euglenoids Fungi and yeasts Brown and golden algae
420	Stems on plants	Psilophyta	Mosses Liverworts Psilophytes Club mosses Horsetails
390	True leaves	Filicophyta	Ferns
345	True seeds	Gymnospermae	Conifers
135	Flowers	Angiospermae	Dicots Monocots

The dating of the various classes can be disputed but the history shows how plants became increasingly more complicated to result in the highly-organised flowering, seeding, leafy plants. The organisation is pre-determined in the chemical structure of young cells, which resemble animal cells, but will change as they become adult. The young cell has the potential to perform many chemical tasks in due course but at this early stage is richly furnished with the enzymes and other proteins which will be needed for the tasks. As the cell divides and becomes specialised it takes up water and chemicals to form sap. Animal cells grow only by division and are therefore always protein-rich. Plant cells grow also by taking in water and chemicals, diluting the protein content to the point where it can become insignificant in terms of commercial or diet protein value. In due course, the thin flexible skin of the cell becomes hard and thick, producing wood and fibre. Hence, although the protein content of green plants may be relatively small away from the germ or growing tip, it has value by its composition and mixture. The cell includes:

Nucleus—in which DNA carries the genetic code and passes it to RNA so that the cell functions are correctly dictated.

Mitochondria—proteinic substances which oxidise food and convert energy into ATP (adenosine triphosphate), the agent in enzyme synthesis.

Chloroplasts—green bodies found particularly in green leaf, which absorb sunlight and convert carbon dioxide into sugar. There are also yellow-to-red versions containing carotene.

Golgi—complexes of protein and fat with contained enzymes, mainly storage of energy.

Reticulum—a platelet structure providing communication within the endoplasm.

Ribosomes—protein with RNA, producing more protein according to instructions imprinted by DNA on the RNA.

Starch grains—increasing in proportion as the cell matures, hence found more in stems, tubers and fruits.

This list is indicative only. The cell contains thousands of substances and is constantly engaged in the manufacture of new substances. The basic reaction is the production of sugar and it has been calculated that the plants of the world produce an annual weight of 150 000 million tons. The sugar is the energy source for the many metabolic reactions, each one regulated by an enzyme which is a protein. In effect, if the cells are caught young, green leaf can provide a valuable selection of proteins, with sugar and with water according to the age of the cells, and with representative samples of most organic substances required in body chemistry. They may also contain substances which are not desirable in human body chemistry, including many toxins which are likely to be proteins.

CULTIVATED CROPS

Cultivated green leaf crops for direct human consumption are mainly mustards bred from a single wild mustard ancestor. The mustard family has proved easy to modify by selection and is now represented by a full range of members from red cabbage to radishes and turnips. The difference is that red cabbage is 90% water and 1.7% protein in the leaf as eaten, whilst the turnip is 95% water and only 0.8% protein in the root as eaten. On the other hand, the soft cells of cabbage green leaf offer no shelf-life whereas the tough cells of turnip give the tissue a long storage life.

Green cabbage is said to have been enjoyed during the Bronze Age. With more certainty, it is known that the Romans ate many members of the mustard family. Red members came during the fourteenth or

fifteenth centuries, followed by cauliflower and broccoli, and subsequently by sprouts. The family has proved so flexible that there has
been no serious effort to find other green leaf vegetables for table use.
As should be expected, the protein content varies according to the stage
of development of the part of the plant which is eaten. Roughly:

	Protein content (%)
Sprouts	3.6
Red cabbage	1.7
Green cabbage	2.2
Cauliflower	3.4
Mustard and cress	1.6
Watercress	2.9

The root crops, which are members of the same family grown for old
tissue which will store, show values of 0.8–1.2% protein.

Obviously, there is no need to confine interest in green leaf to the
mustard family. All vegetable cells, whether they are to become stem,
leaf, flower or fruit, pass through a young stage when they are protein-
rich and not yet bloated by water absorption. There have been estimates
of the dry protein which could be obtained by crushing the liquid from
jungle or thick scrub. The top estimate is 4 tons dry protein from one
acre but 0.5 tons could be a more practical extraction. Protein from
jungle juice is of interest only where the vegetation is already scheduled
for clearance, as for example in the cutting of the Amazon highway.
The juice is far too rich in enzymes for it to have a reasonable shelf-
life, and the high water content makes it uneconomic to dehydrate or to
transport after heat treatment or other wet processing. Also, even within
a vast entity such as the Amazon basin, there are local variations in
vegetation which could lead to occasional sickness or poisoning if the
juice were to be extracted. As far as jungle and scrub are concerned,
when it is being cleared, there is advantage in providing some animal
consumer, which can as a rule use instinctive selection in its consumption, and in waiting for the animal to mature into excellent protein.

Crops which are now grown for non-food applications should be fully
examined for their protein potential. Notably, this concerns natural
fibres, for which crops are grown to maturity for the sake of the long
old cells. Cellulose contents of such fibres after retting are from about
64% for abaca types to over 90% for ramie types. On the other hand,

if arrested at a lower condition of development, fibre plants can be a most useful green leaf protein source, growing as an established crop in famine areas and in areas where there is deficiency from eating only rice.

Cotton plants. Protein availability (%) (based on USA statistics)

(Yield is 850 lb total plant/acre)

Part of plant	Water	Minerals	Protein	Fibre	Fat (oil)	lb weight in total crop
Entire plant	10.0	12.0	17.6	22.0	4.2	850
Roots	10.0	7.2	9.9	48.6	2.8	83
Stems	10.0	9.6	20.5	49.4	3.5	219
Leaves	10.0	12.9	21.6	12.6	6.1	192
Bolls	10.0	4.9	15.9	19.7	4.1	135
Seed	9.9	4.7	19.4	22.6	19.5	218
Lint	6.7	1.7	1.5	83.7	0.6	?

Approximate protein availability from one acre of cotton

	lb approx. dry protein
From:	
Entire plant (total)	150
Roots	8.25
Stems	44
Leaves	41.5
Bolls	21.5
Seed	42.5

The amino-acid pattern of the protein derived from green leaf is subjected to too many variables for accurate definition but some idea can be gained from the following:

	Sprouts	Cabbage	Cauli-flower	Spinach	Turnip tops	Meat for comparison
	g Amino acid/g nitrogen					
Arginine	0.39	0.47	0.26	0.28	0.38	0.41
Cystine	—	0.10	—	—	0.09	0.08
Histidine	0.14	0.11	0.12	0.09	0.12	0.20
Isoleucine	0.26	0.18	0.27	0.25	0.20	0.32
Leucine	0.27	0.26	0.39	0.40	0.39	0.49
Lysine	0.27	0.23	0.34	0.32	0.22	0.51
Methionine	0.06	0.06	0.13	0.11	0.15	0.15

	Sprouts	Cabbage	Cauli-flower	Spinach	Turnip tops	Meat for comparison
			g Amino acid/g nitrogen			
Phenylalanine	0.21	0.16	0.21	0.28	0.31	0.26
Threonine	0.21	0.17	0.26	0.25	0.26	0.28
Tryptophane	0.06	0.05	0.08	0.11	0.09	0.21
Valine	0.27	0.21	0.36	0.32	0.32	0.33

Compared against meat there are obvious deficiencies in green leaf for human diet. For animal feed the advantage is the high total nitrogen content which can be used by ruminants. Most of the examples have about 0.5% nitrogen and also carry a useful collection of minerals and vitamins.

GRASSES

Grasses are a special green leaf which is in effect grown as a crop by seeding pasture for grazing. Pasture is more of a mixture of plants than is realised and its protein potential is a variable which can be controlled within limits by patterns of seeding, history of cultivation and time of grazing or cropping. It is possible to store grass in a reasonably-advanced stage of growth using airtight containers fitted with a one-way air-lock, as for instance in plastics bags with a simple knot at the mouth, the folds of the knot filling with condensation water and becoming an air-lock. In general, however, open grassland is for seasonal grazing when the growth is young, although economic studies have shown it possible to feed livestock by rotation over successive plantings of mixed grass and other greenery under glass or clear plastics, the animal waste providing the food for suitable fertiliser-sensitive greenery.

Grasses are selected according to growth in the climate. One-quarter of the earth's surface is too dry or ice-bound to support grass, one-quarter is capable of supporting only harsh grass which has little feed value other than to thin populations of animals with tough digestions and the remaining half of the earth's surface will support grasses but forest claims priority under natural conditions. Without interference from man, soft grasses would grow only where they would find light through the trees and harsh grasses only would thrive at altitudes above the timber line. This line is about 4000 m high in the tropics, graduating down to zero towards the poles where only lichens can survive the cold and provide food for local animals. In addition to the effect of the timber line, grass suffers other influences in its distribution. The Prairies, Pampas and Steppes have dry winds which discourage trees, and have 70–100 cm of rain per year which encourages grass, which in turn furnishes the surface with a thick layer of vegetable matter capable of retaining an optimum moisture balance in the soil. Deep ploughing or excessive drainage can damage the water balance to produce a dust bowl and at higher water contents in wetter climates grasses give way to mosses and ferns.

There are some 10 000 species of grasses recorded and available for examination as encouraged pasture. One interesting grass is Turtle Grass which grows wild in Central America and the Caribbean. Its relative Canadian Pondweed is grown for fish food and both members of the family can show 13% protein, which is more than in cereal grain. Plots in Florida have been harvested twice per year using a special mower cutting 1 m deep. There could be 4 million acres of Turtle Grass within easy reach and feeding trials have already shown it superior to alfalfa for feeding sheep. Whether cuttings will take in cold water is yet to be discovered but they can be transplanted after rooting into heated effluent water from industry.

Grasses tend to have relatively short seasons in which they are excellent diet with comparatively little cellulose, a substance which is digested only by micro-organisms and then only at a lethargic rate. Other green leaf crops can offer a longer season and a lower cellulose-content, and possibly a higher protein yield per area.

COMFREY

Comfrey is an interesting potential source. It is a common plant in many climates, bearing large leaves which are barely stalked but run down the stem as wings. In Nakuru in Kenya it grew to 124 tons/acre, being cut monthly and thereby suited to continuous cattle feeding. Unfortunately for Kenya, comfrey is sensitive to pyrethrum eelworm and might carry the eelworm into pyrethrum, which is an important crop for Kenya. The largest comfrey plantation is in Rhodesia at 25 acres with a yield of 80 tons/acre for feeding bullocks. A similar yield is found in Zambia for feeding chickens. Comfrey is seen as a potential replacement for fish meal in South America as more fish meal is used to enrich bread, and as a replacement for oilseeds in Africa when oilseeds are improved to become diet for humans, since 100 tons of comfrey supply 3.5 tons of dry protein which is three times the yield of oilseeds on an area basis. There is a claim that comfrey is individual in its tryptophane content of 0.64%, much more than in other vegetables and twice the content of cheese. Conversely, comfrey lacks methionine (0.58% against 0.66% for cheese) and isoleucine (1.15% against 1.28% for cheese or beans). However, the amino-acid balance is probably less important than the fact that comfrey is the only known land plant to take up vitamin B12 from soil, the only other plant doing this being porphyra seaweed as used for laver bread in Wales and dulse in Scotland. Earthworms produce vitamin B12 for comfrey to take up and pass on in feed.

In northern Europe comfrey could give six cuts per year to a yield of 60 tons/acre. It has use as feed for racehorses because the fibre content is low, the ratio of protein to fibre in comfrey being about 3.4, whereas that of most green leaf is from 1.5–2.5, although green maize and lucerne can show a ratio of from 5 : 7 if cut at the correct stage. In Japan there are about 28 000 recorded growers of comfrey for poultry feed although comfrey is rich in carotene and produces a yellow colour in poultry meat. It also reduces the soft fat in geese, which could have commercial significance. One use for comfrey is in composting, the rich supply of nitrogen and potash being liberated very quickly to start microbiological activity.

Part 4

Microbial Proteins

Chapter 23

Algae

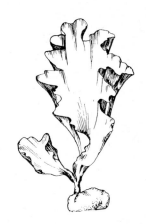

There is reason to suppose that the chloroplasts in green leaf originated as organisms trapped in the coordination of specialist groups into higher organisms. True or not, both are capable of using solar energy directly for chemical manufacture. Red and blue–green algae were the first oxygen-producing plants, following bacteria and preceding fungi and yeasts. Brown and golden algae followed some thousand million years later and were consequently better organised. As indication of the size of the problem of selection, known numbers of species are:

Blue–green—1500
Red—3500
Brown—15 000
Golden—11 000

There is hope that algae will provide low-cost protein from the considerable area of otherwise useless brackish water and from seawater which cannot support fish. Butan Gas Corporation have farms planned for Italy in the salt marshes on the west coast, possibly with the association of fish farming. Other areas of interest are around Sicily and Sardinia, where salt was extracted before other sources of salt became commercial, the area being about 100 000 hectares reasonably free from industrial pollution. The Italian venture will be by introduction but there are existing sources already rich in algae. Sosa Texcoco S.A. in Mexico has started harvesting spirulina growing wild in Lake Texcoco. The algae is supplied to food-processing industries for addition to 10% in chocolate flavoured biscuits and to 30% in other foods, notably in jams and soups and to a concentration according to how much change of flavour will be tolerated. There is related interest in wild algae from Lake Chad in Africa.

There are also various attempts to cultivate algae by industrial methods. The Japanese method has used flat trays with artificial sunlight and the West German trials used basins whilst the Czechoslovakians used sloping troughs. As a rule, industrial methods have produced at a rate of about 10 g dry algae protein/square metre/day but present output figures are not significant. Most of the industrial interest is in scenedesmus and chlorella but it is yet early to forecast which species will be involved.

Scenedesmus has an attractive composition of:

Protein 50–60%
Fatty acids 12–14%
Carbohydrates 10–17%

The remainder of scenedesmus is 3–10% fibre and 4–8% water, both low in comparison to other foods. The low carbohydrate is attractive since it indicates suitability for mixing with low-cost starches such as cassava flour. If the water is clean there is no difficulty in producing clean and pure algae which can be used directly for human diet, the basic requirements being clean water, carbon dioxide which may need forcing into the water, a few minerals, nitrogen, and a system of maximum exposure to ultraviolet light. The algae which appear to have raised most interest are:

Scenedesmus	Spirulina
Chlorella	Nostocales
Chlamydomonas	Anabaena
Coelestrum	Chrysophyta

There have been earlier efforts to farm algae for the fat content before the present surplus of butter and of oilseed oil became evident. These efforts failed for no stated reason but it is suspected that there were problems of dealing with the harvest. However, there are now developments of ultrafiltration and reverse osmosis which should simplify post-harvest handling. One advantage of the spirulina being pulled out of Mexican lakes is its large size, which allows simple filtration and washing and the French Petroleum Institute developed a process for mass-culture of spirulina, reaching 15–18 g/square metre/

day at 65% dry protein content, with equipment designed for 1 ton/day output. The Institute of Chemical Engineering Technology of West Berlin appear to have concentrated on scenedesmus and there is also evidence that nostocales and anabaena can thrive with air as the only source of nitrogen and this may lead to joint production of algae and rice.

Although the selection of species is yet confused, the production conditions are understood. Photosynthesis curves have been drawn and it is not difficult to provide optimum light intensity of the desirable spectrum. The problem is self-shading as the population increases, which is the natural method of controlling growth. Therefore industrial methods need some system of continuous movement to allow the maximum exposure of each organism, since tests have shown that scenedesmus grow twenty times faster in provided optimum light than in natural conditions. Temperature–growth rates are also well known, as are the optimum growth temperatures for common species. This optimum temperature varies according to the intensity of the light, as might be expected from an organism taking energy from both radiation and local heat. So far, emphasis has been on higher-temperature algae because the activity is exothermic and it is considered easier to control temperatures by cooling than by heating. Experience in Bangkok has indicated that overheating is not likely to be a problem in tropical countries, where 30–40 °C is a useful operating range.

The optimum acidity (pH value) for maximum clean growth could be important, according to whether the algae production is to be related to industrial acid waste or agricultural alkali waste, or whether any natural water concerned is acid or alkali. The forced feeding of carbon dioxide into the wet mix changes the pH value, making it important to relate the gas flow to required acidity. Spirulina appear to thrive at pH 9.5 and it is probable that strains can be found to thrive at pH 10.5. Since most industrial sources of fixed nitrogen will be ammonia, urea or amino effluent, an alkaline medium is easy to provide. Since, however, the forced feeding of carbon dioxide will produce acidity any provided alkalinity will be destroyed, but one answer appears to be bicarbonate, which may be satisfactory for chlorella but probably not for many species.

There is no technical difficulty in providing a suitable mixture of carbon and nitrogen for growth in clean water. The simplest mixture would be carbon dioxide plus ammonia plus a few trace minerals. Commercial production, however, is not likely to use clean water since all the clean water will be needed for human consumption. Therefore feedstocks will probably be industrial effluent or sewage, both of which will be supplied with varied and variable composition, uncertain acidity and temperature, and probably containing substances which interfere with algae growth. For the time being it seems advisable to concentrate on natural contamination of water, notably sewage, with a subsequent rearing of fish for sport or meal.

The finer details of equipment for industrial production of algae mass are determined by the medium and the organism. Japanese experience has been with shallow trays using carbon dioxide blown through the fluid. Other workers have used shallow ponds with mechanical stirrers or deeper ponds with circulation pumps. Czechoslovakian workers have used a weir system with the mass flowing over 2-cm steps before being returned back to the higher level to flow again. There is also some discussion of air-bed techniques but opinion is that some system of slow flow of a film will prove to be the most economic.

Reported yields are not indicative of possibilities. Dortmund reported 28 g/square metre/day, Bangkok claimed 35 g and Bulgaria is said to have reached 45 g. It is possible that commercial yields with fine selection of the species will reach 70–170 tons/hectare using sewage. The commercial indication is that cultured algae will be fed directly to fish farms as a slurry but it is practical to produce a dry powder with the composition of about 60% protein and 10% carbohydrate. At 1973 prices, this should give it a price advantage of at least 25% over fish meal and soya. There are few risks of toxicity other than any introduced from the feedstock but it may be essential to sterilise sewage before use.

Japan has at least ten commercial plants processing chlorella into tablets or extracts for the health market. Output is of the order of 500 tons/year and sales depend on CGF, which is promotional identification of Chlorella Growth Factor. With regard to CGF, similar health improvement can come from yeasts and both protein concentrates are probably satisfying some unidentified deficiency. However, the ultimate motivation for algae cultivation may not be the shortage of protein in the world. Algae are efficient as cleaners of water and in the direct absorption of solar energy. With a dire need for clean water and an energy crisis the use of a biological method of dealing with sewage has obvious attraction.

Chapter 24

Fungi

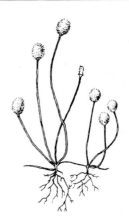

Algae and fungi are the intermediates in the plant evolution scale. roughly 1000 million years after bacteria and 1000 million years before the sophisticated stemmed, flowering and fruiting vegetation. It is common to describe fungi as algae without chlorophyll but this is misleading. Algae are reasonably inactive in the chemical sense, relying mainly on sunshine and warm wet conducive climates for growth, and are not destructive or invasive. Fungi are active parasites relying on destruction for their food and thriving in all descriptions of environment from arctic wastes to the inner depths of animal flesh. The essential fungal structure is a bed of hair-like threads which may, for no obvious reason, fuse to form a mushroom or toadstool by which device the fungus scatters its spores. The hair-like threads find and penetrate cracks and pinholes, gaining entry into tissues which are then consumed from within. Most of the familiar plant diseases—rust, wilt, blight, etc.—arise from invasions by fungi, as do many animal complaints, but since it is not uncommon for fungi to have two or more hosts, it is impossible to effect control until all hosts are identified. Thus, rust on wheat needs the eradication of local barberry before it can be reduced. A significant fraction of the world problem of pollution is due to attempted chemical control of fungi in agriculture, as the ultimate analysis may show more damage from the control measures than from the offending fungi.

In their defence, fungi with bacteria are responsible for the conversion of natural litter into rich moist humus. Their body protein is the first stage in many consumption chains. Perhaps more important to the present context, fungi manufacture a very wide range of chemicals which are of value and may be essential to our survival. Penicillin is a classic example from the antibiotic list but one needs to consider also the list of vitamins, organic acids and trace amino acids which are suspected but not confirmed. Progressive opinion now appreciates that fungi, yeasts and algae can probably provide trace chemicals which are essential to bodily welfare but are excluded from modern diet by over-selection of high-yielding crops and subsequent processing mainly for display values and convenience.

Unwelcome fungi are frequently known as moulds or slimes according to whether they are dry or wet. Slimes are running masses of protoplasm without cell walls, a seemingly unfortunate accident in evolution which provides copy for science fiction, particularly since it feeds by slowly engulfing its victims and will spread anywhere it can find food, water and freedom from enemies. Most of available information on fungi is negative, relating to the control of growth to minimal rates, but there is some positive information arising from the culture of fungi for anti-biotics. Arising from this, the human market would probably accept health foods derived from fungi but it is not probable that they would accept common protein food known to originate in fungi, mould or slime. This doubt amongst human consumers about fungal protein is inevitable after a long public association of fungus with disease. For example, *Phytophthora infestans* was responsible for the Irish potato famine and was identified too late to prevent disruption of the country, and *Claviceps purpurea* was, as ergot on rye, responsible for group madness and prophetic vision during the formative years of Europe. As a general rule, protein from fungi lacks methionine and there could be a problem of excess nucleic acid. Otherwise, fungi are first-class proteins with the advantage that they can be produced rapidly from any organic waste. There is also indicated value in a mixture of fungal protein and fish meal, which has sufficient extra methionine to overcome the deficiency in the fungal protein.

The ability of fungi to break down cellulose is of special interest. The most common natural waste product is cellulose in its various conditions including timber-trimmings, papermill waste and straw from cereal crops. If these major raw materials can be partly digested, or even made weak by chemical attack, it is easy to grow yeasts and productive bacteria on the broken product. Fungi are considered to be the ideal agents for converting useless cellulose waste into a form in which it is sensitive to further micro-organic attack, the microbes from both stages

being harvested as protein. The Swedish Forest Products Research
Laboratory has broken down cellulose insolubles using fungi, as have
Aston University and Tate and Lyle. There has been considerable
development of fungi grown on sugars, taking off the filaments as a
scum for washing and drying and feeding to animals. The scum can also
be used without washing and drying for early addition into compound
or swill. There are hopes of the development of a farm-size protein-
generating unit taking straw, hedge-trimmings and the like for conversion into protein-rich swill for direct feeding, probably using two
stages involving fungi and then yeast.

There are some 40 000 species of fungi available for selection, each
of which has its main area of parasitic activity but is likely to be active
outside its main area. Inevitably, man has employed fungi as parasites.
Spotted Alfalfa Aphid is controlled by deliberate infection and there is
similar biological control of other insects. One interesting employment of
fungi as parasites is in the control of nematodes, parasitic worms which
do great damage to vegetation. A selected fungus can seek the nematodes,
apply a few retaining strands and then consume the meat. However,
fungi include not only parasites which destroy living tissue to rebuild
for personal requirements but also those species which break down dead
tissue for rebuilding and those which can feed on basic chemicals as raw
materials. The frontiers between fungi, bacteria and algae are vague but
fungi have, in general, a much wider range of sources. It is inevitable
that developments have used previous experience of the fungi used to
manufacture medicants and other chemicals such as citric acid, and it is
also inevitable that conceptions of industrial mass production have
examined known industrial substances, but it is probable that the
ultimate pattern of production will use species and raw materials other
than those evaluated at present, notably in combined operations involving
other micro-organisms and revised farming methods leading to animal
and fish protein. Present indication is that emphasis should be laid on
the initial breakdown of cellulose, using fungi which are observed in
natural decay mechanisms, amongst which are:

	Optimum pH value	Optimum temperature °C
Aspergillus flavipes	6.5	28
Aspergillus fumigatus	5.6	45
Curvularia lunata	7.0	31
Gliomastix convoluta	9.0	28

	Optimum pH value	Optimum temperature °C
Humicola grisea	7.7	45
Myrothecium verrucaria	6.0	31
Penicillium chrysogenum	4.2	25
Sporotrichum carnis	4.5	25

This list is only indicative of the optimum conditions to be expected. It is possible that emphasis will be on the higher-temperature species, using exothermic heat from any associated growth of yeasts or bacteria. The potential destructive activity is important and it is worth noting that on pure cellulose myrothecium has a rapid rate of destruction, probably twice as fast as penicillium and three times as fast as aspergillus. On the other hand, aspergillus is familiar from studies of its growth on crops and penicillium is familiar as a common mould with potential in antibiotics, therefore it could be some time before the final pattern of species and raw materials is presented to engineers for suitable plant design.

Meanwhile, it is important to remember that large selected fungi are enjoyed as diet, although modern man has lost the ability to recognise edible versions and has grown to rely on cultivated mushrooms grown for maximum weight. Almost all the cultivated mushrooms are *Agaricus campestris* because this is evidently the most reliable in cultivation. Other mushrooms either do not appear when required or appear in profusion out of season and in bad condition. The near relative is *Psalliota campestris* or common field mushroom, which many prefer for its flavour despite its lack of flesh. Other large fungi of interest include:

Blewits—*Tricholoma personatum*—bearing a yellow cap on a lilac stem, delightful to eat but may be confused with purple agaric.
Chantarelle—*Cantharellus cibarius*—funnel-shaped and delicate apricot in colour, much esteemed by ancients for its flavour.
Common morel—*Morchella esculenta*—with a honeycomb pattern in rich brown on the cap, there being a cavity in the cap and stalk. It is edible but uninteresting in flavour.
Edible boletus—*Boletus edulis*—brown and characterised by millions of pinholes where the gills should be. It is non-poisonous but not a delicacy.
Fairy ring—*Marasimus oreades*—found as rings reputed to be meeting-

places of little people. Pale buff colour and a delicacy of construction. The flesh will dry and reconstitute. Non-poisonous but not exciting in flavour.

Puffball—*Calvatia gigantea*—said to have been given its name by Puck and is reputed to have some affinity with fairies. A large cream-and-brown ball which is edible but tasteless whilst young, becoming unpalatable as the spores develop.

Horn of plenty—*Craterellus cornucopioides*—funnel-shaped and dirty blue with long lines down the stalk. Non-poisonous but not enjoyable.

Shaggy cap—*Coprinus comatus*—with a white-and-yellow cap which could be mistaken for feathers in a bad light. On decaying, it dissolves into a useless black fluid. Non-poisonous but difficult to catch in a condition fit for eating.

Sheathed agaric—*Amanitopsis fulva*—Orange cap with a slight dome and a thin stalk coming out of a cup. Non-poisonous but uninteresting in flavour.

Warty cap—*Amanita rubescens*—with a rusty brown scaled cap and a bulbous base to the stalk. Non-poisonous but not particularly attractive to eat.

These are field mushrooms, or representatives thereof, which thrive on dead field vegetation and can rarely be cultivated. There are also large fungi growing underground and a wide range of tree fungi, many of which are superb in flavour. There could be justification for the development of cultivated tree fungi using granulated wood waste. Volvariella, which is a south-east Asian equivalent to the common European Agaricus mushroom, is reasonably specific to rice straw for its diet but has been grown on mixed rice straw and sawdust. Strangely, the development has been to find a profitable outlet for sawdust, which is a problem material in waste disposal.

Domesticated large fungi are up to 92% water, about 2.5% unavailable carbohydrate, no available carbohydrate or fat, but up to 0.65% total nitrogen. Two-thirds of this nitrogen is as urea and, using a multiplication factor of 6.25, this means a protein content of about 1.8%. The phosphorus content is high and, it should be noted, the phytic acid proportion of the phosphorus is nil, making mushrooms a useful food in mixtures. The riboflavine and nicotinic acid levels are also high.

Chapter 25

Yeasts

Yeasts are described as simple fungi with a limited range of activity or as an offshoot of bacteria which reached ultimate development on a simple diet of carbon, hydrogen and oxygen. The romantic version is that algae took their chlorophyll and photosynthesis into plants and became part of the structure as chloroplasts, whilst yeasts took their ability to find energy in sugars into plants at mitochondria, which oxidise food and produce adenosine triphosphate as an intermediate in carbohydrate manipulation. In less-romantic commercial terms, yeasts are attractive for microbial protein because they are already established as health foods and should in theory bring no problems when they are ultimately supplied as bulk protein foods. Consumer acceptance is a powerful force in planning and capital investment.

Fermentation by yeasts has been familiar since man first neglected fruit and found the result pleasant to drink. The alcohol produced was discovered to be a mild preservative and the carbon dioxide produced proved useful in the expansion of bread mixtures. In the production of alcohol there was increase in the quantity of yeast and this was soon recognised as a substance of good flavour which could be processed and sold as a concentration of vitamins to those who felt the need. From its earliest use, fermentation and the associated yeast were mystical, being allocated suitable gods and ceremonies, particularly after consumption of the final product. The mysticism is perpetuated in modern drinking of alcohol, glasses raised in mock offering to the gods with the wish that all will be given divine preference in health and fortune. Broadly, through the ages yeast and its associates have not produced accepted harm to consumers but have produced a power of good.

This has applied, however, only to the familiar fermentation of carbohydrates including milk sugar. When microbial protein was put forward as a probability in mass production, the raw material discussed was oil, but there was coincidental discovery of a link between oil and cancer, bringing consumer rejection of any food connected with oil. The historic virtues of yeast then took second place to the implied vices of oil, and the opinion was formulated that yeast protein was acceptable providing it did not originate from oil.

In terms of diet, fermentation to alcoholic beverages is no more than the conversion of carbohydrates into a new form. Whether the new form is to be regarded as an improvement or a danger or an instrument of evil is not for this book to decide. Beverages ferment to an alcohol content from about 2% for weak beer to about 11% for wines, at which concentration the yeasts find it impossible to reproduce further and fermentation is slowed almost to a halt. Total solids vary from below 2% for some wines to nearly 6% for some beers. Protein content is 0.1–0.4% other than in strong ale which can reach 0.7%. Calories, which represent the energy value of the converted carbohydrate, per 100 ml, are about 30 for beers and 70 for wines, not including fortified wines which may reach 160 calories/100 ml. To give an effective comparison, fruit squash drink should give about 130 calories. Beers and wines are sold partly on their transparency and the fermenting yeast is therefore removed before sale. It is perhaps a sad reflection on modern society that fermentation is followed by removal of the health-giving protein-rich fraction before distribution of a product carrying relatively little nutrition. Beers and wines in primitive societies are consumed without clarification and are excellent aids to health.

The liquid fraction of ferments has a low food value but the alcohol is a mental relaxant and a physical stimulant. Ethyl alcohol is a narcotic which is rapidly oxidised in the body to carbon dioxide and water and in concentrations above 1000 p.p.m. it intoxicates and irritates. Long exposure produces drowsiness, lassitude and lost appetite, and inability to concentrate. It is a systemic toxin but there is no certainty that it produces cirrhosis or other serious damage, although its consumption instead of food after loss of appetite is harmful and can lead to mental instability and/or blood disorder. Providing there is little inclusion of methyl alcohol any damage is temporary and the association of drink with food is acceptable.

Methyl alcohol is a common associate of ethyl alcohol and it is a stronger narcotic and irritant than is ethyl alcohol. The main damage is to the nervous system, notably as optic neuritis followed by atrophy of the optic nerve. Methyl alcohol is slow to escape from the body and over-exposure can produce coma lasting up to four days, during which time cardiac depression is probable and this can cause death. Digestion is also severely disturbed and, if food is taken it may not be absorbed or even retained by the stomach. Other alcohols are likely to be toxic, notably amyl alcohol which is four times more narcotising than ethyl alcohol.

Common fermentation also produces acetaldehyde, which is another narcotic. Glycerol and succinic acid are also produced but are not harmful. The fermentation process has been well described in literature. It uses enzymes in yeasts and can be adjusted to convert over 90% of certain sugars if the inhibitive alcohol is removed. The fact that the word 'enzyme' originates from the Greek 'in yeast' is indicative of the age of the process. The particular enzyme is zymase, which is an enzyme mixture made more active by phosphates. The first stage of fermentation is combination of the sugar with phosphoric acid before splitting and reforming.

Being familiar and accepted, carbohydrates are obvious targets for the mass production of yeast protein. Common waste carbohydrate is mixed starch and sugar and the starch can be broken by boiling in acid but the remains are not suitable for further fermentation or yeast culture. Starch can be converted into fermentable sugars by enzymes in mucor fungi and it is probable that future processing of carbohydrate waste will use mixed organisms.

The sugars in raw materials are mixed. Malt-sugar is sensitive to the maltase fraction in the zymase, whilst sucrose is sensitive to the invertase fraction. When the C_{12} sugars have been broken into C_6 sugars the other fractions in the zymase convert to alcohol and carbon dioxide. The full reaction is seen to be catalytic, at face value producing no more nor less yeast in the process. In terms of protein output, fermentation for the sake of alcohol and carbon dioxide has no virtue. The target is yeast reproduction without the interference of alcohol or carbon dioxide, which can be regarded as by-products to be removed as quickly as possible. Neither is the liquid fraction of the ferment particularly important other than its influence on the production of the solid fraction.

Yeast grown on carbohydrate has been shown to have an excellent amino acid balance and is suspected as having traces of chemicals yet unknown but thought to be essential. They may prove to be new members of vitamin families or trace amino acids not previously included in lists of essentials. Most of the work has concerned torula yeast, which has a composition varied according to the claimant. Two versions have been included in the following table, alongside other protein foods and the FAO standard for humans:

Percentage of—	Torula yeast		Beef	Soya meal	Wheat	FAO standard
Arginine	4.1 or 5.4		7.7	8.4	4.2	—
Cystine	1.0	1.0	1.2	1.6	1.9	—
Histidine	1.7	2.2	3.3	2.6	2.2	—
Isoleucine	5.5	6.4	6.0	5.1	4.2	4.2
Leucine	7.5	8.0	8.0	7.7	7.0	4.8
Lysine	6.8	8.5	10.0	6.9	1.9	4.2
Methionine	0.8	1.5	3.2	1.6	1.5	1.4
Phenylalanine	3.9	5.1	5.0	5.0	5.5	2.8
Threonine	5.4	5.1	5.0	4.3	2.7	2.8
Tryptophane	1.6	1.4	1.4	1.3	0.8	1.4
Valine	6.0	5.6	5.5	5.4	4.1	4.2

Percentages of amino acid are acceptable in this table, rather than proportion of amino acid per contained nitrogen, because the market is mainly in animal feed which is bought in terms of percentage values. At face value, torula yeast appears to be a straightforward replacement for cereal in feed, bringing the lysine which is needed but requiring methionine. Subject to price comparison there would not seem to be much nutritional advantage in using torula yeast instead of soya meal. The critical deficiency is methionine, which is already lacking in cereal–oilseed feeds and needs to be added as a synthetic at a rate of about 0.5 kg/ton for a fully balanced protein diet.

It could therefore be claimed that there is no point in converting carbohydrate foods, which can be eaten by livestock, into torula yeast, particularly for ruminants who have their own built-in microbial protein factory in the rumen. In this respect, the point is that the yeast is available as over 90% protein, which allows high-protein feeding and also saves money in storage and transport. Even so, in a world which is short of food in the places where it is needed, there is justification for not using food carbohydrates for yeast, but using carbohydrates which serve no useful purpose and can cost money because they exist. Notably, papermill waste contaminates water and needs processing. Such processing can be simple extraction and disposal, which is expensive, or it can be conversion into some valuable substance, such as yeast protein although this is not the only possible derivative.

PAPER WASTE

Care is needed in reading reports of yeast culture from paper products and effluent. Work by Aston University was freely reported as feeding cows from newspaper, pulping the newspaper and growing yeast on the pulp before feeding it to cows. In fact, the Aston work followed the lines of work elsewhere, which involved initial breakdown of cellulose followed by fermentation of the break-down products, emphasis being on small-scale production suitable for farm operation. The main organisms were in fact fungi but news reports converted these to yeasts, which is unimportant because they are relatives.

The application of torula yeast need not be confined to animal feed, as is shown by the fact that the St. Regis Paper Company produce some 10 000 tons/year from papermill waste for human diet as an accepted health food. Commercial production is economic at 50% protein, the rest being water and unfermented carbohydrate. Fibre and non-protein nitrogen should be below 0.5% and can be discounted. Minerals are likely to be about 7% and the vitamin pattern can be varied considerably within the limits of yeast vitamins which are mainly vitamin B complex. The St. Regis yeast has been available as a health food in the USA since 1952 and is based on spruce and birch pulp.

In paper-making the wood is steam-extracted to divide the insoluble cellulose from the soluble polysaccharides which would have hardened to insolubles in the living tree. From a typical wood there can be roughly a 50:50 division of solubles and insolubles, common practice being to use the insolubles for paper and throw away the solubles to pollute local waters. Between 10% and 20% of the solubles are sugars which can be food for yeasts in a standard alcohol process. Torula yeast differs from normal yeasts used in alcohol production in that torula can use most of the available sugar as food, including the pentose sugars. St. Regis claim to produce 65 parts of yeast from 100 parts of available sugars. In terms of carbohydrate conversion this needs to be compared with 6% conversion for pork, 2% for dairy protein and below 2% for chicken and beef. The St. Regis conversion rate, which agrees with rates quoted elsewhere, is 6 to 7 times multiplication (600–700%) of the seeding yeast within 24 hours. As direct comparison, beef multiplies itself 0.1% in 24 hours and soya bean 8% in 24 hours. At face value this means a productivity in terms of protein multiplication of 80 times that of field crops and 6500 times that of beef.

One market advantage of the tree–torula route is the lack of real or imagined toxins and the ease of post-production processing. It is not necessary to kill the yeast but markets demand an inert product and killing is done by heating, preferably dry-heating so that water in cells is converted to steam, expands and explodes the cells. For dry powder it is then feasible to use conventional spray or drum driers to a nominal 100% protein. However, wet slurry has a market in compounding and could prove more important than dry powder as apart from animal feed there is a market for slurry in compounds with cereal or improved soya meal as meat and cheese replacement.

Although tannins can be a problem there does not appear to be a significant restriction of woods which can be fractionated for the solubles to be fed to yeasts. Cellulose Attisholz produce yeasts for animal feed from sulphite spent liquids originating in beech and several countries now have plants after the Attisholz process. One process by Attisholz uses beech and spruce residue after it has been used for alcohol production. The fluid is given heat treatment followed by continuous neutralisation, and is then fed into the yeast fermenter, which is designed as a series of pipes with air injection from the bottom of each pipe to give circulation and an exchange of oxygen for carbon dioxide. The circulation also removes exothermic heat. Final yeast is isolated, washed and dried to a solids content of about 22%. It then passes to further drying by hot air through a spray drier, to a dry yeast at 90–92% which is used in compounding. Output is of the order of 3000 tons/year of 53–55% protein feed.

A very small fraction of the world supply of wood is put to constructive use and it is to be appreciated that the young wood discarded in reaching the structural wood has a higher potential of solubles for yeast fermentation. Paper-making uses relatively old wood for the sake of its high insoluble fraction but even this contains up to a quarter of its weight as solubles. The USA paper industry could produce 25 million tons of yeast protein per year without difficulty, to the delight of those who are worried about pollution of waters. Total plant for the USA paper industry would cost perhaps $6000 million for ten years plant life, or $600 million/year to provide one-quarter of the world protein demand. This would therefore appear to be an ideal situation for commercial development having a large receptive outlet, proven technology, ample raw material and justification for the developments leading to cleaner waters and lower-cost food.

If other paper-making countries are included it is not difficult to imagine yeast production from paper-making equal in output to all other protein routes in the world. Many countries appreciate the significance of replacement of conventional feed, particularly if they import feed during the present period of high prices. There is already a scheme in Finland which could replace all the pigfeed used in Finland by yeast protein. In the United Kingdom there is a related calculation that the paper industry would need to spend £19 million on pollution control, and that if the £19 million were to be spent on a yeast protein project the output would be about 200 000 tons. Since paper-making is at a low level of return on capital the prospects of extra cost for pollution control is not welcomed and any profitable project is sought.

The Finnish development has been developed by the Finnish Pulp and Paper Research Institute, as the Pekilo process to 60% protein concentrate. There is approval for cattle feed and output by the end of 1974 should reach 10 000 tons/year from sulphite papermill waste. Eight companies have combined for the commercial development under the title of SITU and there is now a related process in Sweden starting from cellulose which is broken down by fungi before the yeasts are fed.

In addition, a further development on the following lines is probable. Some paper-making effluents are dilute mixtures of polysaccharides and lignosulphonates. Such mixtures can be used as weak adhesives and there is a small market in flooring, foundry cores, soil stabilisation and concrete. It is evidently possible for fermentation to result in a binding high-protein product which will provide the necessary protein in bound feeds without the added cost of weak adhesives, now bought by compounders. Some 40 000 tons of sulphite paper effluent is evidently used in the USA for feed binding and it would seem logical to upgrade the material from a simple adhesive to a protein-rich adhesive.

There could also be changes in attitude from the energy and oil crisis. As oil prices increase it will be more economic to produce alcohol from fermentation than from oil, and the production of yeast protein may yet be confined to residues after alcohol production. It is also possible that new markets for lignosulphonates will develop to leave wood sugars. These, if purified after a profitable outlet for the lignosulphonate has been found, are valuable for non-nutritive sweetening in societies worried about obesity but more worried about non-sugar sweeteners. The USA paper industry buys about 100 million tons/year of wood substances which are not used or find only low-profit outlets.

The availabilities of polluting raw material from paper pulp manufacture have been well documented. Products can be classified as:

Semi-chemical pulp, which is from a series of mechanical and chemical processes, none of which by itself would produce required pulp. This pulp process holds much of the lignin and hemi-cellulose in the pulp, resulting in more pulp per weight of original wood.

Sulphite pulp, which is by mechanical disruption followed by cooking with sulphite. Common sulphites are ammonium, magnesium and sodium. It may be bleached to become bleached sulphite pulp. Part of the hemi-cellulose is hydrolysed to sugars. About half the wood substance dissolves in the cooking liquid, and a further 5% may become soluble if bleaching is used. Sulphite pulp is therefore the main problem in pollution.

Sulphate pulp, which is by cooking disintegrated wood in a mixture of caustic soda and sodium sulphide. Caustic soda alone may be used, in which case the identity is soda pulp but may be described as sulphate pulp which it resembles. The yield is low, 40–45%, but most of the added chemicals are rescued.

Newsprint, which is mechanical pulp in which losses are only the original solubles in the wood.

Fibre board pulp, which is by defiberising chipped wood in steam. Some of the hemi-cellulose is hydrolysed to sugars, giving a loss as solubles of 8–15% according to the original wood.

In 1970, the pulp industry discharged nearly 4 million tons of suspended solids into waterways, nearly 3% of the weight of the final pulp and paper production. In terms of five-day biochemical oxygen demand, the 1970 pulp and paper industry discharged 6 million tons of BOD_5 of which about half came from sulphite and semi-chemical mills. There was also production of other processing waste. Bark content of trees as supplied is 8–13%.

The pollution problem from paper pulp manufacture is serious. Suspended solids will settle within a few hundred metres in still water but most effluents seek moving water which will accept the very high flow rates of effluent. Sedimented solids change the character of the bottom of waters, particularly by removal of oxygen from the mud. Dissolved substances other than lignin are food for microbes in waterways but the developed microbes may be undesirable and may take oxygen away from desirable microbes or other life.

Fish and other water inhabitants need about 3 p.p.m. of oxygen in their water. Most pollution by oxygen-starvation following effluent discharge is within five-days flow, although obviously the flow is influenced by the discharge rate and the effluent concentration. The lignin is not a serious pollution problem but it is a waste of valuable material to let it run with effluent. One serious pollution result is changed pH value, and this is particularly serious if it is with a sulphur derivative which can change flavours in the water.

Most pulp countries have programmes to overcome or reduce pollution.

Austria produces mainly sulphite pulp by twelve mills, of which seven have recovery systems including yeast and alcohol production.

Belgium has sulphate mills with efficient water-treatment plants. Protein production is not probable.

Canada has about eighty chemical pulp mills but the pollution problem is in the forty-five newsprint mills, of which twenty-nine have sulphite pulp production. Some mills will have to close because waste water recovery cost is calculated to be too high.

Finland produces sulphite, sulphate and newsprint pulps. Fifteen of the seventeen sulphite mills have waste-water treatment and recovery. Most of the future improvement will come from in-plant measures to reduce solids in effluent, including the use of yeasts for protein.

France has forty-one mills producing chemical pulp. Two mills are producing yeast and alcohol.

West Germany has twelve sulphite mills, all with primary treatment units for effluent. Sulphate pulp mills are not permitted and most mills will have secondary treatment for effluent in due course.

Italy has twelve small chemical pulp mills, three of which are on sulphite pulp. Effluent treatment is lacking in the mills but there is some measure of sedimentation of solids after discharge.

Japan has nearly sixty chemical pulp mills and more production is intended. All mills have primary treatment of effluent and most are providing secondary treatment.

Holland has a very small pulp industry and existing mills are provided with efficient effluent treatment.

Norway had twenty-three chemical pulp factories in 1970 but they are being progressively closed. The three biggest mills supply half the sulphite pulp and have alcohol plants.

Spain has twenty-seven chemical pulp mills using straw. The smaller mills have no rescue or recovery units but there is some water-treatment activity in larger mills.

Sweden has sixty-one pulp mills of which thirty-three are on sulphite pulp. Half of the pulp is produced along the coast and, as in Finland, concentration is on coagulation systems.

Switzerland has only one chemical pulp plant which is well furnished with water treatment.

Turkey has six chemical pulp plants but output is expected to rise, mainly of sulphate pulp. The two sulphite pulp plants burn the solids in the effluent.

United Kingdom has three mechanical pulp mills, two semi-chemical and one sulphite mill. Roughly three-quarters of the effluent is treated.

United States has about 200 chemical pulp mills, of which forty-two are semi-chemical, forty-two are producing sulphite pulp. The pollution legislation is exacting and many mills will have to close down if they do not find a profitable outlet for effluent.

The general OECD picture is:

Type of pulp	Number of mills	1970 tons output	Probable 1975 tons output
Semi-chemical	118	· 6 495 000	9 136 000
Sulphite	160	11 497 000	11 948 000
Non-integrated sulphate	6	9 173 000	12 258 000
Integrated sulphate	220	34 313 000	44 882 000
Newsprint	127	18 683 000	22 237 000
Fibre for board	55	2 115 000	2 244 000
Other	2907	53 720 000	69 384 000

Semi-chemical output could increase by 40% whilst production of sulphite pulp could increase by only 4%. Sulphite mills will either have to find profitable outlets for effluent or convert to sulphate, or close down.

There is considerable available raw material from debarking and trimming, not only in pulp production but also in other wood-working industries. In pulping operations the debarking can be wet or dry and the discard may be used for fuel. Italy uses all the discard as fuel and many countries use 70–80%. Switzerland uses only 20% of the discard as fuel and Spain uses none. It is possible that debarking discard accounts for a quarter of solids discharged into waterways for wood-working operations.

With regard to loose fibres, most countries have legislation being applied to reduce the solids content of effluent from papermills. Emphasis is on coagulation with effort to find some outlet for the concentrated solids. Part of this emphasis is to rescue water for recycling operations. There could be a 50% reduction of suspended solids in papermill effluents in the near future.

All countries have some recovery system for waste paper, which can be regarded as potential pulp without natural solubles but with new contamination. The contamination could be a problem in subsequent protein production, much of it being intended to inhibit microbial activity.

WASTE PAPER

Insofar as pulp manufacturers are facing threats of high investment for pollution control, and are already running at a low profit margin on capital, mills will have to seek subsidies or find profitable outlets for their discard. The basic extra cost is that needed to remove or make invisible any suspended solids, and to reduce the discharge of oxygen-demanding solubles so that they do not disturb ecological patterns in the water.

The re-use of waste paper, which has a low pollution potential, has influence and can to some extent offset the cost of pollution control. Waste paper recovery is of the order of:

	Mill consumption (*thousand tons*)	*% of total output* (*utilisation rate*)
Austria	274	25
Belgium	141	19
Canada	690	6
Finland	153	3.3
France	1500	35
West Germany	2480	46
Italy	990	32
Japan	4550	34
Holland	600	40
Norway	97	7
Spain	413	29
Sweden	290	6
Switzerland	216	35
United Kingdom	1900	42
USA	11 000	22

These comparative figures show that waste paper is an available raw material for protein, and the work of Aston and Manchester Universities on fermentation of waste paper is significant. The countries listed could supply about 26 million tons through their existing collection mechanics, which are geared to the value of the waste for recycling. It is probable that the maximum recovery from common societies is of the order of 48%, which could be reached only if the waste had sufficient value as a starter for protein. There is some probability that further studies will show the value of waste paper to be high for protein production, making it too expensive for repulping in papermills. If so, the effluent from paper-mills will be proportionally increased by the extra contamination from virgin wood used instead of the waste paper. Even if the waste paper is not used for protein manufacture it will probably be used for structural applications, again at high value, as metals and petrochemicals become scarce. It is advisable to ignore the influence of waste paper on future pulping operations and to consider the potential pollution as that applicable to all-virgin raw material.

POLLUTION ECONOMICS

The probability of obtaining protein from paper pulp production depends on how far governments assist in the finance; most mills being unable to find the extra capital involved for effluent treatment. In Canada about two-thirds of the needed $30 million is from industry and one-third from the government. In Finland the finance is complicated, part of the cost being with the Paper and Pulp Research Institute, which is industry-financed, and part with SITRA, which is financed by the government. Roughly half the total cost is from the government. In France also about half the total cost is paid by the government. In West Germany, mills pay for their own salvation but there are unpublicised grants from the government for specific investigations. In Japan the situation is confused with no clear idea of how much is paid by industry or by the government. In Holland all the cost appears to be accepted by industry. Industry also takes care of itself in Norway but there are grants which could put most of the ultimate cost on the government. In Sweden there is a fund used by the Environmental Care Project, which could take most of the cost in due course. In the United Kingdom the position is fluid but with all the cost at present taken by industry. In the United States, industry spends about $12 million/year and there could be another $7 million from government funds.

It is of interest to compare the financial implications:

	Expenditure 1971 on research and development against pollution from papermills, $ million	Paper and pulp output. 1970 million tons	$ per ton spent on R & D against pollution
Canada	5.6	18.0	0.28
Finland	1.1	7.7	0.14
France	0.6	5.0	0.12
Holland	0.15	1.7	0.09
Norway	0.2	2.9	0.09
Sweden	2.5	11.7	0.21
United Kingdom	0.2	5.0	0.24
USA	19.0	56.0	0.34

Motivation for pollution control in pulp manufacture and in paper making is the high rate of destruction of valuable clean water, about 1 m^3/ton of paper produced. The 2–4% of suspended solids in effluent are uneconomic to remove from such high rates of flow and low concentrations, and would not be removed if they did no harm to the environment. Removal is by conventional filtration, sedimentation and flotation, which can remove about 80% of the solids. The cost of this primary operation is of the order of half a US dollar per ton of pulp.

The cost of dealing with solubles is higher. The most effective preventative action is elimination of the solubles in the process, which would mean using only pure cellulose for raw material and not introducing any chemicals in the programme. It is fairly common for effluents to be evaporated with subsequent burning of the solids, which loses the sugars but rescues, for example, calcium bisulphite. Ion-exchange techniques are also used, at an approximate cost of $1.5/ton of output. In general terms, concentration techniques to rescue or destroy solubles in effluent add $1.0–1.5/output ton. Taking all into account, the cost facing producers of pulp and paper is of the order of $8/ton output for 80–90% cleaning of effluent water. Obviously, this varies by country, legislation and weight of public objection to pollution. Its significance depends strongly on the prices which can be reached for pulp and paper.

In effect, the paper and pulp industry could have a raw material for protein production at a cost of the order of $10/ton, could use anti-pollution capital to convert this into valuable protein which could sell at perhaps ten times the raw cost.

Assistance from governments need not be by direct grants or payment of investigational research costs. French papermills have direct subsidies for water pollution control up to 10% of investment. In Sweden there are 25% subsidies which can be increased to 75% during recession periods and in unemployment areas. In West Germany there are direct grants for areas of unemployment, up to 25% on a short-term basis. Belgium has a special subsidy which reduces the interest on borrowed capital for pollution control.

Most countries have some form of rapid write-off for equipment, this being reflected in lower tax payments. In Austria, 60% can be written-off in one year. The write-off period in Canada is two years and in Finland it is four years. The write-off period is important since, in academic terms, a protein plant using papermill effluent is anti-pollution equipment but is usually estimated on a ten-year life. If the fermentation equipment for protein from effluent is given a cost of $400/ton capacity and can be written-off against tax in one year, the final product carries a plant cost of only $40/ton. Added to the $10/ton raw cost, this gives an ex-works cost of the order of $50–60/ton, selling against feeds with only half the protein value but four times the price.

Taking the top dozen pulp producing countries the cleaning of water after production of about 60 million tons of pulp has been calculated to cost about $2300 million over the 1971–1975 period, otherwise calculated as a 40% on-cost to intended investment for normal production purposes. Other estimates put the extra cost to the USA alone as $3000 million for only 30 million tons of pulp. Whether the final cost is $40 or $100/ton of output is probably unimportant in the need for clean water. Within the present context the important point to appreciate is that the discard is suitable for in-plant processing directly to protein.

SUGAR

In commercial terms, sugar means sucrose extracted from cane in hot climates and beet in temperate climates. The concept of yeast protein is attractive to sugar producers since both materials can travel together into food compounding and supermarket shelves. Sugar is underproduced by intent to maintain prices in world markets and an alternative outlet would be welcomed. In fact, an alternative market could become essential for survival of the industry if trends continue away from sugar, sugar being accused of causing obesity and bad teeth. The movement away from sweetness in the world includes reduction of traditional puddings and the increased use of rice for savoury dishes. It has encouraged detailed examination of non-fattening sugars as found in the solubles of trees, and the introduction of new protein sweeteners as rivals to non-sugar synthetic sweeteners now under pressure from health legislations. The sweetest product known is a protein monellin derived from a wild red berry dioscoreophyllum, which is completely safe for mammals and has a sweetening power 3000 times that of sugar. Less than 40 000 tons could satisfy world demands for sweetness.

Sugar is probably the easiest route to cultured microbial protein and yeasts are the obvious choice of microbe. With oil and energy becoming scarce it is probable that sugar will be needed for industrial chemicals and the demand cannot be forecast. For food applications the demand estimate is 108 million tons by 1982, when production could reach 115 million tons. The extra 7 million tons will be absorbed in chemical production and there is justification in expanding output. Expansion could be criticised if the market were to be confined to existing food outlets but the needs for chemistry and the possibility of protein production need to be considered.

Apart from the obvious step of ceasing to restrict area and output, more sugar can be obtained by improvements in extraction. Hokkaido Sugar Company have an enzyme process for fuller extraction of sugar beet. It is estimated that fuller extraction of cane, and a shorter period between cutting and milling, would provide at least an extra 9% of sugar. If, as it should be, extra sugar is made available for conversion into yeast, then there are differences of opinion concerning the process. For effective marketing by sugar suppliers a new protein would need to be for human consumption and preferably be obtained from refined sugar, if only to allow adjustment of one raw material for both the sugar and protein markets. Conversely, it seems illogical to refine sugar for conversion and then mix it into carbohydrate and fibre as compounded feed. It is better to take out the easy fraction from cane and beet, saving processing cost in the production of refined sugar, and then use the sugar-rich residue for yeast production. The markets would then have a lower-cost refined sugar and an animal feed containing 25–30% excellent protein with a fair content of sugar and fibre. Under this system of two-product planning, world output of feed could be of the order of 50 million tons/year from an enlarged sugar industry. Increased area and output of sugar is vital to developing countries, second only to coffee in terms of significance in national economics. Developing countries supply about 70% of world sugar and about half of world sugar is under the control of the International Sugar Agreement, the other half being sold by private agreements. There is intention of the United Nations taking over interference with sugar supplies and this could well mean progress in the use of sugar for yeast protein. Taking an extreme example, Mauritius depends on sugar for 40% of employment and 94% of exports, with no skill or capital available for diversification. If sugar output cannot be increased and a reasonable price obtained, it will be necessary to seek diversification within sugar technology using a low-capital process.

Mineral concentrations in sugars (p.p.m.) (As a factor in fermentation for protein)

	Refined sugar	Raw sugar	Molasses
Calcium	15.0	300.0	5800.0
Chromium	0.13	0.3	1.0
Cobalt	0.05	0.4	0.3
Copper	0.2	3.0	15.0
Iron	0.4	20.0	110.0
Magnesium	2.0	90.0	7500.0
Manganese	0.13	—	4.25
Phosphorus	10.0	440.0	850.0
Potassium	20.0	—	20 000.0
Zinc	0.2	8.7	8.3

Protein sweetener. Amino-acid pattern (%) (protein from juice of Serendipity berries)

Arginine	7.0	Threonine	4.7
Cystine	1.8	Valine	4.1
Isoleucine	8.3	Aspartic acid	11.0
Leucine	5.9	Serine	2.8
Lysine	10.1	Glutamic acid	7.6
Methionine	5.2	Proline	8.2
Phenylalanine	5.4	Alanine	3.9
Tyrosine	5.8		

The pure protein sweetener has about 3000 times the sweetening power of sucrose.

World Sugar Production, F.O. Licht opinion

Thousand tons approximate, raw value	1971/2	1972/3	1973/4
Beet sugar			
West Europe	13 601	12 643	13 271
East Europe	25 791	25 583	27 140
Total World	31 562	31 395	32 658

World Sugar Production, F.O. Licht opinion—continued

Thousand tons approximate, raw value

	1971/2	1972/3	1973/4
Cane sugar			
Europe	34	31	30
North and Central Americas	12 449	14 145	14 911
South Americas	9 680	10 582	12 091
Africa	5 302	5 493	5 601
Asia	10 962	12 479	13 102
Oceania	3 207	3 214	3 205
Total World	41 635	45 944	48 940
Total world sugar from beet and cane—			
	73 197	77 339	81 597

European beet sugar production, F.O. Licht opinion

Thousand tons approximate, raw value, 1972/3

West Germany	2268	Yugoslavia	395
France	3050	Greece	131
Belgium	685	Switzerland	68
Holland	772	Finland	93
Italy	1317	Turkey	829
Denmark	349	Hungary	330
United Kingdom	985	Poland	1826
Ireland	175	Albania	19
Austria	407	Rumania	610
Sweden	299	Bulgaria	230
Spain	818	USSR	8500

Protein yeasts produced by Akt. Dansk Gaerings-Industri

Bakers yeast—*Sacch. cerevisiae*—grown on molasses
Fodder yeast—*Cand. utilis* and *Cand. tropicalis*—grown on molasses or sulphite paper-
mill waste
—*Cand. lipolytica*—grown on mineral oil
Whey yeast—*Sacch. fragilis*—grown on whey
Brewers yeast—*Sacch. carlsbergensis*—after debittering
Distillers yeast—*Sacch. cerevisiae*—grown on molasses

Product manufactured from 20% yeast cream. Final product is:

	% approx.
Fat	10
Yeast dry matter	85
Water	5

Protein rating (N × 6.25) is 40–45%

Amino-acid pattern, Bakers yeast, D.G.I. claim

g/16 g Nitrogen

Arginine	4.59	Tryptophane	1.19
Cystine	1.08	Tyrosine	2.76
Histidine	2.06	Valine	4.99
Isoleucine	4.19	Aspartic acid	9.01
Leucine	6.29	Glutamic acid	15.21
Lysine	7.16	Glycine	4.23
Methionine	1.72	Proline	2.95
Phenylalanine	4.16	Serine	4.33
Threonine	4.64	Alanine	6.23

Utilisation values are:

	Without added methionine	*With added methionine*
Digestibility (%)	83.9	81.5
Biological value (%)	49.8	84.5
Net protein utilisation (%)	41.0	69.2

St. Regis Company torula yeast: composition

	%
Protein (N × 6.25)	50–54
Non-protein nitrogen	0.3–0.5
Ash	7.0–7.8
Fibre	0.4–0.5
Carbohydrates	25–30
Moisture	About 5.7

Several grades vary in vitamin composition from low to high potencies in thiamine, riboflavine and niacin.

Oil-derived microbial protein, composition, USA opinion Dept. of Agriculture

	%
Moisture	7.03
Total Nitrogen	6.92
Lipids	18.50
Carbohydrates	21.90
Protein	43.60
Minerals	4.43
as Calcium	0.21
Phosphorus	1.25
Potassium	0.50

Amino-acid patterns, opinion of University of Western Ontario
(unstated units for comparison only)

	FAO standard	Milk	Fish concentrate	Soya	Cotton-seed	Algae carbo-hydrate
Isoleucine	4.2	6.5	4.2	5.8	4.0	3.9
Leucine	4.8	9.9	7.2	7.6	6.2	7.1
Lysine	4.2	8.0	8.2	6.6	4.2	5.4
Methionine	2.2	2.9	2.7	1.1	1.5	1.0
Phenylalanine	2.8	5.1	3.6	4.8	5.2	4.2
Threonine	2.8	4.7	4.0	3.9	3.5	4.4
Tryptophane	1.4	1.3	0.9	1.2	1.6	1.3
Valine	4.2	6.7	7.9	5.2	5.0	6.8

	Fungi/ carbohydrate	Yeast/ carbohydrate	Yeast/ oil	Bacteria/ oil	Fungi/ natural gas
Isoleucine	3.5	5.5	4.5	3.6	5.1
Leucine	6.1	7.9	7.0	5.6	8.1
Lysine	5.4	8.2	7.0	6.5	8.5
Methionine	1.4	2.5	1.8	2.0	1.8
Phenylalanine	2.8	4.5	4.4	2.9	4.6
Threonine	3.4	4.8	4.9	4.0	1.7
Tryptophane	1.4	1.2	1.4	0.9	1.2
Valine	3.9	5.5	5.4	4.5	6.6

Comparison of amino-acid patterns (%), USA opinion Dept. of Agriculture

	61.4% Soya meal	Beef	Milk	Wheat flour	Torula yeast	Oil-derived protein
Arginine	8.4	7.7	4.2	4.2	4.1	8.0
Cystine	1.6	1.2	1.0	1.9	1.0	0.1
Isoleucine	5.1	6.0	7.8	4.2	5.5	3.1
Leucine	7.7	8.0	11.0	7.0	7.6	7.0
Lysine	6.9	10.0	8.7	1.9	6.8	11.6
Methionine	1.6	3.2	3.2	1.5	0.8	1.2
Phenylalanine	5.0	5.0	5.5	5.5	3.9	7.9
Threonine	4.3	5.0	4.7	2.7	5.4	9.1
Tryptophane	1.3	1.4	1.5	0.8	1.6	1.2
Valine	5.4	5.5	7.1	4.1	6.0	8.4
Histidine	2.6	3.3	2.6	2.2	1.7	8.1

St. Regis Paper Company torula yeast, amino-acid pattern

Based on 16% nitrogen (100% protein)

Arginine	5.4	Lycine	8.5
Alanine	6.1	Methionine	1.5
Aspartic acid	8.6	Phenylalanine	5.1
Cystine	1.0	Proline	0.5
Glutamic acid	14.5	Serine	3.8
Glycine	4.4	Tryptophane	1.4
Histidine	2.2	Threonine	5.1
Isoleucine	6.4	Tyrosine	4.3
Leucine	8.0	Valine	5.6

Chapter 26

Bacteria

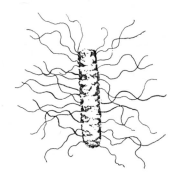

As far as is known the first organisms on earth were bacteria-like, created by accidental coincidence of chemical reactions which could coexist in a cooperative organisation capable of reproduction. Later came specialist organisms such as algae, which concentrate on the employment of ultraviolet light, and yeasts, which are concerned with reactions of carbon, hydrogen and oxygen. Bacteria are the primary scavengers, growing in number on diets according to their individual preference and breaking down organic substance to manufacture their own body protein. Any organic substance can be related to some destructive bacteria which will feed and multiply to provide excellent first-class protein if the substance is provided with the right conditions of moisture, temperature and atmosphere. There is no general specification of conducive circumstances, activity being found in environments from high in the sky to deeply contained within animal tissues. The industrial provision of a conducive circumstance is made easier by the non-sexual reproduction of bacteria and by the ability to manufacture protein without light. One incentive towards the industrial production of bacterial protein is the fact that bacteria convert cellulose, which is the most common waste organic substance available.

INDUSTRIAL PRODUCTION
Capital investment for industrial production needs a fairly assured market and inhibitive attitudes need to be studied. Science fiction has drawn

attention to the possibility, if not probability, of mutation and specialisation of cells converted from small-scale to mass production. Each vegetable cell carries within itself the blueprint of a complete plant. An orchid seed is a collection of undifferentiated cells. If it is deposited in a conducive environment it will enlarge and then, for reasons which are not fully understood, will produce a leaflet and a rootlet and subsequently a new orchid. There is a genuine fear that bacteria in mass will likewise mutate and specialise, possibly not to become a fearful monster as invented in science fiction but perhaps to a new organic mass with undesirable reactions when consumed.

There is also an associated fear that any developed specialised cells from compressed bacteria may prove to be immortal. As a natural rule, specialised cells develop until they have produced a body member or organ and then cease reproduction beyond that needed for replacement. Unspecialised cells reproduce without limit whilst they have the necessary food and energy and conditions. The second-stage fear is that compressed bacteria will produce a specialised mass capable of reproduction without end using circumstances which are not those provided for the original culture. The concept is that a leak from a bacteria factory might find conducive circumstances in the local plants and animals, bringing disaster to the local environment and subsequently destroying humanity.

There is a further fear that new relationships may be established between bacteria and plants or animals if bacteria are forcibly cultured. Close relationships already exist, as for example the nitrogen-fixing bacteria on certain roots and the bacteria which are part of ruminant digestion. This particular fear is encouraged by the total damage inflicted by very slight infection in highly-bred plants or animals, particularly if the cultivation is intensive. It concerns mainly bacteria and fungi, a classic example of fungal influence being bakanae, or foolish-seedlings, in plants. This is a rice disease but if the extract of the fungus, gibberelin, is fed to other plants there is peculiar growth. Flowers appear out of season, cabbages grow 4 m high and radishes swell to weights of over 15 kg or stretch to over 1 m long. In this respect, bacteria are feared more than fungi because bacteria were identified in early history as carriers of death and destruction. They carry this unfortunate image despite their essential value to world society and the good they do to plants and animals.

It could therefore be difficult to convince consumers that since they enjoy the bacteria in cheese, and have populations of bacteria already within their bodies, they should eat industrial bacterial protein. It could also be difficult to convince authorities that it is safe to have bacteria factories within their areas of jurisdiction. Almost certainly, industrial bacterial protein needs to be confined to animal-feed markets for the time being, and to be established in selected areas where there is sufficient scientific education to overcome the inferences from science fiction. The reason why bacterial protein should be factory-produced is the failure of agriculture to meet demands. Agriculture is restricted by climates, soil chemistries and the results of interference with nature by man. It cannot possibly supply sufficient protein without drastic changes of attitudes and there are environments in which it cannot be productive, whereas industrial microbial protein, notably bacterial protein, can be produced without regard for climatic variations or soil chemistries and this can be done on any scale of operation from very small to very large. A remote wind-lashed island or a dense concentration of urban humanity or any other social situation can be the site of a factory with output dictated by capital investment and engineering skill.

Bacterial protein, Chinese Petroleum Corporation, Taiwan, claim

---

Most successful bacteria—*Pseudomonas* 5401 (ATCC 21094)
Feedstock—n-paraffin
   Ammonia or ammonium salts
   Air to provide oxygen
Fermentation at 36–38 °C, pH 7.0
Maximum cell concentration—16 g/litre after 24 hours fermentation
With feeding rate 12.5% of volume of culture per hour, a cell concentration of 10 g/litre could be maintained
With feeding rate 25% of volume of culture per hour, a cell concentration of 8 g/litre could be maintained
Yield of dry cells—105% of original fuel oil
Protein content of dry cells—73.62%
Product analysis—

	% unwashed	% washed
Protein	71.21	80.0
Oil	2.07	1.17
Moisture	9.96	—
Ash	9.28	5.63

Amino-acid pattern comparison %

	Pseudomonas on gas oil	Pseudomonas on fuel oil	Unidentified yeast
Arginine	4.98	4.68	2.37
Aspartic acid	7.24	8.47	5.63
Alanine	6.37	6.41	3.36
Cystine	0.43	—	—

Bacterial protein, Chinese Petroleum Corporation, Taiwan, claim—continued

Glutamic acid	8.67	10.05	7.57
Glycine	3.75	4.26	2.45
Histidine	1.21	1.87	1.03
Isoleucine	3.84	4.33	2.35
Lysine	4.29	9.06	3.89
Leucine	6.57	6.74	3.60
Methionine	1.27	0.81	—
Phenylalanine	3.29	3.39	2.17
Proline	2.94	2.36	1.59
Serine	2.96	3.07	2.52
Threonine	4.08	3.77	2.54
Tryptophane	1.16	0.91	0.27
Tyrosine	2.74	2.30	1.56
Valine	3.48	5.08	2.60

Feeding trials. Bacterial protein against soya cake

	Days tested	Feedprotein	Conversion rate (g fed per g growth)
Rats	28	Soya cake only	7.436
	56	Soya cake only	7.169
	28	Bacteria only	5.361
	56	Bacteria only	7.184
	28	50:50 mixture	4.496
	56	50:50 mixture	6.152
Chickens	28	Soya cake only	2.498
	56	Soya cake only	3.226
	28	50:50 mixture	2.352
	56	50:50 mixture	3.203
Laying hens	90	Soya cake only	3.230 (per unit weight of egg)
	90	1 part bacteria 2 parts soya cake	3.055
Pigs	20	Soya cake only	3.842
	60	Soya cake only	3.799
	100	Soya cake only	4.169
	140	Soya cake only	4.372
	20	50:50 mixture	4.689
	60	50:50 mixture	4.547
	100	50:50 mixture	4.273
	140	50:50 mixture	4.536

Factory-produced bacterial protein for animal feed has been anticipated by nature in ruminants. They have populations of bacteria in their
rumens and it is common to develop these populations by feeding urea
instead of protein. One ton of urea will replace 5–6 tons of conventional
protein feed, but only as a source of nitrogen. Hence, conventional agricultural substances are also needed by the animal and the favoured
system is to dust grass with urea so that it is eaten by the animal and
also acts as a fertiliser for the grass. The use of urea as common feed
for sheep and grass was known in 1918 but application in forced feeding
is recent. The urea is fed only to adult animals and is rated as 45–46%
protein equivalent, one unit of urea to replace eight units of oilseed
cake. There is some danger of urea agglomerates but there is development of starch-bound urea to avoid this danger. Starch-bound urea is
produced by mixing with cereal flour and extruding hot, so that a starch
gel covers each urea granule. It then delivers to the bacteria in the rumen
a parcel of individual compound particles for complete consumption. A
further development is a reaction product of ammonia and phosphates
for feed.

Urea needs to be fed to the animal in small doses over a long period
of growth. It is not effective when fed in high concentration or as a
sudden change of diet, and whether it will become a major item in feed
depends mainly on world chemical requirements arising from oil shortages. There could be more important uses for urea than the feeding of
cattle which can eat other substances. On the other hand, 100 000 tons
of urea can replace oilseed grown on 1 million acres of agricultural land
which might have a better function in direct feeding of people instead
of animals. Since, however, the possible intake of urea by a cow is
limited, it may prove more sensible to cultivate bacteria under ideal
conditions outside the cow and then feed finished protein to the cow.

There has been some confusion in the approach to bacterial protein.
As an industrial process it has attracted interest in companies who are
related to hydrocarbons and therefore emphasis has been low on the
more-fundamental routes using waste cellulose for its carbon content
and urine or similar waste as a source of nitrogen if nitrogen gas cannot be fixed by the selected bacteria. About 1970, there was indication
that plant cost for bacterial protein would be of the order of £150/ton
capacity with plant suited to outputs from 1000–200 000 tons/year. This
was calculated to last ten years before replacement and to give a protein
cost about level with that of protein extract from oilseeds.

Cellulose as a raw material for bacterial protein is limiting in its range of suitable bacteria and it can be expected that earlier success will be with lower carbohydrates, notably the excess sugar which is available when growers allow production to be maximised. Louisiana State University produced excellent bacterial protein at 50–60% dry protein as a powder for animal feed. The raw material was sugar-cane waste which can be accepted as cellulose with sufficient retained sugar to encourage rapid growth of bacteria and thereby make it easier for the cellulose to break down. Many establishments are now looking seriously at two-stage processes—bacterial breakdown of the cellulose followed by fungal attack—this evidently being more productive than bacterial attack in these circumstances. There is an instinctive selection of fungi and yeasts for sugars, more being known about fungi–yeast fermentation of sugars than about bacteria in the same type of reaction.

The selection of bacteria for dealing with cellulose is confused partly because previous research has been aimed at reducing bacterial activity on cellulose textiles, but now has to consider the encouragement of bacterial growth on crude cellulose waste. It is also confused because some bacteria exist with two or more names or change their name after an original name has become familiar. Some of the familiar bacteria are:

Strongly active*	Active
Cytophaga globulosa	*Cellvibrio fulvus*
Cytophaga hutchinsonii	*Cellvibrio vulgaris*
Cytophaga myxococcoides	*Cytophaga rubra*
Myxococcus cytophagus	*Corynebacterium fimi*, which may
Myxococcus hutchinsonii	be known as *Bacterium fimi*,
Spirochaeta cytophaga	*Bacterium liquatum*, *Cellulomonas fimi* or *Cellulomonas liquata*

There are also a large number of bacteria which may yet be fitted into the mentioned groups or be proved worthy of inclusion. The above list is by no means exhaustive.

BACTERIAL ACTIVITY

Bacterial activity is reduced in acid conditions, which is why canned meat needs more sterilising heat than canned fruit needs, and why yoghurt has a shelf-life. Most of the useful bacteria thrive between pH

---

* All of these are alternative names or alternative forms of *Sporocytophaga myxococcoides*.

5.5 and pH 8.5. They have a specific optimum pH and a specific optimum temperature. Those consuming cellulose include:

	Optimum pH	Optimum temperature °C
Bacillus thermofibrincolus	8.2	65
Cellulobacillus varsarviensis	7.6	29
Cellulomonas biazotea	6.4	28
Cytophaga hutchinsonii	7.5	25
Cytophaga polonicum	7.4	23
Itersonia ferruginea	7.2	26
Sorangium compositum	8.3	35
Sorangium nigrescens	8.3	35
Spirochaeta cytophaga	7.3	30
Vibrio amylocella	7.6	37

Although cellulose is the main component of general agricultural waste there are commercial quantities of protein waste, mostly fur and feathers. The bacteria consuming such protein include:

	Optimum pH	Optimum temperature °C
Proteus vulgaris	8.2	36
Bacillus subtilis	7.7	37
Bacillus mesentericus	7.8	37
Bacillus megatherium	7.2	35
Bacillus mycoides	8.0	30
Pseudomonas pyocyanea	7.9	37
Pseudomonas fluorescens	7.8	25
Bacterium alkaligenes	8.0	37

Activity is also related to moisture content above a threshold minimum requirement. For pure cellulose there is slight activity below 10% moisture but significant activity at higher levels. If a culture can be expected to develop, for example 1.5 million bacteria at 9% moisture, the progression is likely to be:

Moisture content	Bacteria population after, say, 3 days (millions)
9	1.5
10	125.0
15	500.0
20	1100.0
30	1500.0

Under normal circumstances, bacteria take three to eight days to produce serious damage to cellulose or waste protein. As has been shown in studies of the biodeterioration of waste paper, much depends on the pH value and moisture level, paper remaining intact in so-called 'lifeless' dry soils. In the breakdown of protein waste, *Bacillus subtilis* can produce serious damage after only two days whilst *Bacillus mycoides* may not show any visible activity for five days or produce serious damage before eight or nine days. For both cellulose and waste protein there may be advantage in using mixed cultures, not only mixtures of bacteria but also mixtures including fungi or yeasts or algae.

BACTERIAL PROTEIN

There would be advantage to the world if processes were developed for bacterial protein from fats, since surplus fat is associated with increased protein output from natural sources. In this the problem is partly that fermentation of fats produces unpleasant flavour but a more serious problem is that fats do not mix with water. Some of the problem has been solved in the development of hydrocarbon oil fractions as sources of protein, although there is now opinion that hydrocarbon routes are better related to gas fractions, notably methane. The ICI route converts the methane to methyl alcohol and uses this as feedstock for the bacteria. A process by the Formosan Petroleum Corporation started by selection of soil organisms, of which Pseudomonas 5401 was chosen. This grows well on lower fractions of oil with added ammonium salts at 37 °C and pH 7.0. Yield is slightly higher than the weight of the original feedstock with a final protein content of 74%. Absorption of the supplied nitrogen is 90% and, alongside the 74% protein in the final product are 2% oil, 10% moisture and 9% minerals.

Bacterial growth is commonly used to decompose waste oil and this may indicate a future route to protein. Union Carbide in Puerto Rico dump bacteria-rich molasses with added phosphates and ammonia into processing tanks. The offending oil–water mixture is pumped in at 3000 gallons/min and suffers two stages of bacterial cleaning before being pumped into the local bay. Currently, oil–water mixtures are being cleaned at a rate of 4 million gallons/day, which may give some indication of the size of possible protein plants.

The pattern of amino acids in bacterial protein varies with the route but even within a route there is variation according to who makes the analysis and claim. It is probable that bacterial protein will have a reasonable balance but can be lacking some methionine and/or trypto-phane. General opinion is that it will, when produced in bulk, replace mainly fish meal in feed. Its potential use in human diet was reduced by rejection of bacterial protein in Japan, public memories of toxins from industry having influence on government approval of projects. Mitsubishi intended a plant at Niigata, rated at 5000 tons/year using methyl alcohol, for completion in 1973. On the other side of the world, ICI have plans for 100 000 tons/year by 1978, also using methyl alcohol, and Shell have similar plans. Hoechst are also active with methyl alcohol. Sumitomo, Dainippon and others are involved in a £19 million project in Rumania calculated to deliver 120 000 tons/year by 1975.

Esso routes concern methane and two organisms identified as ATCC 21438 and 21439, which are pseudomonas, and another three organisms identified as ATCC 21232, 21235 and 21236, which are corynebacteria. Corynebacteria are said to be active on methane without conversion to the alcohol. Fermentation is in aqueous salt solution with excess oxygen, with the following salt pattern:

	g/litre
K_2HPO_4	2–8
$(NH_4)_2HPO_4$	8–12
Na_2SO_4	0.3–0.8
$FeSO_47H_2O$	0.01–0.03
$MgSO_47H_2O$	0.3–0.8
$MnSO_47H_2O$	0.01–0.03
NaCl	0.01–0.03
—Plus water to 100%	

Other nutrient mixtures can be used, including those with phosphorus supplied as phosphoric acid, which helps to adjust the pH value. Temperatures are of the order of 25–45 °C and pH values are 5.5–8.5, which is relatively unspecific. After growth the bacteria are cooked to kill at 120 °C for 30 mins.

The use of corynebacteria is of interest in that patent 1300654 by Kabushiki Kaisha Tekkosha concerns the same bacteria as a source of lysine. Relatively pure acetic acid is used as the feedstock for a variant under the reference NRRL B-3671, and it is interesting to add that Hoechst in Europe also ferment acetic acid. Carbohydrates may be used instead of, or alongside, the acetic acid and it is claimed that lysine can be produced to 2%.

Chapter 27

Oil

The carbohydrates which are consumed by microbes to produce protein are simple multiples of CH_2O. Hydrocarbons differ from carbohydrates by their lack of oxygen and if microbes are expected to grow on hydrocarbons they have to be forcibly supplied with oxygen, which can present a problem in the handling of large volumes of ferment. There is also a problem in supplying nutrients to microbes in a hydrophobic liquid, and a further problem when the grown microbes need harvesting and washing before killing and subsequent consumption. Protein from oil is a more difficult route than protein from carbohydrate and it does not have an assured market. There is an implied link between oil derivatives and cancer which, even though the link is not confirmed and despite the fact that no raw material is carried through with the microbial protein, inhibits consumer acceptance. Even without the implied link between cancer and oil derivatives, there would be instinctive preference for protein manufactured from carbohydrates because they are familiar food substances. Any derivative of carbohydrate, be it bread or cultured protein or beer, is acceptable to the common consumer. Oil is not a familiar food and its common derivatives are offensive to common consumers. The rejection is unfortunate because protein from oil fractions could be highly significant in world economics, and there is no technical reason why such protein should be rejected.

The composition of crude oil varies considerably in different fields and it may be directly associated with natural gas. The crude is divided into fractions according to boiling points. Demand for the lighter end of the mixture is high, and cracking is used to break down some of the heavy fraction for light hydrocarbons. When necessary, coal can be used as a source of almost any chemical found in oils. The chemicals of primary interest for fermentation are the normal paraffins, chains of CH_2 units suitably terminated by extra hydrogens. Other hydrocarbons can be fermented but the results may not be according to market demands and the refined other hydrocarbons may be too valuable for proteins. It is important to understand that the hydrocarbons involved are refined fractions, not unprofitable hydrocarbon waste although there may be developments with such chemicals in the future. To some extent, proteins are competitors to motor cars in the oil business and when oil becomes scarce this can have influence. The fact that Union Carbide and others use bacteria to break down oil waste before dumping does not by necessity mean that similar oil wastes are low-cost raw materials for microbial protein.

Evidence relative to results when hydrocarbons meet microbes can be suspect, partly because previous effort has been aimed at preventing microbial growth, not accelerating it, and partly because published results must concern a limited range of microbes. It is probable that trials involving a small variety of organisms ignore significant species and also prevent synergism. Such trials probably relate to hydrocarbons in their pure and excellent condition, without breakdown by age and ultraviolet or by the inclusion of catalysts. Enzymic breakdown of hydrocarbons is an established fact, the rate of breakdown reducing as the chains become longer and more side chains are included. Enzymes are active only in aqueous media and they need to be brought into intimate contact with the substance to be degraded. Hence, a large hydrocarbon molecule which is richly furnished with side chains cannot be penetrated by enzymes even if they make contact, which is unlikely since such large hydrocarbons are certain to be highly hydrophobic. Normal paraffins are attacked up to $C_{32}H_{66}$ but resist microbes from C_{36} upwards. If, however, the paraffins are branched then even as low as C_{15} will repel microbial attack, whereas a straight chain with twice this number of carbons will be sensitive. For straight chain paraffins there seems to be a threshold at about molecular weight 450, above which microbes do not attack and below which there is attack but it may not be sufficient for microbial protein production.

There now appears to be a possibility of using higher hydrocarbons as diet for microbes, preferably yeasts, by mixing with carbohydrate. Rice-starch grains are extremely small and they can be compounded into hydrocarbons up to two-thirds of the final mixture. Initial microbial attack is on the carbohydrate, which is lost to expose a very large area of hydrocarbon in a structure which resembles a microscopic sponge, each cell of which is lined with water-sensitive microbe-infected remains of starch grains. Contact is intimate and the microbes, preferably as a mixed population, can attack and thrive. There is also a possibility of development of systems using non-polar solvents. As mentioned above, attack by microbes on straight paraffins is below the C_{35} threshold, and above C_{35} such paraffins become insoluble in non-polar solvents.

When one discovers that even a single dimethyl group in a paraffin will discourage microbial activity, it is remarkable that very large and branched molecules exist in nature and are freely attacked by microbes. In these there seems to be some weakness from amide bonds and ester groups. Subject to more investigation it may prove possible to grow microbes on low-value hydrocarbon fractions by the provision of such sensitive points in molecules. At present, however, the hydrocarbon fractions of value to potential protein factories are also valuable elsewhere, and are likely to become more valuable as the oil–energy crisis develops.

The concept of microbial protein from oil dates from the 1940s and the development work by BP, who have processes based on n-paraffins and distillate gas oil. The n-paraffin is extracted from crude oil and subjected to continuous fermentation. The gas oil is also subjected to continuous fermentation but with a proportion of n-paraffin fermented before other hydrocarbons are separated from the biomass. A small-scale plant rated at 4000 tons is operative at Grangemouth and there are two production units intended—100 000 tons rating in Sardinia and 16 000 tons at Lavera. In the n-paraffin route the fermentation is under aseptic conditions with only the selected organism active. In the gas route only the selected organism is allowed to predominate, mainly by adjustment of the pH and temperature. The n-paraffin is presently inexpensive and is almost entirely consumed in production. The gas oil is also inexpensive but it needs a subsequent stage of solvent extraction after fermentation, which can be expensive. A suitable mixture of minerals and nutrients is fed as a continuous stream with water into the fermenter, to be joined by n-paraffins before sterilisation. After cooling, oxygen is fed into the mass as air bubbles, with ammonia to provide the nitrogen. Reaction is exothermic, calling for cooling to the optimum 30 °C. Fermentation produces a yeast cream at about 15% solids, which is then dried by spraying to about 5% moisture content. The Lavera plant, using gas oil, follows this basic route but does not sterilise the initial mixture and includes a solvent extraction stage. Where gas oil is used, the harvest is pumped to a centrifuge to recover gas oil and water before the yeast cells are passed for drying. Final traces of gas oil are removed by counter-stream solvent extraction.

The final BP product has 62.5% dry-weight protein from n-paraffins, or up to 70% from gas oil. Methionine is deficient but otherwise the product could replace soya or fish meal.

The final product should comprise:

Percentages	From n-paraffin	From gas oil
Moisture	4.2	5
Nitrogen/dry weight	10	11
Protein (N × 6.25)	62.5	68.7
Lipids	8–10	1.5–2.1
Ash	6	8

The amino-acid pattern is roughly similar for n-paraffins and gas oil.

	From n-paraffin	From gas oil
Arginine	5.1	5.0
Cystine	1.1	0.9
Histidine	2.1	2.1
Isoleucine	5.1	5.3
Leucine	7.4	7.8
Lysine	7.4	7.8
Methionine	1.8	1.6
Phenylalanine	4.4	4.8
Threonine	4.9	5.4
Tryptophane	1.4	1.3
Valine	5.9	5.8

One problem met by BP and others was the lack of official testing procedures when they introduced microbial protein. A toxicity testing scheme was devised by CIVO in Holland, relative to the feeding of the protein to animals for short, medium and long periods. There were also tests to discover if any link existed between oil-derived protein and cancer, or if any interference with reproduction could be found. At the time of writing there has been no ill effect in thirteen generations of rats and twenty-three generations of quail. ILOB, also in Holland, also evaluated the new proteins in feed as replacement for conventional cakes and dried milk, with no dire consequence in five generations of pigs and poultry.

Although this examination has been more than that given to any other feed protein, there is hesitation amongst approval authorities. France prohibited microbial protein without specific authorisation, whilst the United Kingdom allowed use unless given specific prohibition. The approval/prohibition situation is complicated by the lack of an agreed test, and is likely to become more complicated as more routes are commercialised. Shell and ICI have developments relative to protein from natural gas by bacteria, with methyl alcohol as an intermediary stage between the methane and the protein.

The 1973 oil crisis had been forecast for at least thirty years and its major disruption was in finance. Revenue from oil to Arab countries could show a surplus of \$20 000 million by 1975 and double this by 1980. The actual sum is less important than its potential value as capital for microbial protein from oil, with production in the Middle East. It is obviously attractive to such barren oil countries to have industrialised food production, which could solve many human problems but could also provide a platform for new animal-protein ventures.

Amino-acid patterns, microbial proteins

mg/g Nitrogen	Bacterial protein by Esso–Nestle	Candida utilis yeast	BP yeast from n-paraffin	BP yeast from gas oil	TPI Rhizopus fungal protein	UWO Graphium fungal protein	IFP Spirulina platensis algae	IFP Spirulina maxima algae	Chlorella algae
Isoleucine	225	239	281	331	206	318	390	375	244
Leucine	350	475	438	488	278	505	556	540	438
Lysine	405	300	438	488	323	530	285	282	427
Methionine	87	69	113	100	93	112	165	152	93
Cystine	38	—	69	56	88	—	59	60	75
Phenylalanine	180	538	275	300	194	280	283	275	305
Tyrosine	—	388	219	250	172	—	302	283	248
Threonine	250	338	306	338	224	106	326	320	208
Tryptophane	56	150	88	81	76	—	100	101	85
Valine	280	238	338	363	240	410	420	410	347

Part 5

Protein Economics

Chapter 28

Variations in Production, Distribution and Consumption

The object of protein supply is to provide an acceptable protein-rich diet in constant quantities using reliable distribution. Every word of this broad specification is weighted with variation and most of the variants cannot be translated into simple arithmetic terms.

The intoxicating concept of growth and efficiency which has qualified industrial development obscures the fact that output is dictated by local conditions of production, and that the monetary value of output can bear little relationship to actual benefit and contribution to local welfare. Societies have developed patterns of supply and demand according to their historic circumstances, unique to the locality and not subject to a common worldwide technology. Most areas have failed to appreciate their potential and have consequently not met their patterns of demand. Frequently, the failure has been aggravated by the introduction of foreign technology, particularly when the foreign technology relies on mono-culture and intensive production of harvest weight rather than variety and quality. In any locality, potential agricultural output has an optimum output, above which there is damage to the environment and below which is under-employment of resources. One important factor in protein supply is the preservation of the conducive situation so that supplies are continued, with natural renewal and without exhaustion of production facilities.

Demand patterns are based on the fact that each person needs up to 100 g/day of first-class protein which needs to reach stomachs after a long and difficult negotiation of social and technical obstacles. The protein needs to be related to other food components. It can be of animal or vegetable origin, or mixed, and it matters little where the protein originates if the amino-acid pattern is correct. In general, animal protein is sensitive to biodeterioration and there can be technical obstacles to efficient supply. Also, most of the social objections to food concern animal proteins, making it easier to supply vegetable protein into a superstitious society. On the other hand, animal protein is nearer than vegetable protein to the human protein it is intended to fortify, making it advisable to provide at least some animal protein in diet if the technical and social obstacles can be overcome.

It is also advisable, where possible, that animal protein should be delivered to the consumer urgently and without the use of preservation or compounding techniques. The value of preservation and compounding depends on the experience and skill of operators, and on the education of consumers, making it possible for such techniques to be a hazard. If so, there is economic justification for a fragmented output pattern, flesh being produced at small-farm level rather than in centralised mass-production. In societies which are richly furnished with small traders and middlemen there is economic justification for all possible protein to be produced by the consumer for his own use. Unproductive profit margins between fields and stomachs inflate prices and discourage consumption.

Unfortunately, most vegetable proteins are seasonal and need to be tied to a storage system. Losses in storage, of quality and quantity, are inevitable but vary according to the crop and excellence of the storage. In basic subsistence agriculture it is normal to store at farm level for one year including seed for the next season. If the agricultural pattern is with one main crop there can be a failed season, making it essential to carry at least two years of stored product, whereas in a mixed agricultural pattern, a poor season will reduce overall quantity but it is rare for all crops to suffer significant loss in one season. Hence, the quantity to be stored depends mainly on the pattern of production, preference being for a mixed production pattern with storage quantities calculated to the next crop. The safest production mixture is one which includes representatives from all vegetable groups—cereals, pulses, roots, etc.—with available animal protein for ceremonial occasional meals and as reserve protein which can be killed any time. Obviously, milk and eggs should be included in the mixture where possible, as constant supply and because the cows and chickens can be killed off if grain stocks are spoiled by moisture or are stolen by enemies.

Variations in production, distribution and consumption are extreme. Situations are far from identical in Calcutta, Detroit, Kano and places in the Arctic which are too remote to have names. For the majority of humans there is no possibility of an idyllic subsistence life with its constant production and consumption of fresh and excellent protein. Most humans are non-agricultural and they have to rely on distribution and the giving of money in exchange for food. In this respect, the nutritional value of the bought food is incidental, value being measured in terms of derived pleasure and satisfied appetite. The type and quantity of food which is bought depends partly on the available cash-in-hand with each consumer, but also on the alternative needs and facilities for spending the cash. During the early 1970s in the United Kingdom, inflation caused a reduction of *per capita* protein intake, partly due to consumers buying domestic products instead of food, because the prices of these were likely to rise rapidly. The same period of inflation in India produced widespread malnutrition because retail prices increased to make more of the population unable to afford sufficient food. It is important to differentiate between market depreciation arising from lack of purchase power and that arising from desirable alternative uses for the purchase power.

In a money-conscious society, any retailed item of food carries the cost of initial production and subsequent handling to the point of sale. To bring the item to the consumer requires the services of intermediates who need a profit margin so that they too can become consumers. There is for each item a threshold retail price, below which either producers or handlers will lose money and consequently will seek alternative activity. Within the general pattern of food, proteins are higher priced than are carbohydrates. If, therefore, a consumer is faced with proteins or carbohydrates during a period when money is tight, the choice will be carbohydrates because the price threshold can be lower. Suppliers will favour carbohydrates when money is not tight, because the low price threshold allows high profit margins by selling carbohydrates in the same price range as proteins. Almost all market conditions favour carbohydrates before proteins, particularly since carbohydrates are easier to process and store than are proteins.

It is fairly obvious that world emphasis cannot be switched from carbohydrates to proteins without a drastic reduction of the threshold price for protein. Whether agriculture can offer lower production cost for protein is doubted, particularly if agricultural workers are to be given improved welfare. Therefore, an industrial route to manufacture is indicated as desirable, preferably of a product which can offer the same convenience as carbohydrates in processing and storage. The target threshold price would appear to be that of common wheat or rice according to the feeding habits of local societies.

Urbanised societies have high land prices, high labour costs and high overheads regardless of the use of the land and labour. Agriculture can be profitable only with high-yield high-value crops or animals, preference being for market-garden crops for local sale. Bulk proteins therefore need to be imported, selecting materials which can be handled and stored within the facilities available. Broadly, the imported proteins need to be inert and insensitive, and to be malleable so that economic flat-sided uniform packages can be stacked and carried. Processed cheese fits into the requirement whilst natural cheese does not. Compounded meat fits but fresh bloody meat does not. Milk powder for reconstitution and UHT long-life milk fit into the system but fresh milk is completely unsuitable.

Such a diet is restrictive and it lacks certain desirable traces which are mainly provided by local horticulture. It is preferable that the imported foods should come from many sources, not only to ensure that some of the missing traces are included but also so that buyers can seek the lowest world prices and prevent monopolistic pressure. The conventional pattern of supply has been low-cost production of raw foods in low labour–cost areas, shipment of the raw material to the proximity of consumers, processing and storage near to the point of consumption. Several trends have emerged during the past few years to disturb the convention. Low labour–cost areas rightly consider that if profit is to be made in processing then the profit is better with the producer. Freight costs have increased, making it sensible to remove unusable fractions from commodities before they are shipped and to upgrade product values before shipment so that freight rates are in effect reduced. Most important, societies have learned that they cannot afford to rely on foreign sources of essential raw materials. In other words, processing is being moved away from the ultimate consumers and to the original producers and future trade can be expected to develop as a movement of processed commodities, not of raw materials. As a side issue, this change also transfers processing waste from the proximity of the consumer to the proximity of the original producer and future industrial projects relative to protein from waste need to be with this transfer in mind.

Societies are mixtures of social groups which can be listed as:

1. The fortunate affluent few who buy at will with little regard for retail prices and have no need to suffer malnutrition, although most suffer from unwise diet.
2. Affluent consumers who have sufficient purchase power to eat well but may be under pressure to spend their money on non-food, notably on housing, travel and speculative investment.
3. Consumers who have only sufficient purchase power for comfortable survival in their prevailing environment, and who are notably sensitive to retail prices of food.
4. Consumers who lack money in hand but have access to local agricultural products.
5. Impoverished consumers who do not have access to local agricultural products but need to buy imported food.
6. Consumers in the care of authorities who accept responsibility for the purchase of food and the selection thereof.

The problem groups are those which do not have sufficient affluence to justify imported foods, and do not have access to local agricultural products. Within this group the most serious problem is when the lack of access is due to inability of the territory to produce crops or animals by conventional agricultural techniques. For such groups there is an urgent need for revised culture techniques and the introduction of industrial routes to protein. Where populations are thin, as in most arid environments, the main need is for a revised approach to crop and animal production, using educated control of the climate and acceptance of unusual plants and animals. Where populations are dense the only logical system of local protein production appears to be factory-farming of microbes and a scientific recycling process for human waste.

Where local agricultural production is possible it is important that domestic requirements should be met before exports are developed, particularly since the stability of future export markets can be doubted, as illustrated by the probability that Scandinavia will cease to be a market for feed grains when microbes-from-paper-waste have developed for animal feed. It is vital that any export business is built on a foundation of local demand which can be manipulated to suit variations in export quantities. It is likewise vital that local supplies of protein shall be free from interference by any foreign authority. The vagaries of local diet are, therefore, a primary consideration and religion in its broadest sense is probably the most influential factor.

Half a century ago it was reasonably possible to forecast many demands for food by study of the pattern of religious faiths in a community, but dogmatic religion is now less important in society, having been replaced by insecure adhesion of individuals to specific religious conventions. Fidelity is more to the group and its culture than to a divine supervisor. The groups which strongly influence buying habits are:

Vegen—Eating only pure vegetables.
Lacto-vegetarian—Dairy products and vegetables only.
Kosher—Food from an orthodox source, with complications relative to meat and milk.
Kedassia—As for kosher but the food source needs to be licensed.
Moslem—Meat from prescribed slaughter, but no pig.
Mormon—No fermented or stimulating food.

Groups which influence buying but are not regarded as religious groups include:

Diabetic—Low carbohydrate and low fat.
Slimmers—High protein and low calorie count. Within this group is to be considered the significant number of people who have to be selective in diet to prevent heart failure or gastric disorder.

Religious influence on local diet, when it was formulated, had direct association with local food production facilities and limitations. It has rarely been allowed to change with circumstances and modern diet patterns do not coincide with the ability of a region to supply types and quantities of food, even for long-term residents of a region. Furthermore, groups have migrated and mixed to a situation in which specific religions can no longer be related directly to geographic locations.

PRODUCTION
Any area capable of supporting human life will support some form of animal life which is suitable for food. On the understanding that a domestic market can be developed, the economics of meat production are dictated by the conditions of supply of feed, the routes being:

1. Freely available feed as grazing land or as substance unfit for humans but fit for scavenging animals.
2. Feed produced as a crop.
3. Bought feed.

Free range
Free-ranged animals need low-cost area and reasonable supervision, the only significant production cost being that represented by the area and labour. The area needed per unit weight of final protein is proportional to the unit size of the animal, rodents and chickens showing more productivity than sheep, which in turn show more productivity than cows or buffalo. The selection of the animal depends partly on the available vegetation and partly on the relative wetness of the soil. It further depends on the unit bulk required for slaughter. Small animals can be killed in rotation to provide a constant supply of meat, but large animals require a rotational distribution system, neighbours killing in turn, or a collective preservation or marketing organisation.

The problem with collective disposal is that handlers and middlemen can take profit to excess. Even if they take a reasonable profit the final price of the meat is higher than that of direct supply. With notable exceptions, the herding of animals on open pasture is better with small animals which can meet requirements in one killing event. However, small animals need confinement whilst large animals can be herded with a little supervision. Under most circumstances the economic animals are of the size of sheep or goats or geese. Sheep are favoured for their docility and ability to provide wool before they expire. Goats are favoured for their flexibility of diet and geese are favoured for their scavenging capabilities. In some areas, geese are also favoured for their ferocity against intruders, human or otherwise.

Enclosed
By the laws of supply and demand, land values increase as populations become more dense. Land is needed for housing, roads, social services and any industry which is allowed to develop by the increased local markets. Likewise, labour costs increase as populations become dense, there being more types of activity available for labourers to use in agreements of sale of time and effort. It then becomes essential to use confined rearing of meat, with private production of food for the animals or with bought feed. Feed can be bought out of local crops or as imports but imports can only be with equivalent exports, which can be part of the reared meat or some other goods using triangular trade. The use of imported feed is inevitably more expensive because it introduces third and fourth parties to act as traders. The use of local crops also adds to the meat production cost, by the introduction of third and fourth parties, but it does confine the collective profit to the society producing the meat.

Also, the use of local crops allows the society to benefit from the labouring efforts of animals before they are slaughtered. Hence, the preference in animals is for large animals which can work before they die, the buffalo being an excellent subject for development. In economic terms, whereas a free-range animal is qualified by high labour in production, an animal in mixed farming is replacement for labour whilst it lives, probable dairy protein during its life and meat after slaughter. The cost of this labour–milk–meat package is the provided food, which the beast helps to produce through its energy and its fertiliser production, together with the cost of care and security and the cost of an associated meat distribution system because large animals provide too much meat per slaughter for one farmer.

Mixed

In terms of protein, meat from mixed farming is unavoidably more expensive than is vegetation, there being a loss factor in feeding food fit for humans to animals for ultimate consumption by humans. The loss factor is not easy to define because not all food fit for humans is acceptable by humans, and the use of ruminants makes it practical to convert foods which are not fit for humans. Also, the use of scavenging animals rescues food fractions outside harvesting facilities, and also converts items of feed not counted in the general economics (kitchen waste and a vast range of titbits found by the scavenger in its wanderings).

It is comparatively rare to find environments which will provide facilities for fully-balanced mixed farming. The variables involved are many and are constantly being changed by situations in world economics and politics, and by progressive local improvements in welfare. As a general rule, any environment can be shown to favour one aspect of agriculture, with graduated disfavour of other aspects. The economics of local agriculture are dictated by the graduation pattern and the relative scales of favour and disfavour. In theory, each environment should have a basic economic agricultural pattern, above which overproduction of one commodity pays for the supply necessitated by underproduction of another. In practice, there is confusion in all agricultural patterns, arising mainly from unsatisfactory planning followed by uneducated interference and efforts to transplant experience without detailed study of the environmental factors. Unsatisfactory planning has resulted in excessive monoculture, with consequent neglect of a basic economic agricultural pattern. Uneducated interference has caused damage to the environmental factors, notably depreciation of ecological balances and soil qualities. Transplanted experience has carried infection and infestation, bringing the threat of universal contact between all hosts and parasites and a planetary need to use chemical control with consequent increase of pollution and reduced output of world protein.

There has also been introduced an influence of encouragement of cash crops for trade with associated discouragement of subsistence crops for local diet. The classic example is probably natural fibres, notably jute. Before synthetic fibres, jute was a profitable cash crop with a sure market in all trades needing sacks. It could be sold at high profit to pay for imported foods and jute areas could afford to allocate land to jute instead of to food crops. The introduction of stretched polyolefine synthetics has destroyed the market by providing a technical equivalent at half the jute price and jute areas now face famine because the land is used for non-food. The basic choice is between 1600 lb/acre of jute with a lost market and 900 lb/acre of rice which has a ready outlet in feeding local people. There is no justification for good agricultural environments in famine areas being used for non-food.

Intensive
Mixed farming in affluent societies is capital-intensive, organised to eliminate manual labour and to maximise standardisation of everything from species selection to final packaging. The inevitable outcome is industrialised agriculture, which is highly capitalised monoculture using synthetic environments to produce extra yield. So far, industrialised agriculture has concerned only conventional plants and animals but there is now some evidence that other sources of protein should be, and will be, developed. Costs in industrialised agriculture are related in the first stages to land prices and equipment costs, subsequently to energy and feed costs. Hence, the fortunes of projects are dictated by foreign events such as an increase in the price of oil or the failure of Peruvian fish meal. Also, since output by industrialised agriculture is above local requirements, any project is likely to be remote from local society. It can be placed anywhere, according to the local costs of energy and feed. The main requirement is an assure outlet for the mass-produced product.

Existing industrialised agriculture can be regarded as an interim stage. Plants and animals which have evolved through natural environments are unlikely to succeed in synthetic environments. Given time, man could evolve his own species range of plants and animals which have life histories and chemistries suited to artificial environment, and there is some hope that this will be brought about by genetic manipulation and rearing from individual cells.

The ultimate stage in industrial agriculture is the culture of micro-organisms instead of conventional plants and animals. The growth of microbes on formulated media under controlled conditions is a process which fits into industrial attitudes and organisations. It can be defined in terms of initial capital, running cost, output, profit margin, risk factor, and any other terms needed by planners and economists to implement a programme. Furthermore, microbial protein can be produced on a plant scaled to meet local conditions, and it can be without regard for climate or other agricultural influences. Initial capital is high, at about £150/ton capacity, but initial and subsequent costs are not influenced by the location. Unlike traditional agriculture, microbial-protein production can carry the same plant and technology into all areas. Hence, it can benefit from cost reduction through standardisation and the transfer of experience, and should in due course supply the least expensive form of protein.

Chapter 29

Agricultural Outputs

Recorded world meat output was 98 million tons in 1970, 101.5 million tons in 1971 and 103 million tons in 1972. Whether this indicates more efficient recording or a steady increase of 2–3 million tons/year is yet to be discovered. Traditional methods of raising meat rely on 3- to 5-year development periods, so that the 1971–1972 high retail prices for meat will result in more meat in 1974–1975, although the demand for meat could develop at a rate which will maintain the high retail prices.

Cereals are harvested to an annual world total of about 1250 million tons according to records. This is roughly 350 million tons of wheat, 300 million tons of rice, 300 million tons of maize, 150 million tons of barley, plus a remaining assortment including oats, rye, sorghum, etc. The wheat is a temperate crop suited to estate farming over wide areas. The rice and maize is the labour-intensive fraction whilst the barley and others meet individual circumstances of growth. In theory, this spread of growth requirements should optimise total cereal production and it was thought that world cereal output could not fail. However, it has now been realised that the southwards drift of the Sahara is likely to continue, and that droughts need not by necessity be local but can affect cereal crops of all types and in all countries at the same time. A variability of perhaps 5 million tons is possible from climatic failure, giving a probability-range for world cereals of 1200–1300 million tons from existing facilities.

Recorded output of oilseeds needs to be dated since it is growing. 1972 output was a little short of 120 million tons, 7 million more than in

1971 and 10 million more than in 1970. The growth of oilseeds appears to coincide with a fall in root crops, 524 million tons in 1972 after a fall of 10 million from 1971 and a fall of 35 million from 1970. It has been claimed that oilseed feeding compound is replacing roots for livestock, with twelve times the protein content of roots, but this claim is doubted because roots are directly fed whereas oilseed compound is bought feed.

Recorded pulses total about 44 million tons but this is probably only dried and stored pulses and the total for fresh vegetation reaching ultimate consumers is a possible 600 million tons not counting that sold into processing industries.

If the various protein sources could be evenly distributed, and handling losses were eliminated, world agriculture could provide a daily protein *per capita* dry weight of:

From animal sources	40 g/day
cereals	60
non-cereal vegetables	45

The fact that this total is well above the *per capita* needs is indication that there is failure of distribution, not failure of production. It is now realised that transport facilities and distribution systems cannot be introduced at a rate which will satisfy the growing demands of increased populations and higher standards of living. The effort is, therefore, to develop agriculture alongside outlets, and to associate agricultural development with industrial protein production and green leaf protein extraction. Some trials with green leaf protein have shown yields of 3000 kg/hectare/year, as compared with 500–1000 kg from conventional agriculture.

It has been common opinion that a little animal protein is essential in diet, and that vegetable proteins need to be well mixed if they are to provide a satisfactory amino-acid pattern. Recent developments of high-protein high-lysine cereals and other vegetables have simplified diet problems, and there are indications of more variation in regional diets. It is not probable, however, that total protein production from agriculture will increase to meet demands. In fact, a decline could become evident as more areas suffer damage arising from the growth of populations and the continued concentration into urban communities.

The problems facing world agriculture are many and the answers are not easy to find. Some of the problems can be listed:

1. World inflation has made any transport expensive and it is becom-

ing uneconomic to carry low-value goods. Commodities need to be upgraded in value to justify freight rates, making obsolete the historic system of shipping raw foods, with their high content of discard, for processing in the affluent consumer areas.

2. The possibility of price rises from speculation make it unsafe for any agricultural project to rely on imports, particularly of feed or fertiliser. The only safe future projects will be those based on closed-cycle operation which can be carried out in complete isolation.

3. Genetic improvements will make obsolete most of the existing animals and plants. There are already crosses between buffalo and conventional milk cows, and new species of plants. These are only the first results of new genetic technological developments using direct interference with genes and reproduction from cultured tissue.

4. Good agricultural land is being taken for non-agricultural purposes and the remaining agricultural land is becoming too expensive for conventional mixed farming.

5. World ecological balances are being disturbed to a degree whereby no area, however remote, will function as an agricultural source of protein without corrective interference. The majority of agricultural areas do not have the education or capital for such corrective interference.

6. Labour is becoming increasingly expensive, and unwilling to suffer rural conditions and the implied indignity of farm working. Future agricultural projects need to be with minimum labour content. Any labour involved needs to be either unskilled but with relatively high wage rates or highly skilled with very high wage rates, according to how much automation and mechanisation can be introduced into the farm involved.

7. Crops and animals can be expected to decline in quality, partly because higher yields are needed and this reduces quality and partly because growth environments are becoming more fouled by pollution. The levels of pollution in some areas could make certain crops or animals unsuited to the locations. Levels of heavy metals and effluent hormones are probably the most serious consideration.

8. Dramatic and unpredictable changes have become common in production costs and market conditions, such changes now taking place within periods shorter than those necessary for forward planning, certainly of projects demanding planning five to ten years ahead.

9. World trade in commodities has become entangled in a network of obsolete codes of practice, legislations, levies and support measures.

The farmer is no longer master of his own fate, but is a servant of trade and economic legislation. Farming has ceased to be an attractive activity.

Reducing these problems to a single economic focus, the reason why world agriculture is failing to meet demands is acceleration. The cost of transporting has increased at a faster rate than has been anticipated in broad economic planning. Changes in raw costs have been more dramatic and unexpected than could be allowed for in primary planning. The new species have arrived sooner than was thought possible and have replaced slow evolution by instant revision. Good land is being extracted from agricultural production too quickly for new land to be cleared and provided with communication. Pollution has spread more rapidly and over a wider area than was expected. Farm labour has lost its traditional character of stability and reliability, becoming more in line with the self-demanding mercurial labour generated by industry. Most important, probably, control and organisation has found it impossible to keep pace with changes of circumstances.

Urban and rural population growth. FAO statistics

	Millions			% of total		
	1960	1970	1985	1960	1970	1985
World	2981	3635	4948	100	100	100
Urban	986	1358	2198	33.1	37.4	44.4
Rural	1995	2277	2750	66.9	62.6	55.6
So-called developed countries	976	1090	1275	100	100	100
Urban	565	699	928	57.9	64.1	72.8
Rural	411	391	347	42.1	35.9	27.2
So-called developing countries	2005	2545	3673	100	100	100
Urban	421	659	1270	21.0	25.9	34.6
Rural	1584	1886	2403	79.0	74.1	65.4

Urban populations by regions. 1970. FAO statistics

	% urban
Europe	63.6
Western Europe	74.4
Eastern Europe	54.0
Southern Europe	50.8
USSR	57.1

*Urban populations by regions. 1970. FAO statistics
—continued*

	% *urban*
North America	74.3
Oceania	67.9
Africa	22.3
Northern Africa	34.9
Tropical Africa	15.3
Southern Africa	45.6
Latin Americas	56.2
Central America/Caribbean	48.7
South America	59.9
East Asia	29.6
South Asia	20.7

Nutrition intakes. Urban and rural. Various countries. FAO statistics

Between 1960 and 1970. (Dates not specific)		*Calories*	*Total protein*	*Animal protein*	*Vegetable protein*	*Fats*
Tunisia	Urban	2550	67.7	15.0	52.7	77.5
	Rural	2315	63.7	7.4	56.3	55.2
Trinidad	Urban	2850	83.6	43.3	40.3	95.8
	Rural	3011	81.7	31.8	49.9	84.0
Chad	Urban	2113	73.3	23.9	49.5	52.2
	Rural	2467	90.1	10.5	79.6	62.9
Dahomey	Urban	1908	52.0	10.0	42.0	46.2
	Rural	2142	51.0	7.0	44.0	47.4
Morocco	Urban	2521	70.0	19.0	51.0	—
	Rural	2888	84.0	12.0	72.0	—
Brazil	Urban	2428	74.0	30.7	43.3	63.0
	Rural	2640	79.2	29.7	49.5	60.0
Bangladesh	Urban	1732	49.5	12.1	37.4	25.0
	Rural	2254	57.4	7.9	49.5	17.2
Pakistan	Urban	1806	58.4	9.8	48.6	40.0
	Rural	2126	69.8	7.9	61.9	40.3
Korea	Urban	1946	62.8	10.9	51.9	19.5
	Rural	2181	66.9	5.1	61.8	15.8
Japan	Urban	2038	71.0	30.0	41.0	32.0
	Rural	2170	70.0	24.0	46.0	25.0
Panama	Urban	2101	71.0	38.0	33.0	59.0
	Rural	2089	60.0	27.0	33.0	50.0
Nicaragua	Urban	2108	72.0	35.0	37.0	60.0
	Rural	1986	64.0	23.0	41.0	46.0
Costa Rica	Urban	2330	67.0	31.0	36.0	67.0
	Rural	1894	54.0	19.0	35.0	44.0

Grammes per person per day

Chapter 30

Industrial Protein

In simple theory, industrial routes to protein are more reliable and economic than agricultural routes, if only because they escape the variability of weather. Industrial routes cultivate organisms under artificial conditions which imitate and subsequently improve on natural environmental conditions. Traditional plants and animals are presently used but there are developments of cultivating new crops including micro-organisms. However, since traditional plants and animals were selected or developed to meet prevailing natural conditions it is not probable that they will thrive to advantage under artificial conditions and it is probable that they will be replaced by new species which could not thrive under natural conditions but will thrive under the protective conditions of scientific control. In view of the rising cost of area, the primary requirement of a subject for industrial protein production is ability to grow in cramped quarters, needing no activity other than the consumption of food and the breathing of air. The second requirement is a rapid conversion of supplied food into body weight, preferably at a standard rate so that harvests and executions can be organised to coincide with demands. The third requirement, which could be the major problem in species determination, is ability to resist disease despite the lack of valuable traces in their diet and the restriction of movement.

Economic factors are controlled mainly by the selection of species and there are certain moral issues to be studied. Young humans suffer an education which includes the development of a love–hate relationship with animals due to become meat. Selected animals are personalised and

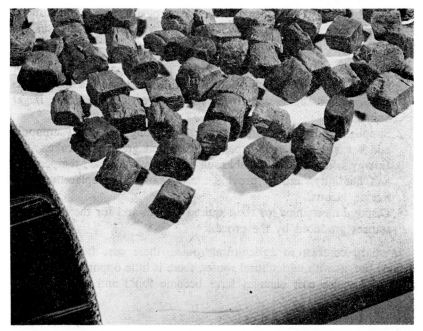

Fig. 1. Mixed Kesp chunks coming off the production line.

there is a developed obligation to provide comfort and affection, and to respect the dignity of the animal even unto death. Unfortunately, the personalisation stems from prior atonement for the subsequent act of killing and is directly related to the desirability of the final meat (some societies show the same prior affection for vegetation and ardent gardeners are known to love their tomatoes more than their family). Ultimate economy in industrial routes to protein is therefore inhibited by impossibility of satisfying consumer demands for familiar substances whilst satisfying consumer demands for personalised comfort of the protein source. Whether a chicken or pig needs free movement and a natural sex life is not the point of issue, but many consumers feel that doomed animals should be given conditions which would be enjoyed by humans, this being illustrated by fairly widespread rejection of products of factory farming. In fact, bodily comfort is an asset in rates of growth and it is strongly doubted if animals (or plants) suffer distress under correct scientific rearing. In this respect it is to be noted that there is evidence that vegetables respond to mental stimuli and are now

19—WPR * *

considered to develop according to conditions of distress or contentment. The various environment specifications have been detailed in the sections on individual protein sources. The common cost factors are:

1. Initial capital-intensive plant, which can be reaction kettles for microbes, perpetual illuminated waterfalls for algae, serviced banks of cages for small animals or rows of serviced pens for larger animals.
2. Supplied feed, which can be from a vast range including ammonia and waste cellulose or expensive balanced granulated cake.
3. Energy to replace the variable sun energy by controlled temperature and humidity, and to provide motive power as replacement for human labour.
4. Disposal mechanics for the required protein and for the other substances produced by the process.

In sharp contrast to agricultural routes, these cost factors can be defined but, as with agricultural routes, there is little opportunity to plan forward because cost changes have become rapid and unpredictable.

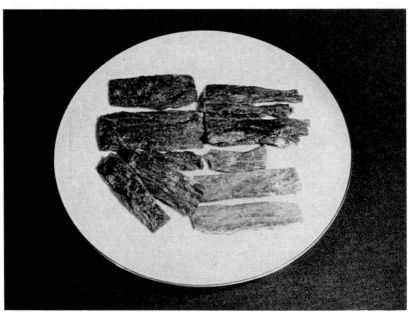

Fig. 2.   Japanese simulated meat.

Hence, the economics are more reliable as the planning period is reduced, giving favour to short-life animals or vegetables. It is safer to plan ahead with chickens than with pigs, and safer with pigs than with cows. Likewise, it is safer to plan with lettuce in controlled greenhouses than to plan ahead with fruit trees.

Capital equipment and feed are dictated by the requirements of the organism and can be standardised. Engineering and feed compositions are identical for the organisms whether in hot wet Ghana or icy Siberia or stormy remote islands or in the middle of urban Calcutta. The variable is the energy, which needs to supply optimising heat and to motivate devices in differing conditions. There is also variation in requirements for disposal, particularly in the disposal of effluent. An extreme example is the need to introduce processing of waste instead of dumping at sea where sea-dumping would attract sharks. More common is the need to process excrement to avoid pollution, and mention should be made of the problem of finding outlets for chicken feathers.

The economic advantages of industrial routes are:

1. Area and volume are low in terms of units of protein produced.
2. Locations can be dictated by market requirements and can be with complete disregard for climatic variations.
3. Much of the cost can be reduced by standardisation.
4. Results can be assured because growth depends on the application of conditions which are imitations of conditions which have given success elsewhere. Within this advantage is the ability to scale up production from pilot schemes, and to vary output with comparatively little influence on per-unit cost.

The disadvantages facing economic planners include:

1. Certainty of economic success depreciates as planning periods increase. With high initial capital it would be better to plan well ahead but the stability of energy and feed prices is suspect, with little flexibility within planned systems for changes of energy or feed. It is difficult to switch from electrical to water power at short notice without losing the stock in hand. It is likewise difficult to switch from mainly-oilcake feed to mainly-microbial protein feed without exhaustive feeding trials.
2. The organisms which provide the most acceptable proteins are those which are likely to instigate objections to factory farming and producers can face serious rejections.

3. Production must be associated with a certain and effective disposal organisation. Since the protein is produced at a high rate with no periods of hesitation and no facilities for matching output to erratic demands, the disposal organisation needs to be constant, not related to seasonal or accidental demands. Free-range chickens can be killed as required but battery chickens need to be killed at a stated hour of a stated day. In effect, industrial routes need a supporting freezing industry or a dehydration industry.
4. Technical developments are inhibited by non-technical factors, including personal objections to eating unfamiliar food and to buying familiar food in a revised form.
5. With few exceptions, production relies on uncontrolled supplies of embryo stock, energy and feed. It is comparatively easy for a project to be made economic or uneconomic by some person or authority not directly concerned with the production.

PROTEIN AND FOSSIL ENERGY SOURCES

The relationship of orthodox forms of energy to human vitality is complex, giving rise to interesting but suspect calculations that a human body radiates with the energy-equivalent of a 60 Watt light bulb and labours with the energy-equivalent of half a kilowatt upwards. On this basis, human labour costs 200 times the price of fossil energy, which is why machines have largely replaced men.

In effect, any organic substance has to be evaluated in terms of its ability to provide body energy or some other form of energy. Up to about 1700, the choice was between human energy and animal energy with the animal frequently providing body energy for later use as human energy. Since 1700, there has been progressive employment of fossil fuels, augmented in recent years by nuclear energy. These have proved so convenient and effective that many natural sources of energy, such as sun and tides, have been neglected. Broadly, the division of energy sources is into those which are material and may have sensible uses other than burning, and those which are movements of air or water which have no evident use other than conversion to heat or light or controlled force. The material sources further divide into those which are replaced by nature within a reasonable period, and those which when used are never to be seen again.

One of the many calculations of fossil energy reserves indicates that total reserves are only about 1% of the yearly delivery of energy from

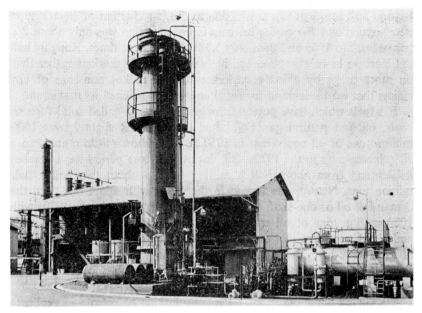

Fig. 3.   Protein from petroleum.
Pilot Plant Fermentor at Lavera Refinery, France, which is operated by BP's French associate.

the sun and are much lower than the energy potential of wind and tide movements perpetuated by solar radiation. There would certainly appear to be no justification for using materials for their energy content before they have been used for some useful structural or chemical function, of which this context has an interest in the potential conversion to protein. Notably, the potential of oil as a raw material for protein is of urgent interest after prices rose from $1.75 to $10.0 within two years and completely changed the economics of oil usage.

The commercial development of oil dates from the late nineteenth century, when lamp oil was needed to replace the expensive and smoky animal fats and vegetable oils in common use. The lighter petrol fraction had no obvious outlet until the arrival of the motor-car, after which it became the major consideration in oil politics. Petrochemicals were, and are, small consideration in the general pattern of oil consumption, almost all of it being converted into heat with notable loss.

From about 1925 to the middle 1960s, energy consumption increased at an annual rate of about 3.3%. The rate subsequently accelerated beyond 5%, much of which was due to the introduction of electricity to new populations. *Per capita* increase in consumption was only about 2% per year up to 1965 and then only 3.3% up to recent times. Roughly half the increase in consumption can be blamed on new markets rather than on more usage by existing customers, which makes nonsense of any claims that world demand for fossil energy has reached its maximum.

The fuels which have potential for protein are so-called solid fuels or coals, oil and natural gas. Solid fuel demand was slightly over 1000 million tons of oil equivalent in 1950 and has shown little more than a 50% increase up to the 1970s. Oil, during the same period has increased its demand from about half a million tons to about two and a half million tons. Natural gas started in the 1950s with about one-third the demand of oil or one-sixth the demand of coals, ended in the 1970s with 1000 million tons of oil equivalent or two-thirds the demand of coals and about two-fifths that of oils. As might be expected, there is a direct link between *per capita* energy consumption and the Gross National Product of a population but this link is too variable to have serious value. One variation is the proportion used by a population for vehicles. In the United Kingdom in 1971 the consumption of petroleum products in vehicles was about 20% of total energy consumption but in the United States gasoline for cars accounted for about half the total energy consumed.

All consumption patterns can be expected to change as energy costs increase. Supply patterns can also be expected to change as higher selling prices introduce new sources previously thought not worthy of effort or capital. Unconventional sources of oil, such as shales and tar sands, have more oil than conventional oilfields but the degree of extraction depends almost entirely on the price of oil. There is an estimate that total world oil is 10 million million barrels, of which 38% is not likely to be discovered and only 25% would be within reach for extraction. An alternative estimate puts the oil within reach at 850 000 million barrels, of which about one-third has already been used. According to the reference, we have oil for any selected period from 10 to 200 years. The vagaries of estimation apply particularly to the United States, which has sufficient oil to last until 1985 using present extraction technology.

Present extraction technology, geared to a price of one dollar per barrel, leaves three barrels in the ground for each barrel sold. Using gas or water as backing pressure, now that the oil price warrants the capital expenditure, increases extraction to about 60%. Using back pressure and a solvent to draw the oil out of the rock could give total extraction, which would supply the United States for about sixty years at the present consumption rate (which would probably not be held if oil prices rose to allow more expensive extraction). A very high price for oil would justify extraction from unconventional sources, which would probably allow America to survive for another two centuries at least.

It is not probable that the future price of n-paraffins from oil will be sufficiently low for protein culture outside the oil-producing countries. In fact, since the main future demand would be for this fraction of the oil it is doubted if even the oil producers would find protein-from-oil economic. The 1971 pattern of oil production was:

	Million barrels	% of total
USA	3478	19.9
USSR	2701	15.5
Iran	1657	9.5
Saudi Arabia	1642	9.4
Venezuela	1295	7.4
Kuwait	1068	6.1
Libya	996	5.7
Iraq	622	3.6
Nigeria	556	3.2
Canada	483	2.8
Indonesia	326	1.9
Total 11 main producers	14 824	84.8

Future patterns will include the influence of the fact that 61% of known reserves are in the Middle East. Tar sands could prove to have stocks which rival those of conventional oilfields, although extraction beyond a few hundred million barrels per year is unlikely before 1985. The stocks of oil held by shales can be variously calculated according to the oil-strength of the rock investigated. With rocks richer than 10% petroleum by weight there could be up to 20 million million barrels, which is twice the early optimistic estimates of conventional oil.

The general conclusion regarding oil and protein is that the selling prices of n-paraffin fractions will make it difficult for protein manufacture from n-paraffins to be economic. There should, however, be a surplus of other fractions generated in the world demand for light fractions. Hence, the petrochemical industries could find a comparative reduction in their raw material costs if they avoid the n-paraffin fraction.

Protein manufacture would therefore develop more rapidly if it could use one of the unrequired fractions.

As a point of interest relative to fuel stocks, the calculation of total coal in the world is 10 million million tons and this could last at least 2000 years. At the present stage of research and development, coal is not a probable raw material for protein culture.

Natural gas, to complete the trinity of fossil fuels, is an exceedingly probable raw material for protein culture. Estimates of world stocks are impossible since the richer sources are now thought to be well below the 3000 m depth, in sedimentary formations not yet visited. Despite the development of special vehicles it is logical to use gas near to the point of extraction, preferably converting it into a liquid or solid form which can be handled in conventional vehicles. The use of the gas as feedstock for microbes is one of many possible conversion techniques, development being controlled mainly by the price relationship of protein to other derivatives of methane. In this connection it is only a matter of time before the development of a process for converting methane gas into a liquid fraction to use in internal combustion engines. Processes for converting the methane into protein as organisms already exist and are sufficiently developed to promise perhaps a million tons of protein-from-gas by 1980.

At the time of writing, early 1974, microbial protein has a ready market in animal feed at a price of the order of £200($450)/ton dry weight protein, mainly as replacement for soya or fish meal. It is fairly obvious that a protein project will be able to pay relatively high prices for petrochemical raw materials, although it is likewise obvious that protein projects will seek the least expensive feedstock, which petrochemicals will not be.

Chapter 31

World Protein Supply and Demand

SUPPLY

The sun pours out 5×10^{23} horsepower, which is 3.8×10^{23} ergs/sec. The earth collects only one part in 20 million of this energy, and manages to lose half of this in atmospheric disturbances. Most of the energy flows from the tropics to the poles, from whence it is radiated away to be lost for ever. A little is caught in passing by vegetation using photosynthesis. The annual fixation of carbon by vegetation is thought to be of the order of 56×10^9 tons. Most land-based plants convert about 1% of radiation reaching their surfaces but the more plentiful and efficient marine algae are said to convert up to 7% of available radiation. Conversion in the first stage is to carboyhdrate, about 140×10^9 tons/year, which could become 35×10^9 tons of protein. This would be 10 tons *per capita*/year or 500 times the quantity needed. This is a suspect and rather pointless calculation but it serves to indicate the vast potential available from natural generation. Natural generation in accessible places can be increased by providing more green leaf per unit area, by reducing the energy loss in evaporation, by retention and conversion of selected parts of the solar spectrum, and by emphasis on vegetable proteins rather than on animal proteins. At least 30% improvement of yield can come from mulching to retain water in the soil and enclosure of plants to reduce evaporation from leaves and to provide a higher conversion temperature. The probable practical maximum for protein production by exposed crops in an excellent climate is of the order of 4 tons/acre of dry weight protein. Crop protection might increase this to 6 tons but there would be drainage of the soil chemicals and heavy manuring would be essential. There is a calculation that man can reach good arable land to an extent of about one acre *per capita*. Other animals can also reach the acre to consume part of the harvest, and it can be taken for granted that not all the harvest would be taken in before it deteriorated. All such calculations of harvest per area *per capita* are highly suspect. A more practical realisation is that only about one-tenth of the surface of the earth is suitable for arable farming, and most of this is outside the regions which show the highest existing and expected populations.

Direct calculations of the potential output of natural protein are further complicated by the interaction of food chains. There are three basic food chains:

1. *The predator chain*, comprising initial absorption of solar energy by plants which are eaten by animals. Large animals eat smaller animals.
2. *The parasite chain*, in which small animals eat large animals or rob large animals of energy.
3. *The saprophyte chain*, in which microbes use dead tissue as sources of food.

As a rough approximation, each change of state of the food is at 10% efficiency, a man eating fish needing 10 kg of fish to manufacture 1 kg of human protein. The 10 kg of fish need 100 kg of zooplankton, which in turn need 1000 kg of original plant plankton. In fact, chemicals are constantly being passed up and down the chains with heavy losses, sometimes jumping a stage and sometimes following a saw-edge pattern of movement. It is impossible to give even a vague calculation of total world protein potential without considering the influence of climates and accessibility. Furthermore, production at sea is within a layer some 200 m thick, which allows radiation to reach a higher number of organisms than is the case on land, where production is only over a single layer of surface. There is therefore justification for perpetual mixing of the upper reaches of sea water to increase the producing depth, associated with a perpetual extraction of organisms so that other organisms may have more room to develop.

Of calculations, the most effective is that man can now reach useful land to an extent of about one acre *per capita* and that the land could be made to produce up to 4 tons dry weight protein/acre. Climatic conditions reduce this to a hypothetical 2 tons/acre on dry land but it is probable that marine sources could give a compensatory 2 tons *per capita*.

There is no doubt that man will push his frontiers on dry land outwards into the ocean depths, so increasing the effective area. Also, microbial protein could, if need be, deliver 100 000 tons/year/factory acre, although other areas would be needed to furnish the raw material for the microbes. There is no reason for statements that man is reaching the limit of availability of protein from natural sources, although he has reached the limit of available supplies using existing methods of production, handling and distribution.

The vegetable fraction of food produced from original sun energy starts with sugar and finishes mainly with cellulose, the ultimate carbohydrate polymer. It is not probable that man will ever be able to catch more than a small proportion of the transitory sugars and starches. Even under controlled conditions up to two-thirds of the carbohydrate needs to be harvested as high polymer, which is not suitable for human digestion and has little value in stock feeding. It is possible to use the cellulose fraction for microbe production to give protein, possibly with a two-stage process involving initial breakdown of the cellulose followed by yeast culture on the breakdown products. Alternatively, cellulose can be hydrolysed by boiling in sulphuric acid to render sugars, which can then be feedstock for yeasts. 1973–1974 costings show that acid routes should give a sugar cost of about £30/ton from low-cost cellulose with a plant cost of about £1.5 million for a 70 000–100 000 tons/year project and a subsequent fermentation plant could cost about £1 million for 100 000 tons/year. Spread over five years the final dry protein cost should be of the order of £20/ton plus the sugar cost of £30. On present costing it is probable that waste cellulose could be converted for a selling price of £50/ton dry weight protein, one-quarter of prevailing dry protein costs using fish meal or soya.

An alternative route is to feed the vegetation to livestock and accept only 10% conversion. A higher conversion rate is practical by confinement of the livestock and it is possibly by confinement to rescue the waste products for algae culture. The ultimate rescue is probably division of the excrement into solubles and insolubles, the solubles being passed on for algae culture and the insolubles dealt with as waste cellulose. The details of production depend on local circumstances but all need to utilise the entire pattern of chemicals in the original vegetation, including those which have passed through animals and are in effect partly pre-treated ready for fermentation. The concept of food from excrement is not disgusting, it being an improved version of the natural route through field droppings, saprophytic degeneration and subsequent use of the by-products in new vegetation.

The marine picture is not quite so simple. On land, man has physical contact with the products of photosynthesis and can extract desirables before converting indigestibles. In a marine environment the ultimate product at present is fish protein and supplies depend on the degree to which breeding of fish can be encouraged. It is pointless to extract vast quantities of virginal fish but likewise pointless to leave old fish to die and rot or be eaten by other fish. The taking out of adult fish to a maximum extent is acceptable if young fish can be left to breed, stocks being self-compensatory if depletion results in an increase of the proportion of young fish. Selective catching is unlikely and it can be forecast that world fish stocks will decline, particularly if drag-netting and vacuum systems are allowed to develop. The available waters are:

	Surface million km^2	Volume million km^3
Deepwater—		
Deepwater Pacific	165.25	707.555
Deepwater Atlantic	82.22	318.078
Deepwater Indian	73.44	291.030
Deepwater total	320.91	1316.663
Intercontinental—		
Arctic	14.06	21.453
Australasia	8.14	9.873
Americas	4.31	9.373
Europe	2.97	4.318
Intercontinental total	29.48	45.017
Inland—		
Hudson Bay	1.23	0.158
Red Sea	0.44	0.215
Baltic	0.42	0.023
Persian Gulf	0.24	0.006
Inland total	2.33	0.402
Shelf waters—		
Bering	2.27	3.259
China	1.25	0.235
Japan	1.01	1.361
Andaman area	0.80	0.694
North Sea	0.58	0.054
Saint Lawrence	0.24	0.030

	Surface million km²	Volume million km³
Shelf waters—*contd.*		
Irish	0.10	0.006
Others	1.83	1.420
Shelf waters total	8.08	7.059

World total area is 360.8 million square kilometres over a total volume of 1368.471 million cubic kilometres. The average depth is 3783 metres but only the top 200 is of direct interest until plans for stirring the deeps are realised. Of the 500 million square kilometres of earth surface about 70% is water. From this, catches are of the order of:

	Million tons
Europe—	
Norway	3.1
Spain	1.5
Denmark	1.4
United Kingdom	1.1
France	0.75
Iceland	0.7
Poland	0.5
West Germany	0.5
Portugal	0.5
Italy	0.4
Holland	0.3
Total Europe	12.1
Africa—	
South Africa	1.1
Angola	0.3
Total Africa	3.8
Americas—	
Peru	10.6
USA	2.8
Chile	1.3
Canada	1.3
Brazil	0.5
Mexico	0.4
Total Americas	17.9

	million tons
Asia—	
Japan	9.9
China	6.9
India	1.8
Thailand	1.6
Indonesia	1.2
Korea	1.1
Philippines	1.0
Taiwan	0.65
Vietnam	0.6
Burma	0.4
Bangladesh	0.4
Malaysia	0.4
Total Asia	28.2
USSR	7.3

Catchings are largely dictated by local preferences other than where the fish is caught for canning or for meal. Consumption in so-called developed countries is of the order of 20 g animal protein *per capita*/day. In developing countries, mainly because distribution systems are lacking, it is of the order of 9 g animal protein *per capita*/day. These are averages and have no significance because consumption is not evenly spread. Of more significance is that only about 5% of USA animal protein is of marine origin, whilst 63% of Japanese animal protein consumption is of marine origin. The average proportion in the world is of the order of 12% as fish in the total animal protein. As meat prices continue to rise it can be forecast that more fish will be exhaustively caught and stocks will decline rapidly. It is not improbable that the fish content of average animal protein consumption will rise to 20%, particularly if freezing methods are extended into developing countries.

The grand total of about 70 million tons caught in the world can be roughly classified as:

	Million tons
Herring, sardines, anchovy	19.0
Cod, haddock, seapike	10.7
Various bony fishes	6.7
Tunny, bonito, mackerel	4.9
Salmon and trouts	3.0

	million tons
Flounder, halibut, sole	1.4
Sharks and rays	0.5
Molluscs	3.2
Other shellfish	1.7
Sea animals	1.0
Freshwater fish	8.9
Various unidentified	8.6

There is intensive effort to develop the catching of unfamiliar fish, with the hope that fish fingers and reconstituted ground fish will help to hide the new diet when it reaches the consumers. There could be benefit from emphasis on catching the more vicious predators, notably shark, which are rivals for the stocks of plankton-eating fish.

The Peruvian disaster has disturbed the pattern of meal production but the 1971 breakdown is indicative:

	Fish meal production in million tons 1971
Peru	1.95
Japan	0.70
USSR	0.40
Norway	0.40
USA	0.35
South Africa	0.30
Chile	0.25
Denmark	0.25

In a normal year, fish meal output is about 6 million tons. It could increase rapidly, from improvements which make it suitable for human diet and from wider appreciation that most marine life is suitable for fish meal and that there is no need to confine meals to small fish of the anchovy type, particularly since using the small fish means seasonal operation, which is uneconomic. It is therefore probable that existing types of fish meal will be upgraded for human consumption, being replaced by plankton meal and microbial protein in animal feed.

It is not probable that the consumption of traditional fish will rise to any significant extent. In general, catching costs related to probable catch weights indicate higher retail prices, but at the time of writing, cod in the United Kingdom is over 70 pence/lb and has met consumer rejection.

Per capita consumption of fish per year is roughly 70 kg in Japan, 10.5 kg in Europe and only 5 kg in the USA.

The main problem in fishing is that opportunities for low-capital projects have already been realised and are showing production costs which can result in only higher retail prices. Lower retail prices, which would maintain the market, are only possible by heavy investment, which appears to be unwise in view of pollution of waters and failure of nations to agree on controls. It is fully realised that most of the capital-intensive schemes will rapidly destroy stocks and that returns on capital will not justify short-term operation. The main hope of increasing supplies of marine protein is to ignore the existing familiar finned fish, to possibly reduce catches thereof to safeguard future stocks, and to concentrate on extraction of other marine life which has so far been neglected.

With the understanding that the accuracy of statistics is a function of the honesty and education of those who supply information, world agriculture in contact with authorities can supply the following dry weight protein:

	Million tons
From Meat	20
Dairy products	10
Eggs	3
Cereals	75
Roots	⎱5.25
Pulses	⎰2.2
Oilseeds	40
Fresh vegetables	18
Fish	14

There is double-accounting in this table because much of the vegetation and about one-tenth of the milk is used for animal feed, to be repeated after loss under the heading of meat. Offsetting the double-accounting is an undetermined unrecorded output from private gardens, hunting and unpublicised fishing, and the gathering of wild vegetation. The final total reaching human diet is probably about 150 million tons dry weight protein, of the order of 135 g *per capita*/day.

FACTORS WHICH INHIBIT SUPPLY

In all sources the inhibition to increased output is the lack of education which could be applied to increasing areas and reducing losses. Vast areas in Siberia, Amazonia and Africa have yet to be opened for cultivation. Even within easy reach of existing skilled farmers there are significant areas which are both unproductive and undecorative. The problem is not only the lack of education but is also the lack of willing people to educate. Agriculture as an occupation has a bad image in almost all societies, and it frequently warrants such an image by virtue of the poor pay and uncomfortable working conditions.

Labour problems could seriously reduce the total world availabilities of proteins. In early 1974, European dairy farmers claimed impossibility of operation because grain had increased in price. Cereals had increased from about £30–£70/ton, and comprised some 85% of feed—the other 15% being protein cake which had shown a similar price rise. The real problem was that dairy farmers could not find labour to convert to grazing, or to bring in daily fresh vegetation, but were restricted to bought stored feed. A reduction of dairy farming, as operated by European farmers, means a reduction of beef output after an initial glut of beef as herds are thinned by removing heifers. Much of chicken-and-egg protein output also relies on bought feed, the increase in price of which cannot be offset by setting the birds to open-range scavenging. Broadly, any fraction of the protein supply which relies on imported raw material has been made suspect by inflation. Fractions which rely on local raw materials should increase output to take advantage of the higher prices and to replace expensive imports.

Declines in fractions of the world protein supply will be in flesh proteins more than in vegetable proteins. It is much easier to apply mechanisation to plants, which stay in one place from seed to harvest and can be ignored for a few hours to allow labour to work reasonable hours. Animals are mobile, sensitive and inconsiderate in their times of giving birth or needing food. Also, if protein quantity is the target the fact that livestock need six times their growth rate as food input (and perhaps more under common conditions of rearing) is important. In terms of efficiency of production of human flesh from available protein it is ridiculous to feed milk powder and protein-rich feed to animals, simply to convert the chemicals at high loss to another form of edible protein.

Expansion of output can be expected in vegetable proteins, partly from the considerable effort of governments and international agencies, partly from natural increases in working populations but mostly from improvements in crop selection. If, for example, high-protein cereals become universal they will add an extra 60–70 million tons dry weight protein to the total, which is equivalent to a three-fold increase in meat output.

The key to future protein supply patterns is the rate at which consumers are given, and are educated to accept, foods which are not conventional diet. Deflavoured and reflavoured animal feed is an obvious selection for development, including imitation meats made from vegetable protein concentrate. Microbial protein and cultured algae also need to be included as substances which can be manufactured where other crops will not grow. In theory, good agricultural land should be used mainly for high-protein crops for human diet, poor agricultural land should be used for houses and factories, including factories to manufacture cultured protein from the waste produced in the houses and factories. Systems already exist for the conversion of urban waste into excellent protein at a cost which is of the order of one-quarter that of high-protein animal feed.

Unfortunately, protein output is frequently the last consideration in the allocation of land and the application of labour. *Per capita* output of agricultural products increases in so-called developed countries, where sophisticated methods can be used, but the output is restricted to maintain prices. *Per capita* output in many so-called developing countries has fallen, because population increase has favoured urban social groups in which the extra people are either industrial or idle. Comparing the middle 1950s to the early 1970s there have been falls of *per capita* production in agriculture of:

	Fall %
Philippines	1
Argentina, Morocco, Paraguay and Peru	4
Indonesia	5
Cuba, Syria, Tunisia	9
Chile	10
Uruguay	14
Dominica	17
Algeria	36

The reasons for the mentioned declines are many and they cannot be blamed entirely on urbanisation. The serious declines can be related to political disturbances and some of the less-serious declines were helped by fruitless agricultural schemes without efficient planning.

In theory, agricultural output should increase proportional to the expansion of populations and proportional to the rate at which fallow land can be cleared and improved. The theory is made invalid by the high rate of increase of urban population and an associated movement of agricultural labour into industry. Population growth rates are, roughly:

Under 1.5%—USSR, Europe and North America.

1.5–2.5%—China, Oceania, Central Africa, Caribbean, Israel, Japan, South Africa, Korea, Mongolia, Vietnam.

Over 2.5%—South America, East Africa, West Africa, Near East, Northwest Africa, Central Americas, and most of Asia not mentioned as below 2.5%.

About one-quarter of the world population is increasing at a rate of below 1.5%. Another quarter is increasing at a rate between 1.5% and 2.5%. The other half of the world population is increasing at a rate above 2.5%. World population is by no means evenly spread over the available land. Allowing a generous 1 hectare/person as a mean *per capita* necessity for food production, Europe, China, the Caribbean and most of Asia are fully populated. USSR, the Americas and coastal Africa could withstand an eight-fold increase of population to occupy all available land. Oceania and central Africa could probably increase fifteen or twenty times before they ran out of land.

Per capita *production value, various countries, 1970, World Bank opinion*

	Population (millions)	Gross National Product $ bn.	GNP per capita ($)
United States	204.8	974.2	4760
Sweden	8.0	32.5	4040
Kuwait	0.8	2.9	3760
Canada	21.4	79.1	3700
Switzerland	6.3	20.8	3320
Denmark	4.9	15.7	3190
France	50.8	157.4	3100
West Germany	61.6	180.3	2930
Norway	3.9	11.1	2860
Australia	12.6	35.5	2820
Belgium	9.7	26.3	2720
New Zealand	2.8	7.6	2700
East Germany	17.2	43.0	2490
Holland	13.0	31.7	2430
U.A. Emirates	0.2	0.5	2390
Finland	4.7	11.2	2390
United Kingdom	55.7	126.7	2270
Czechoslovakia	14.5	32.3	2230
Austria	7.4	14.8	2010

Per capita *production value, various countries, 1970, World Bank opinion—contd.*

	Population (millions)	Gross National Products $ bn.	GNP per capita ($)
Israel	2.9	5.7	1960
Japan	103.4	198.8	1920
USSR	242.8	434.9	1790
Libya	1.9	3.4	1770
Qatar	0.1	0.2	1730
Italy	53.7	94.6	1760
Puerto Rico	2.8	4.7	1650
Hungary	10.3	16.5	1600
Poland	32.8	46.0	1400
Hong Kong	4.0	3.8	970
Cyprus	0.6	0.6	950
Malta	0.3	0.3	810
Bahrain	0.2	0.1	550
Lebanon	2.7	1.6	590
Zambia	4.1	1.6	400
Oman	0.6	0.2	350
Turkey	35.2	10.9	310
Rhodesia	5.3	1.5	280
Jordan	2.3	0.6	250
China	836.0	121.9	160
Kenya	11.2	1.7	150
Uganda	9.8	1.3	130
Sri Lanka	12.5	1.4	110
India	538.1	57.3	110
Pakistan (then including Bangladesh)	130.2	12.8	100
Ethiopia	24.6	1.9	100
Rwanda	3.6	0.2	60

DEMAND

Demand is a function of numbers and *per capita* purchasing power, with the proviso that *per capita* purchasing power may be delegated to authorities buying on behalf of individuals. It is much easier to define than to satisfy. Each person needs a basic ration to become a healthy contributive member of world society. Without this basic ration the person is a liability and a danger, insofar that a sick person promotes social disorder and is sensitive to infections which can spread amongst more fortunate members of society. Sickness from protein deficiency is made more effective under modern conditions of mental confusion and stress. If earlier man had protein deficiency he fell sick and probably died without influence on more than a few others. If modern man has protein deficiency it is the humanitarian concern of all others, but is also a potential hazard which needs to be eliminated (the hazard, not the man).

Above the basic protein ration, each person needs a supply to compensate for inevitable waste in consumption and to provide raw material for the cultural aspects of diet. With sufficient protein already produced, and further supplies not difficult, there is no logic in a strict parsimonious diet when extra food can bring joy to a troubled world.

Affluent societies

Affluent societies are those with high *per capita* incomes relative to prices, whereby individuals collect material assets and spend a reasonably low proportion of income on food. Food is bought from highly-organised distribution systems, with several handling stages, each of which adds a contribution to the final retail price and supplies of food are through trade and processing industries. Up to the mid-1960s the form and presentation of food was almost entirely dictated by the manufacturing and processing industries. Through the 1960s there developed a situation in which larger retailers took over responsibility for the form and presentation of food. Manufacturers and processing industries found it advisable to send out a product under many brand identities, whereas previously the product had existed only as one well-known identity.

Consumers in affluent societies enjoy a mixed diet which is over-rich in carbohydrate and fat. Refined sugar is a major component used to supply instant energy and most of the protein is derived from cereal, which introduces more carbohydrate. Protein deficiency is comparative, the main problem being overdoses of carbohydrate and fat which reduce the effectivity of protein consumed. Excess fat comes partly from the habit of frying food, and there is a difference in diet pattern between those who use solid fat and those who use liquid vegetable oils.

Protein deficiency associated with low calorie intake is common in affluent societies, arising mainly from ignorance and from the spoiling of good food by bad cooking. There is also deficiency arising from limited time allowed for feeding, notably amongst office workers who also suffer from lack of movement in environments of constant mental stress. Genuine protein deficiency in affluent societies would not be eliminated by any provision of extra supplies, although protein-rich quick beverages and protein-rich bread for sandwiches would help. One result of poor diet in affluent societies is the introduction of health additives which, in theory, offer the traces and vitamins which are missing from normal urban diet. It is indicative that the current outlet for yeast is as a health additive.

Over the past half century in affluent societies there has been a movement away from the family as a social unit. In Europe the movement was instigated by independence of individuals during the 1914–1918 war, when young men were torn from families to fight and young women replaced men in industry. War was followed by economic chaos, which caused migrations and family ruptures, to be followed in due course by another war, generating more independence, and a subsequent period of economic reorganisation. The result of this brief history is a division of purchasing into two types.

1. Purchase by the individual for his or her own consumption.
2. Purchase by a representative of a group, which may be a family, from a common income and for common consumption.

In the first type of purchase, which is mainly impulse buying, the proportion or character of any protein involved has no significance. Purchase is of convenient satisfaction, the price being examined by the purchaser in terms of convenience and satisfaction compared against similar products. Diet is mainly a function of the occupation of the consumer, suitably modified by any social activities. Food is mainly pre-packed and purchase is of the package, not the food.

Purchase on behalf of a group, which may be a family, is mainly by elder generations who compare asked prices against remembered prices for the same product. The purchaser is fully aware of the contents of a package and will seek lower prices for like goods regardless of the packaging or advertising. Slow increases in retail prices are acceptable but rapid increases bring consumer rejection. When United Kingdom prices for butter increased in anticipation of EEC membership there was a general swing towards margarine. Likewise, high meat prices in the USA and Europe brought consumer rejection.

Inflation during the early 1970s encouraged the purchase of semi-capital manufactures, and discouraged the purchase of food. There was a general reduction of food intake, which probably did more good than harm in affluent societies, and a reduction in the proportion of protein in diet. Since most consumers in affluent societies buy roughly twice their minimum requirements of protein, the reduction of protein purchase after inflation could be insignificant providing the carbohydrate and fat intake does not increase in compensation. Taking the United Kingdom as an example, protein intake up to 1970 was about 28% above the recommended intake. In 1971, this fell to only 24% above recommendation and it fell even further in 1972–1973–1974.

There have been many detailed studies of the relationship of prices to demand in the inflationary period of the early 1970s. Most need to be treated with extreme caution since they are narrow in their investigation and are based on statistical information more than on human reactions. Distribution within affluent communities favours inert preserved and processed foods, the supply of fresh food being difficult but carried out because a significant market exists. It is possible to define a steady state of supply including fresh and inert foods, 1970 being a reasonably stable year before the disturbances of speculation by merchants and the oil crisis. A typical steady state exampled by the United Kingdom was an average of £37 income/household, of which a little short of £31 was spent on goods and services. About a quarter of expenditure was on food, which equates to £2.11 *per capita.* Of this, £0.60 to £0.65 was on seasonal fresh foods and about £0.55 was on inert packaged foods. The total United Kingdom food bill was a little short of £7000 million, roughly divided as:

	£ *million*
Bread and cereals	900
Meat	1970
Fish	240
Oils and fats	320
Sugar and sugary products	650
Dairy products	1050
Fruit	410
Vegetables	780
Beverages	410
Manufactured food	220

The provision of a satisfactory protein diet to elderly consumers has its own problems. Elderly people spent their formative years during periods when less was known about nutrition and there was limitation of variety amongst foods. They find it difficult to adjust, particularly to the lack of personal service in modern distribution. Frequently, shopping is done on their behalf but a very large proportion of elderly people have to shop in strange circumstances which are largely not designed for old or infirm consumers. As a rule, elderly people are limited in their purchase power and the money which they do have is made less effective by the difficulty of finding small portions. In the United Kingdom in 1971, almost 9 million elderly people spent £1342 million on food, much of which was ill-spent on protein-deficient foods or on excessive portions of which much was wasted by non-consumption. The United Kingdom situation is worthy of study since it is roughly a compromise situation between the various extremes in other countries.

Of the United Kingdom elderly people:

43% have difficulty in walking
30% have arthritic hands which limit carrying
50% shop 2 or 3 times per week
15% shop 4 to 7 times per week
2% never go shopping
33% have help with their shopping
28% found difficulty in reaching shops
50% use small shops, of which two-thirds prefer small shops
68% use supermarkets, of which 50% prefer supermarkets
33% found small shops expensive
1% found small shops inexpensive
3% found supermarkets expensive
16% found supermarkets inexpensive
90% complain that there are no seats in shops

Poor societies

Affluent societies resemble each other because affluence brings mobility and communication. With a few notable exceptions, poverty is caused by a local circumstance and the impoverished are unable to escape their environment or seek curative technology through experience of foreign societies. Also, affluence brings education and technical imitation, whilst poverty is directly associated with ignorance. Protein is lacking in diet because consumers do not have the money to buy it and do not have the capital to generate purchase power amongst consumers, and do not have the education to develop local sources or to imitate foreign producers.

The need is not only to supply protein. If protein is supplied without associated improvement in welfare and education the result can only be extended misery and an increase in population, which means more protein deficiency in more people. Obviously, protein needs to be supplied as charity during the period of development of purchase power but the main target must be the introduction of development capital and education to manufacture a higher level of welfare which will generate its own satisfactory supply of protein. Agriculture is only one sector to be granted vitalising capital, and it may not be the most important. The late 1973 allocation of funds by the UNDP is indicative:

	Total grant ($m)	—of which, for agriculture ($m)
Afghanistan	20.0	5.270
Barbados	2.5	1.025
Bolivia	15.0	4.900
Botswana	5.8	1.614
Congo	7.5	3.115
Dominica	7.5	2.235
El Salvador	5.0	0.820
Guyana	5.0	0.191
Iran	20.0	5.436
Lebanon	10.0	4.005
Maldives	1.0	0.261
Mexico	20.0	3.572
Morocco	20.0	4.327
Pakistan	18.5	5.638
Papua New Guinea	5.0	0.281
Paraguay	7.5	0.732
Rumania	7.5	0.685
Rwanda	10.0	1.990
Sierra Leone	7.5	1.708
Sudan	20.0	5.942
Swaziland	5.7	1.192
Turkey	20.0	4.375
Upper Volta	10.7	4.087
Uruguay	10.0	1.720

It should be stressed that UNDP funds are not the only source of capital but they are indicative of the extent to which agriculture has significance in fund allocation. They reflect long-term planning, being too slow in formulation to include aid for events such as the Sahara drought. Disaster funds came mainly through UNICEF, including direct material aid which cannot be effectively costed.

There is a significant difference between protein deficiency in affluent societies and protein deficiency in poor societies. In affluent societies the deficiency is developed in adults who choose unsatisfactory diet. Infants are well fed during the critical first few months and through the following five formative years, and faulty diet is unlikely to produce a damaged brain or body chemistry in the children of an affluent society. In poor societies there is protein deficiency or unsuitability from the time of birth. The deficiency results in imperfect brain formation, leading to inferior mental ability in the later adult. This leads to a perpetuation of protein deficiency through ignorance regardless of the availability of protein supplies.

Recovery from protein deficiency in affluent societies is mainly a problem of correcting personal diet, after which the person regains health. Recovery from protein deficiency in poor societies is a medical problem because there is body damage, and a social problem in that deficiencies will be perpetuated if the social structure is left in its traditional shape.

There are two extremes of individuals who are subject to protein deficiency:

1. In an affluent society, the person who is under high and continued stress including genuine fear of his own environment. Such a person selects diet for its convenience and speed of consumption, and absorbs food during periods of mental tension. Nervous instability is increased by pollution (notably by metals and carbon monoxide) in air, food and water.

2. In a poor society, the person who is generated and reared in circumstances of poor protein supply and poor education. Such a person selects diet according to historic familiarity. Any innovation is suspected, mainly because the subject lacks the education to appreciate any applied reasoning.

These are extremes, but they are sufficiently numerous to confuse the issue. Such consumers are not in a fit mental condition, and need attention other than the straightforward supply of protein.

As far as the majority of consumers are concerned, there are two main demands. The first is a low-priced protein food which will be bought as basic nutrition at a price which is directly related to the available income, and as an alternative to high-price flesh protein. The second demand is for protein food to be consumed as part of the pattern of social life, tailored according to the conditions of consumption. In effect, the former is essential chemical requirement so that the body can function. The latter is, for want of a better description, food for the soul. Essential as it may be, the provision of basic protein rations is only a first stage in the development of a healthy person.

Mixed societies

Affluence and poverty are relative terms, as are developed and developing, educated and ignorant, well-fed and undernourished, and all the other divisional classifications used to describe people. Societies are intimate mixtures of degrees of wealth, learning and health. Some are dominated by identifiable groups who can be given attention but it is important to realise that all characters of individual can be found in most societies, including characters who are deficient in protein. One common deficient character is the urban office-worker living alone, drinking too much alcohol and eating too much refined carbohydrate, too busy to eat cooked meals during the working day and too lazy to prepare balanced diet during the evenings. Another common cause of protein deficiency is mental stress, which arises from many causes including the hypothetical need to accumulate wealth.

It is a well-known fact that urbanised man and woman seeks status in the competitive atmosphere of excessive proximity. To maintain this status the individual seeks and performs tasks which are beyond normal ability, inducing mental stress and compensatory extra physical effort and self-denial. The body is denied the food and recovery periods which are essential for correct function, leading to disorders of digestion and blood chemistry which make the self-denial more damaging.

The theoretical *per capita* protein requirement is from about 35–150 g/day according to body weight, condition and activity. It can be shown that recorded world output of protein could provide an average of 135 g and unrecorded output is considerable. It has been stated that there is a problem in distribution which denies each individual his or her ration. It can now be appreciated that there is a further problem unrelated to questions of supply and distribution. Individuals in the midst of plenty are likely to suffer protein deficiency because they exist in false environments and are engaged in activities which inhibit protein absorption. Hence, although United Nations statistics and other arithmetic statements of situations have value, they do not give an accurate picture of the overall problem and can hide social factors.

In Western Europe the average protein intake per day is of the order of 85 g of which 60% is of animal origin. In Eastern Europe the intake is near 100 g with one-third from animals. In North America the intake is 95 g with two-thirds from animals, Australia and New Zealand being similar. In so-called developing areas of Africa, South America and Asia the intake is from 50 g–100 g with the proportion from animals mainly 25% but reaching 60% in some meat areas. It is impossible to generalise in the confusion of tribes, nationalities and geographic circumstances of Africa, South America and Asia. It can be accepted, however, that there are parts of the world which are, for various reasons, denied their fair share of world protein. A rough estimate based on average intakes and populations shows this misplacement of protein to total about 21 million tons dry weight protein per year, or from 100 million tons upwards of protein foods.

If farm labouring can be encouraged the most satisfactory way of inducing populations to absorb any new protein supplies is to develop agricultural outputs in the famine areas, if only because the output will be of familiar foods at reduced prices since they are from domestic production. Such a world scale of increase of agriculture would require a 100% increase of meat, or a 200% increase of dairy products, or a 25% increase in vegetable output including the introduction of the new high-protein cereals and roots. It is obviously more practical to concentrate on the vegetables, particularly since many of the unfortunates are vegetarian and most of the areas lack facilities for storage and distribution of sensitive meats or dairy products. Also, vegetable harvests can be made to increase in short development periods whereas animal routes need a long development period.

There are two outstanding problems:

1. To provide more protein where needed, partly by extraction from oversupply elsewhere and partly by new sources. The notable required transfer of protein is dairy protein from the surplus production in so-called developed countries, which could satisfy 5% of the urgent demand. Increases in agricultural output may or may not satisfy the requirements but there is more potential in microbial and other new proteins using industrial routes.

2. To mould societies or sectors of societies so that any supplied or generated protein is absorbed. This means the introduction of familiar proteins or the up-grading of familiar food by the addition of protein. Present opinion is that microbial protein has the ability to be used in compounding, notably in bakery products, and has the weak flavour to be compounded in high proportion without local objection. Also, microbial protein avoids the religious complications, even if it carries the psychological complication of 'eating germs'. Part of the moulding of social conditions includes the provision of a low cost imitation meat, probably based on textured soya or pulse, which can be used to force reductions in fresh meat prices.

Chapter 32

Speculation

Speculation is a necessity in civilisation. It is anticipation of events and related forward planning, and concerns all stages of the food chain from the initial crop, which is planted or reared according to anticipated profit, to the eventual buying of food for consumption, the purchaser buying early if a price rise is forecast. It is the economic backbone of trade and industry and is the theoretical skeleton of distributive structures. In a lazy world, changes in supply and prices have been slow and could be related to reliable previous events. Most sectors could follow harmonised patterns of speculation, leading to collective development with very few economic or social disasters. In the extreme example, the demand for chipped flints declined progressively from the stone age to the present day and its rate of decline to the few remaining flint-knappers was predictable at all stages. Likewise, the demand for shoes could be anticipated with accuracy using personal income as a guide.

During the early nineteenth century there was development of marketing and persuasion of identified groups to buy. There was also much cross-linking of activities so that supply and demand became a complicated subject, leading to the present state of affairs in which food is absent from supermarket shelves because there is a famine of plastics for packaging and because there is a shortage of oil for the initial ethylene and styrene. The influence of oversupply or undersupply now extends far beyond the visible applications of the material involved.

This influence has become world-wide. The current drift of the Sahara southwards can be regarded as a repeat of the prehistoric East African famine. This early famine destroyed half the population, introduced cannibalism into mythology and religion, and spread the Bantu throughout Africa after they had overcome their fear of crossing the Zambezi. The later famine, in the 1970s, destroyed 0.75 million tons of edible vegetation and most of the livestock. There is, however, no fertile land for the unfortunates to take over and the problem becomes a world problem with influence on world food stocks. As far as the world grain trade is concerned, there is a reduction of stocks and an increase of demand, which is motivation for grain withdrawal because future prices will rise. The removal of stocks in anticipation of price rises is a further reduction of supply, which promotes more speculative buying for storage, and the situation gets out of hand.

It is now realised that events in any part of the world have influence on situations in all other parts of the world. It is also realised that shortages and gluts are given false proportions by extraction or release of supplies. Furthermore, since mankind has grown to rely on imported supplies for his survival, selling prices can rise or fall with dramatic severity in response to comparatively slight shortages or excesses. It is now freely accepted that the conventional laws of supply and demand do not apply in a communicative world which contains speculators. Arising from this, there is realisation that societies need to produce their own food in isolation from supplies which may be restricted for economic or political reasons. This applies particularly to food processing industries, in which the cost of raw materials varies from 50–80% of the retail selling price. If raw costs double without warning such processing industries cannot survive, it being impossible to pass on obvious large price increases to consumers without some reduction of demand.

The relationship of shortages to price rises can be illustrated by Peruvian fish meal. The normal catch of 2 million tons is a small quantity in world protein for animal feed but it was anticipated by world agriculture and the migration of the anchovy upset economic planning. It signified a probable shortage which could be used by speculators as reason for increasing prices of alternative protein feeds. Peru faced a situation of having orders for 400 000 tons of meal at a contracted price of $165, at a time when they could not supply. By the time the anchovy might have returned, but did not, the world price had risen to $265 with Peru still committed to 400 000 tons at $165. If the anchovy had sufficient neglect for a few years the outstanding debt would be no problem but each year of neglect means a higher loss per ton of the eventual production. It could be that the Peruvian fish meal industry will not recover.

The relationship of shortages to price can also be illustrated by United Kingdom white fish supplies which are influenced strongly by the inflation of meat prices. In 1972, the United Kingdom landings dropped by 29 000 tons to 860 000 tons, about 3%, but the wholesale value rose 10% and retail prices rose 15%.

Another illustration concerns grain in 1972. Crop conditions deteriorated in most countries, there being coincidence of wheat and maize failures from drought and/or ill-timed wet weather with rice failures from non-arrival of monsoons. India had to buy grain contrary to expectation and there was an unanticipated demand for 30 million tons from the USSR. Even so, the shortage was within world stocks and could be described as a paper shortage, not an actual shortage, and one good harvest could refill warehouses. Unfortunately, there was heavy buying by unspecified merchants, which means merchants buying for speculation not application, and the early 1973 prices showed annual increases of 70% for wheat, 55% for maize, 65% for barley, 65% for rye, 80% for oats and 50% for sorghum.

Speculative purchase of goods for temporary storage and delay of application until prices rise from created shortage is destructive and inflationary. It encourages further justified purchase ahead of requirements by users who must have known raw costs over a planned period. This takes capital out of the economy, locking funds as reserve stocks when they could be applied to new equipment or labour for expanded production. The 1972 speculation in grain has caused:

1. Encouragement of grazing instead of using bought feed, bringing about an associated change of pattern of animal rearing.
2. Revision of economic calculations to include a present 50% and a further feared 50% rise in raw costs, inducing inflation since calculated margins have been increased to allow for the further increases. Such revisions concern all sectors of society, including distributive trades.
3. A reduction of working capital, more being held as stocks or in reserve against future unanticipated demands.
4. General distrust of trade as an instrument of supply of essential goods.
5. Increased effort to find new sources of protein, notably green leaf and microbial protein.

6. Political tensions arising from failure of countries to meet contracts and from the imposition of controls which subsequently were shown not to be necessary.

7. Distrust within trades arising from enforced reductions of freight rates by as much as 25%.

Much of the inflationary pressure from trade speculation comes from the uncertainty of the degree of future price rises. If all raw materials could promise a common price rise of, say, 25% it would be sensible for projects to be planned on a basis of 25% rise in raw costs. When the probable rise in raw costs may be anything from 10–200% it is logical for planners to use 200% in calculations of operating costs, and therefore of eventual selling prices. Hence, even if the first-stage inflation is only 50% there will be second-stage inflation of 200%. This type of inflation can only be halted by removal of the uncertainty of raw costs. It is not probable that world raw materials can be controlled other than by reduction of the demand to below harvest-and-stock levels. In the case of protein food, this means an early introduction of very low-priced alternatives.

The vagaries of raw costs can be exampled by changes in price of the following:

August 1972–1973, USA % increase		October 1972–1973, West Germany % increase	
Cotton	160	Wheat	145
Wool	125	Rye	170
Rubber	145	Soya	90
Copper	80	Cotton	175
Zinc	150	Wool	80
		Rubber	70

A planner who has little time to study the finer details of economics might well read the above tables as indicative of a general increase of about 150%, with 200% as a safe anticipation. Such a planner would not be in a position to realise that his local price increases need not necessarily be similar to world price increases, nor would he differentiate between:

1. Non-renewable raw materials, notably the metals, with regard to which any speculative storage is safe because world supplies have a finite limit and prices can be expected to rise sharply.

2. Renewable agricultural products, such as natural fibres, which face competition from other materials. The logic in speculative storage of such materials depends on the alternatives. In natural fibres there is trade speculative storage to take advantage of higher prices when oil reductions bring price rises for synthetics.
3. Renewable agricultural products in which supply is a function of annual area and weather. In academic terms there is no logic in speculative storage of such crops because the cost of storage will lead to lower margins for a later sale, particularly when old crops are sold against the higher-quality new crops. In practical terms, there is logic in speculative storage of such crops if the storage cost over a year is less than the price rise of the product.

Obviously, there is advantage to the supplier in holding back production and disposal so that prices rise. The real danger to suppliers is that consumers will observe uncertainty in their future supplies and will seek alternatives. In any event, consumers will reduce purchases because the higher prices will encourage better product utilisation. It is fairly safe to predict that per-consumer demand for future raw materials will decline roughly at the rate at which prices rise. Per-consumer demand for finished products can be expected to decline with more determination as prices rise. In theory, raw costs should be allowed to increase at the prevailing rate of increase of purchase power, giving the buyer a slight incremental advantage since there is a time lag between purchase of raw material and purchase of finished product.

Householders use speculative storage of dry goods and wet goods in a domestic freezer. In most affluent societies there has been a dramatic increase in semi-bulk buying for household use, and in the use of home freezers. The average home freezer can hold protein food to a value of perhaps £70, which is bought in advance of price rises. The actual financial gain by a housewife in semi-bulk buying and in home freezing is relatively small, but the retaining of private stocks by the housewife enables her to reject prices and refuse to buy for up to three months.

Speculative storage at the production end of the food chain is inflationary and it encourages devaluation of the product as consumers seek alternatives. Speculative storage at the consuming end of the food chain is deflationary. Both confuse the issue of supply and demand by displacing the date when statements are effective. When the United States issued a statement of grain availabilities for 1972 it should have had a one-third reduction to cover purchases by unidentified buyers, this third of availabilities being displaced in time to the subsequent period of inflated prices. Likewise, when the United Kingdom meat industry claimed that retail sales were not reduced by higher prices, the statement should have included the fact that housewives and anyone else with spare freezer volume were buying meat in anticipation of further price rises.

As a general rule, price inflation at a rate of 3–4%/year passes without comment amongst consumers. The price rises during the critical 1972–1973, September to September, period included:

	% *rise*
Canadian No. 1 14% wheat	145
Canadian No. 2 rye	170
Canadian No. 2 oats	75
USA Yellow maize	95
Sugar	25
USA Soya beans	275
Indonesian copra	185
Nigerian groundnut cake	75
United Kingdom wool	55
Argentine beef	45
United Kingdom bacon	52
USA packaged frozen fish	30
USA tinned sardines	3
USA tinned tuna	8
USA fish meal	100

As will be seen in this table, speculative storage inflated the prices of animal feed more than the prices of finished products. Even so, the increases of end-product prices are sufficient to raise rebellion amongst ultimate consumers. The result of speculative storage at both ends of the food chain, as far as links in the chain were concerned, has been at least 100% increase in input cost, more expensive conversion, and refusal of the market to accept 50% rise in prices. Damage to the structure of processing and distribution has been mainly to trust between primary suppliers, handlers, converters and ultimate consumers.

USA wheat, intentions and realisations

Million acres and million tons	1970/1	1971/2	1972/3	1973/4
Winter wheat				
Intended area	38.3	38.1	42.2	43.2
Harvested area	32.7	32.4	34.9	38.5
Intended production	28.0	28.3	35.1	34.8
Harvested production	29.7	31.1	32.3	35.9
Spring wheat				
Intended area	13.2	15.5	14.8	14.6
Harvested area	10.9	15.3	12.4	15.1
Intended production	9.9	9.8	5.7	11.5
Harvested production	7.1	12.9	9.7	10.7

World agricultural recorded output

Million tons	1971	1972	1973
Wheat	353.82	347.38	364.34
Rice	309.10	295.18	317.50
Maize	305.61	302.90	313.17
Barley	151.45	152.44	157.59
Root crops	554.36	535.75	554.45
of which potatoes	293.17	280.69	292.74
Pulses	43.58	43.60	45.18
Other vegetables	267.11	269.06	273.27
Grapes	53.98	51.59	55.27
Citrus fruit	38.97	40.69	41.68
Bananas	31.62	32.92	32.73
Apples	20.96	19.45	20.44
Nuts	2.74	2.76	2.87
Meat	106.92	109.04	109.52
Milk	405.60	412.08	415.46
Eggs	21.95	22.36	22.59

Rice production, geographic distribution, FAO opinion

Thousand tons	1966/68 (average)	1970	1971	1972
Far East	246 882	281 365	281 437	268 424
Latin America	9 897	11 798	10 688	11 797
Africa/Near East	8 486	9 192	9 610	9 495
North America	4 211	3 801	3 890	3 863

Rice production, geographic distribution, FAO opinion—contd.

Thousand tons	1966/68 (average)	1970	1971	1972
Europe	2 449	3 101	3 214	3 217
Oceania	218	268	319	270
Total	272 143	309 525	309 158	297 066
Price index (1957/59 = 100)		104	86	99

(Price index for 1973 was 142)

Meat production, geographic distribution, FAO opinion

Million tons in 1973

North America	25.00	Near East	2.20
Western Europe	21.20	Far East	4.00
Oceania	4.00	Asia	15.70
Africa	2.95	East Europe plus USSR	20.90
Latin America	10.90		

Milk production, geographic distribution, FAO opinion

Million tons in 1973

North America	60.65	Near East	12.10
Western Europe	123.00	Far East	39.10
Oceania	13.40	Asia	5.45
Africa	6.40	East Europe plus USSR	120.00
Latin America	27.00		

Cereal production, geographic distribution, FAO opinion

Million tons in 1973

North America	280.23	Near East	43.08
Western Europe	150.04	Far East	227.23
Oceania	17.63	Asia	229.74
Africa	40.23	East Europe plus USSR	257.11
Latin America	76.16		

Oilseed production, geographic distribution, FAO opinion

Thousand tons in 1973

	Cotton-seed	Ground-nuts	Rape	Soya	Sun-flower
North America	4700	1540	1260	43 880	330
Western Europe	340	20	1430	6	780
Oceania	60	50	20	40	80
Africa	1070	4490	13	70	50
Latin America	3030	1280	50	5830	960
Near East	2880	516	2	22	590
Far East	3700	7180	2390	815	—
Asia	3210	2637	1200	12 004	70
USSR	5040	4	940	874	7500
Others	100	339	12	130	240

Typical price movements, September 1972 to September 1973, in world trade

	Units	1972	1973
United States hard wheat	$/60 lb	2.14	5.16
Canadian rye	$/56 lb	1.19	2.86
Canadian oats	$/34 lb	0.84	1.69
United States yellow maize	$/ton	28.0	55.3
Argentine sorghum	£/ton	30.0	52.2
Caribbean sugar not to USA	c/lb	7.06	10.34
USA sugar	c/lb	8.76	9.01
Dutch onions	£/cwt	2.38	3.08
Central American bananas	$/40 lb	3.00	3.00
South African oranges	£/box (about 62 lb)	1.85	2.34
South African grapefruit	£/half-box	2.16	2.44
German apples	DM/100 kg	78.00	71.00
United States soya beans	£/ton	59.4	115.7
Nigerian groundnuts	£/ton	109.00	166.8
Indonesian copra	$/ton	138.00	360.00
Groundnut cake (Nigerian)	£/ton	59.6	121.8

Price movements mid-1972 to mid-1973, selected countries

All prices converted to US cents/kg

		1972	1973
Copra	India	54.3	78.3
	Singapore	12.3	30.4
	EEC	13.7	31.3
Cottonseed	India	10.0	20.1
	Japan	9.9	14.8
Groundnuts	India	27.0	56.4
	EEC	26.2	35.7
Linseed	Argentina	6.6	14.8
	United States	9.8	21.6
	Canada	11.5	27.8
	India	24.4	35.5
	United Kingdom	13.9	33.5
Rapeseed	Sweden	18.3	19.3
	India	29.4	38.4
	EEC	12.6	30.5
Soybeans	United States	12.2	36.7
	United Kingdom	14.4	20.2
Groundnut cake	France	10.9	36.1
	United Kingdom	12.5	39.1

Price movements, Rice, 1971–2–3

$/ton	Average 1971	Average 1972	Early 1973
Intergovernment contracts			
Burma 42% brokens	76.7	83.2	135.0
Thailand 35% brokens	81.0	96.2	135.0
Thailand 10% brokens	111.6	—	142.0
China 35% brokens	83.4	79.3	117.5
Private trade			
Thailand 5% brokens	129.1	150.7	203.3
Thailand husked 100%	130.4	151.2	202.4
Thailand brokens	67.4	94.5	123.0
Pakistan Basmati	202.4	—	400.0
Italy 3% brokens	80.4	171.3	346.8
FAO price index			
Private trade	83.0	105.0	150.0
Bilateral contracts	90.0	93.0	131.0

Chapter 33

National Situations (Selected Countries)

At the time of Neanderthal man, more than one-third of the people died before they reached the age of twenty and less than 10% lived more than forty years. Of Asiatic Sinanthropus, half died before they reached fourteen years, 10% died before they reached thirty and only 10% outlived forty years. Death was mainly by war, infanticide and casual battle. When man learned to live with his neighbour on settled farms, populations grew at a steady 0.5–1.0%/year. When he discovered the value of fossil energy, and introduced mechanical invention, there was almost no control over population growth rates and life expectancy extended to sixty years in most societies, three score years and ten in more comfortable surroundings.

About 10 000 B.C. the world held about 20 million persons maximum, 2 million minimum. The actual number can never be known but was probably near to 5 million. A nation was then a group of perhaps 400 people who had a vague idea that other people existed but rarely made contact. By A.D. 1750, populations were mixing freely and there were fixed frontiers, even if the geographic lines were disputed. By then, there were probably 750 million people, distributed as:

	Million
Africa	100
Americas	15
Asia	500

	Million
Europe	120
Oceania	2
USSR	30

There was then widespread utilisation of fossil fuels and a general introduction of technology. By 1850 the total population had reached 1200 million and by 1950 it had reached 2500 million. The multiplication over the 200 years had been:

	Multiplication
Africa	2.0
America	22.0
Asia	2.5
Europe	3.0
Oceania	6.5
USSR	6.5

In effect, there had been a movement of people and culture out of Eurasia, which held 80% of the world population in 1750, notably into the Americas. It was possible to divide nations loosely into those with original culture, farming and food, and those with a foundation of originals under a new, energetic, population which had foreign culture, agriculture and food. The exodus from Europe was the largest mass movement in history, particularly since much of it was as controlling minorities in new countries.

From 1950 onwards there was progressive development of independent nations but the frontiers were political and artificial. There was also a reversal of the migration pattern, particularly with foreigners seeking education and work in Europe. It can be presumed that there will be an ultimate similarity amongst the people of all nations but at present each has to be regarded according to its history of migration and commercial exploitation. The following examples illustrate the point:

ANGOLA AND MOZAMBIQUE

Portugal regards Angola and Mozambique as part of Portugal but there is a racial attitude which is illustrated mainly in the degree of education and responsibility found amongst natives. White authority is maintained by military power in some areas whilst black authority is maintained elsewhere by similar military power. It seems impossible to develop economic stability whilst the region is thus divided, particularly since the heavy cost of military operations prevents effective investment. On the other hand, progress was initiated by the realisation that economic development must take place if full-scale war is to be avoided. The pattern of production is mixed with emphasis on agricultural products. It is fully appreciated that the agricultural and fisheries potential is vast but there is a serious shortage of investment capital and a steady refusal by Portugal to let foreign investment become seriously involved. South Africans have come into the country to raise cattle and there is a constant flow of workers into South Africa, frequently by illegal movement across the borders. The question is asked whether Angola and Mozambique will in future be dominated by Portugal or South Africa, or whether true independence will be realised against all economic odds.

Protein production could be realised by all known routes but will probably develop around beef cattle. The rate of beef development will depend strongly on how quickly nomadic herdsmen can be converted into settled farmers but it will also depend on the degree of entry of South African capital. Another controlling factor is water distribution but this is already a major interest, not only for farming projects but also to develop mineral interests. Protein crops are also probable and there could be interest in upgrading coffee waste by growing yeasts.

ARGENTINA

The Pampas of Argentina is probably the world's richest natural grazing area and cattle have been ranged for over a century. Selected areas have sufficient water for arable crops but neither arable crops nor beef have developed at a rate indicated by the available terrain and climate. Mostly, this has been because producer prices for cereals and beef have been kept low and neither land nor equipment have been preserved in good order. Farmed areas are reducing as the law is applied which dictates that the property of a man must be divided equally amongst his children when he dies.

Agricultural practice is far from efficient and some yields are the lowest in the world. There is a national deficiency of phosphate which should be fairly easy to overcome but there is also a national aversion to chemical treatment of the soil. Foot-and-mouth disease is endemic amongst the cattle and it has proved impossible to vaccinate the 50 million cattle three times per year.

The potential for protein from Argentina is almost exclusively through traditional agricultural routes which could increase output several times if producer prices were adjusted to encourage activity. The meat output would certainly have to be related to processing, even if this comprised no more than deboning and defatting before deep-freezing.

BLS (BOTSWANA, LESOTHO, SWAZILAND)

The three former protectorates which form BLS are defined as independent but are ruled by clients of South Africa. They are enclosed by South Africa and over half their revenue is related directly to the customs union with South Africa dating from 1910. In 1910 it was intended that BLS would later be incorporated into South Africa but this did not occur and, in fact, South Africa reversed the intention by offering independence to its own ten native tribes. Hence, there is a political brotherhood between BLS and the Bantu but, because South Africa dominates, comparatively little economic coordination.

BLS needs a European outlet for production, to replace the preferential United Kingdom market and to escape dependency on South Africa. Such an outlet can only be agreed if BLS can offer equal rights to its European market and to its present dominating partner South Africa, but South Africa is unlikely to allow removal of its privileges or to relax its control of the BLS economy and there are examples of South Africa restricting development within BLS, such as the destruction of the plan to produce fertiliser in Swaziland from imported nitrogen. This project stopped because it was claimed that such a scheme would make South African farmers dependent on foreign suppliers. A project for milling of maize in Lesotho was likewise stopped but was later rescued by another milling company. It is therefore not probable that there will be significant industrial development in BLS and agriculture can be expected to be kept at a low level of productivity and efficiency. The small countries cannot compete against South Africa and South Africa shows no intention of promoting development.

Botswana has about 700 000 people. Half the country is unproductive Kalahari desert and most of the rest is poor agricultural land. Cattle are reared but the main revenue comes from workers who migrate into South Africa. The potential revenue is in minerals including a very large diamond pipe likely to produce stones for another century at least. With such wealth to be developed it is doubted if agricultural development will attract much capital when better land is available elsewhere and within reach. No significant developments of protein are expected but, for political reasons the cattle industry could be given public support, possibly with private neglect.

Lesotho is the smallest and poorest of the BLS countries. There are mountains which could be used to develop a tourist industry but no other economic prospects. The soil is poor and incapable of supporting the population, despite the fact that able-bodied Basuto migrate to work in South African mines. Broadly, the only resource is cheap labour and there has been some effort to introduce industry which will not damage South African interests. It is probable that Lesotho could develop as an African Switzerland with similar tourist facilities and a mixture of light industries. There is some effort to modernise agriculture but this depends on ability to stop soil erosion and to develop horticulture more than agriculture. The potential for protein in bulk is not high but there is a need for industrial protein production, possibly microbial or algae protein, to replace shortfall in conventional agriculture.

Swaziland has the highest *per capita* income of the BLS countries. Population is towards half a million and there is no need to send workers into South African mines. The economy, through land ownership, is mainly in the hands of South Africans and is fairly balanced between minerals and agriculture. Sugar and wood pulp are important sectors and both could become sources of industrial protein by fermentation, particularly since the Sahara is evidently moving south and producing more famine areas as it moves.

BRAZIL

Brazil is a big country and is concerned with big development projects, such as the Urubupunga hydroelectric scheme and the Amazonian highway. Few countries can rival Brazil in terms of untapped resources including the population. Land and labour are more abundant than is capital but agricultural developments are slower than might be expected. Coffee dominated and was profitable until stocks had to be increased to maintain prices and much profit was lost in the deterioration of such stocks (which at one time equalled total world demand for one year). It was then realised that growing surplus coffee was a waste of good land and diversification should be encouraged. Coffee output was reduced and the new low output figure coincided with the 1969 frost and then drought, further reducing output. There is opinion that coffee beans will become a minor item in shipment and that most future coffee shipment will be of extract. This is doubted but it has led to trials with coffee waste as cattle feed, there being some possibility that coffee waste could develop to be as important in animal feed as is soya, particularly if soya is directed more into human diet through simulated meat.

Residue from instant coffee manufacture is being used in mixed feed. The average composition is 24% oil, 10% protein and 36% fibre. This composition makes it of interest only to ruminants and the only significant reason for its use is the low price.

The opening of Amazonia is important. The area is 5% of the earth's land area and has been neglected beyond a few attempts to develop rubber (including the only failure by Ford). Hydroelectric potential is more than the total electricity used in the USA. There are 10 million hectares available for arable crops and probably nine times this area available for herded animals, but the problem is, as might be expected, the size and cost of any project which could be effective. The intended highway will involve up to 3000 miles of road through difficult country and meeting structural problems not previously experienced. It is not yet known, for example, what influence a twenty-mile cleared ribbon through dense jungle will have on climate and ecology although it is known that there will be changes which will dictate the structure of the road.

Urbanisation is rapid, with Sao Paulo absorbing half a million people from 1500 miles around within fourteen years. In such a rapid growth it is inevitable that a gap should develop between the rich and poor within urban limits and a further gap between urban poor and rural poor. Thus Brazil comprises a confused mixture of social conditions ranged from primitive Amerindians to very rich urban property dealers.

The potential for protein production is vast. Green leaf protein would be an obvious development were it not for the fact that arable crops grow rapidly. Algae protein would be equally obvious if there was less potential for high-value fresh vegetation. Microbial protein is attractive for its rapid high profit to new industry but it will need to be related to animal husbandry. In general, there is potential for any route to protein production with productivity tied to the rate at which capital and labour can be recruited and to the pattern of skill which can be introduced into the economic structure. Almost certainly there will be an influx of foreign influence and Brazil can be expected to grow into a major developed country with an international character of the type realised in the United States.

Statistics are too temporary to have significance in Brazil but some measure of the rate of growth can be appreciated from the fact that Sao Paulo state had slightly more than 8000 tractors in 1950, over 61 000 in 1960, and now at least 160 000. Exports from Brazil are now worth about $5500 million but should reach over $20 000 million in about five years and inflation has run at about 20%/year but may now be nearer the target of only 12%. Development has been far too rapid and riches have come to a very few whilst many are worse off and the greater proportion of population has seen no change.

Foreign direct investment is responsible for only about 5% of the economic effort but foreign money is buying into Brazilian enterprises at an increasing rate. The question asked is how long Brazil can continue its growth at 10%/year, and its higher domestic inflation rate, before something unknown yet but certain to be drastic comes to pass. One answer is that growth must continue because Brazil is the richest potential source of raw materials and agricultural land left to be developed. Rapid growth brings its own inflation and the government of Brazil have already faced rebellion from the milk industry. Since the milk industry managed to obtain its demanded price increases by withdrawing its supply, there is a good chance that the meat industry will make a similar threat. No one can forecast because there is a situation of growth and inflation which is unique. Over the past five years, one-quarter of wage-earners showed an increase in purchase-power whilst the other three-quarters showed a decrease.

Whatever happens in the wage-earning areas of Brazil is of little interest yet to those clearing the Amazon. Here, the workers are contracted at minimal wages from local populations or the north-east. Even in the more sophisticated agriculture of the south the workers are badly treated but are probably better off than the people in urban slums. In Sao Paulo, infant mortality rose from 6.3% in 1960 to 8.8% in 1970. With such a society the remark that Brazil is self-sufficient in meat should be treated with reserve. An extensive cattle project is intended to produce export beef within four years but there are problems. Feed is lacking in the August–November period, foot-and-mouth is already evident and will stop many export markets, available cattle are showing low reproduction and high mortality, and there is a shortage of money for deep-freeze facilities. Present cattle are in the Rio Grande do Sul region or in the Sao Paulo region. Rio Grande specialises in European breeds whilst Sao Paulo has Zebu cattle. There are probably 85 million head now in Brazil and some 315 cattle projects approved for the Amazon.

The cattle projects so far recorded have an investment value of about $400 million, with money from all parts of the world. In about five years these projects alone should carry 5 million head and provide 200 000 tons of beef/year. Slaughterhouses are intended at suitable points along the new highway. The existing cattle in Brazil are mainly sick from malnutrition, parasites and foot-and-mouth. There are forty-six authorised slaughterhouses and in 1972 Brazil exported 120 000 tons of beef worth $130 million. About two-thirds of the cattle are mixed milk-and-beef but only a third are in milk and some of these are being slaughtered whilst meat prices are high. It is possibly characteristic of Brazil that milk cows are dry or being killed for meat whilst dried milk is being shipped from New Zealand and Holland to feed the starving poor.

The entire Brazilian agriculture needs higher productivity and organisation according to regions. There are so many climates and soils that the country can hardly be examined as a single unit. Exports now account for about 8% of production and it is impossible to calculate the influence of the home market because wealth is so uneven. Coffee, sugar and cotton are important now but the future appears to lie in meat and soya. Forecast increases include 6% for sugar, 3% for cotton, an ambitious 47% for soya and a massive 100% for wheat. Most other crops are expected to increase 10% and coffee is expected to decline by 30%. Brazil is the world's largest producer of sugar, producing over 6 million tons with almost half for export and a production of 10 million tons before 1980 will be easy if markets arise. Annual soya production is now about 5 million tons after climbing at a rate of more than 1 million tons increase per year since 1970. As with sugar, increased output will be easy if the market is available.

In all crops and herds there is low productivity, area being increased rather than yield per area. Sugar productivity is only slightly above half that in South Africa and the USA. Maize productivity is less than half that in other countries and soya productivity is also low. Whether Brazil should aim for productivity when there are vast areas to be opened can be questioned.

In terms of potential protein it is worth looking closer into the opening of the Amazon. The intention is to drive a highway some 5300 km from north-east Brazil to Peru and to house up to 2 million poor inhabitants of the north-east along the road. Each settled family will get 100 hectares and a house and some money for equipment, and will be paid a basic wage and an allowance for jungle cleared. In theory, the first year will be used to grow subsistence rice and beans and then cash crops are expected. In practice, few of the intended peasants have shown much interest or ability and big business is beginning to move in. The average size of the cattle projects already mentioned is 57 000 hectares and at least one holding group is trying to buy 2 million hectares. If they succeed, strictly against the constitution, there are projects to about 36 million hectares intended by big business. (This is almost three times the size of England.)

The probability is that the opening of the Amazon will not proceed as planned, mainly because developments have to be too rapid for reasonable social improvement. In isolation, large landowners have introduced their own social structures including slavery. Also, the native populations are being denied their homelands and may yet revolt or become instruments of disruptive forces from outside Brazil.

CARIFTA COUNTRIES

The Caribbean countries are too near to North America, and have too pleasant a climate, for them to escape affluent tourism. It can be taken for granted that land prices will inflate progressively and that labour will find more attraction in service industries or industry than in agriculture. Since Trinidad became established as a significant refining point for oils there could be rapid development of petrochemical-based industries. The expected need is for labour-intensive activities which require little land, particularly conversion industries leading to high-value products which will reduce the effective influence of high freight costs.

With regard to protein, it is not probable that the area will be able to compete against larger land areas in the agricultural production of bulk crops, although it will have a ready market for high-value crops including products such as ginger and spices. Whether protein from oil is worth producing is doubted, the profit potential being lower than that of high-value crops and the market pattern lacking a significant outlet for low-cost protein. It is considered that the area is not suited to animal protein production because land is expensive and the climate is violent. There is no doubt that fishing could develop but the indication is that such fishing would have to concentrate on supplies for tourists and near export markets. There could be a profitable development of marine protein other than finned fish but there is doubt that local financiers will seek unusual adventures when familiar activity shows such a ready profit. Overall, Carifta countries are unlikely to develop as major protein suppliers othe rthan in the provision of products for early consumption with high prices.

CYPRUS

Cyprus has an unhappy political history, it being difficult to regard the island as much more than a joint off-shoot of Greece and Turkey. There are 120 000 Turks and 650 000 Greeks and almost no one else. The 1973 drought brought disaster to agriculture, with total failure of the cereals. Up to the drought, Cyprus had shown an 8.4% rate of economic growth against an intended 6.8% and therefore the disaster hit hard because it came at a time of maximum expansion. There could be collapse of agriculture, partly from the disruption of the organisation but also because there is a lack of water. Another factor is the fragmentation of land, seasonal labour and a general acceptance of back-yard techniques in farming.

The damage from the drought included buying grain at inflated prices. Wheat in February 1973 cost $95/ton and barley cost $76.5/ton. By the end of 1973 the wheat price had risen to $218 and the barley price had risen to $142. The collapse of agriculture after the drought probably cost Cyprus 10% of the GNP, which is roughly equal to the increases of GNP in non-agricultural sectors.

It would appear advisable for Cyprus to forget about basic crops and to concentrate on high-value crops using controlled growing conditions. The island seems to be ideal for the production of microbial protein, using fruit as a platform of development of fresh fruit for export and waste for fermentation to yeasts. Fermentation is a familiar technique in Cyprus, the claim being that the Queen of Sheba was an early customer for Cyprus wines.

DUBAI

Dubai has about 75 000 people living in 1500 square miles and is a port. It survives through trade and is sensitive to world influences on commodities. Good relations are necessary with neighbours and with foreign countries, including Iran which is a subject of territorial dispute but is also a market for smuggled goods out of Dubai, and a source of labour. A quarter of imports are on behalf of the state. Of the other three-quarters, at least 80% are probably for illegal entry into other countries, although the lack of records makes it impossible to accuse anyone of smuggling.

About one-third of the population is engaged in trade and about 17% are in communications. Administrators and unofficial government agents probably account for another 16%. The rest of the population is likely to be fully absorbed in a vast project relative to industries behind the port, probably based on petrochemicals but including almost all manufactured goods. It could prove profitable for microbial protein to be manufactured, if only to take advantage of the existing trade organisations, although there is doubt if any manufacture is necessary behind the largest port in the Middle East.

EAST GERMANY

Within the Comecon network, East Germany provides industrial products for other member countries. Since the other countries have mainly new demands the pattern of products from East Germany varies, with over half of the items being results of modern technology. Output depends on the availability of labour, which includes dilution from East Europe, Agriculture has been neglected with some justification insofar that in an integrated economic system it is better to locate industry in poor climates and agriculture where the sun shines. There are, of course, inevitable problems as Bulgaria, Hungary and Rumania transform from agricultural to industrial countries, particularly when such agricultural countries find lucrative markets other than East Germany for food.

There could be political complications if investment paid too much attention to agricultural needs but it would be in accordance with the system to invest in microbial protein. This, it could be said, is an automatic associate of feeding-grade urea as already supplied. Feed based on crops or agricultural protein for human diet is more the concern of other countries within the agreement and there is sufficient reverence for the agreement for investment in agriculture to be inhibited.

EEC

The agricultural structure of the EEC is complicated by administration. The Treaty of Rome in 1957 was followed by the European Atomic Energy Community (Euratom) and by the European Coal and Steel Community (ECSC). The original intention of the EEC was to formulate a common code relative to economic affairs, money, politics and legislation. The original six countries were Belgium, France, West Germany, Italy, Luxembourg and the Netherlands. On 22 January 1972 provision was made for entry by the United Kingdom, Denmark, Ireland and Norway. In September 1972 a referendum in Norway refused the offer to join the EEC but since Norway has only 200 000 farmers this refusal will not influence EEC agriculture. The 1973 budget for the EEC was £2100 million, 81% of which was for the Agricultural Guidance and Guarantee Fund (EAGGF or FEOGA).

The agricultural structure is dominated by the Common Agricultural Policy (CAP) which could change in due course but is now sufficiently complex and confused to prevent any early fundamental change. There is a Special Committee on Agriculture related to the Council but the main agricultural interest is at the Commission, which is financed by levies on imported agricultural goods, customs duties and up to 1% of value added tax after January 1975. At present, up to January 1975 there are direct contributions from member governments. In theory the Commission relies on:

1. Agricultural organisations represented at community level
2. Agricultural Structures Committee
3. Management Committees for product groups
4. Agricultural Fund Committee
5. National experts

These supply opinions which may or may not be used to formulate Directives (which are international law) and recommendations (which are not international law).

New members of the EEC have been given time to adjust their structures over a five-year period. Their financial contribution will increase progressively between 1973 and 1977 to full contribution from January 1978, although it is accepted that this date could well become 1979 or 1980. The full contribution will correspond to the proportion per member of gross communal product, viz:

United Kingdom 19%
Denmark 2.42%
Ireland 0.6%
Norway, if subsequently joins, 1.66%

Obviously, these proportions will alter and the UK contribution is expected to become at least 20%. From 1980 all members will contribute

90% of their agricultural levy and customs duties and VAT to the proportional extent of any deficiency in the fund. New countries will adopt the EEC support system but will set their own basic and intervention levels with progressive increases up to the EEC levels by 1978. UK deficiency payments will be phased out during the period.

Hence, for the transition period, there will be relatively free trade but subject to levies and compensatory payments but the levies will be progressively reduced. At the same time, there will be a universal drift of populations away from agriculture. This drift will vary according to the country. Italy reduced the agricultural population 1969 to 1971 by 340 000 but reduced by only 31 000 during 1971 because 1970–1971 was a depression period and the economy could not stand the rise in unemployment.

Much of the economy of farm operation depends on crop selection. Over the past decade, there has been a decline in production in Europe of rye, oats and potatoes, an increase in barley and maize and a slight increase in sugar beet although this is not likely to show much further increase. For the next few years the indicated growth area in agriculture is that related to fresh meat, including the feed but not including milk and dairy products.

Beef production in the original EEC countries is based on dairy cattle and any increase in beef will result in an increase of dairy products. The probability is that if EEC regulations remove the price-equalisation system in the UK for milk, then some areas of the UK will turn more to beef cattle, particularly in the south-west, and there could be a notable increase in beef exports from the UK into the original EEC. At present the original EEC countries import about 8% of beef requirements, not counting 1.5 million head shipped live into Italy (the proportion of these for slaughter is not recorded). There are special arrangements for the importation of cattle for fattening.

Pigmeat in the EEC has shown continued increase in consumption and this is about 53 lb/head for most countries including the UK. Supplies are from within the EEC from farms with 6 pigs (Italy) to 107 (UK). Demand could increase by 20% by 1980 and herds are increasing. Pigmeat products are calculated on a basis of original carcase price plus a set margin for processing. This margin is another subject of dispute which can be regarded as an unpredictable variable.

Sheep supplies for the EEC are dominated by France (68%) with Italy supplying about 18%. French flocks average 50 head, whilst the UK herds average 225. There are probably 19 million sheep in the EEC, capable of supplying to three-quarters of its demand. UK production of sheep meat is about 277 000 tons/year against only 171 000 tons for the rest of the EEC. It can be anticipated that the UK will supply the necessary meat. Sheep rearing has low priority in the original EEC and wool is regarded as an industrial product not included in agricultural manipulations. Inter-country trading is free for sheep meat within the EEC but imports have a tariff of 12–20%. It is inevitable that one outcome of UK entry into the EEC will be the organisation of the sheep industry and any present comment would be unwise. One important factor is the probable introduction of ewes which will reproduce throughout the year instead of only in a specific two-month period.

There is also free trade in poultry. UK consumption has increased recently to the general EEC level of about 23 lb/head. The EEC is self-sufficient and there is a subsidy for exports. New members will have advantage over old members because they have cheaper feed and compensatory payments will be paid to cover cost differences. Hence, old members will have an export subsidy if they sell to the UK and the UK will have an export levy.

One of the major complications of the UK joining the EEC concerns grains for feed. The total cereal area in the new EEC is nearly 70 million acres with:

35.5% of production in France
19.5% in Germany
17% in Italy
15% in United Kingdom.

The ten countries are 87% self-sufficient (the UK is about 60% self-sufficient) and imports are essential from Canada, Australia and the USA. It is not thought likely that human consumption of wheat will rise within the EEC, but imports are expected to continue for many years, although there is an occasional local surplus which is removed from the market by denaturing for animal feed. A surplus could develop and there is an urgent need for attention to storage methods so that surplus can be held back against famine harvests.

Most of the original six EEC countries have increased barley instead of soft wheat and oats, whilst UK barley has declined in favour of soft wheat. The future prospects for barley depend on the degree to which cereals are replaced in feed and it should be noted that the use of non-cereals in feed is already established in Germany and Holland. In general, oats are being allowed to decline in favour of barley and maize. Maize production through the EEC is increasing, including some 4000 acres in the UK. The United Kingdom presently imports about 3 million tons of maize/year, over half from the USA. The feed value per acre of maize is higher than that of other cereals but the present price is low. It can be expected that the Commission will introduce some regulation which results in higher farm prices for maize.

ETHIOPIA

The social structure of Ethiopia has changed very little in 3000 years. It is probably the poorest country in Africa, with only about 40% of production capable of being expressed in financial terms and over 90% of the population incapable of reading or writing. Many Ethiopians distrust education, discourage initiative of any kind, and consider that young people should be neither seen nor heard. With the paradox which is typical of the country, the structure is sensitive because absolute power is in the hands of a very few, whilst at the same time the structure is immobile and insensitive because the population refuse to recognise or accept change.

The majority live in feudal serfdom. Ninety per cent of the population are agricultural on land owned by the church, the government or by large landlords who have suitably served the throne. Tenants pay landlords from 30–75% of their crops as rent for the land, and have no security of tenure. Legislation to improve the situation is frequently discussed but it is difficult to establish effective law and order in the midst of ignorance and illiteracy. One of the reasons for the discussed legislation is the pressure from foreign countries refusing to continue aid if reforms do not result from the aid. In 1967, Sweden helped in the Chilalo Agricultural Development Unit on condition that Ethiopia carried out land reform by 1970. By 1970, no such reform had been made obvious and there was no evident point in Sweden providing more aid. Similar situations could be reported relative to other countries providing aid to Ethiopia.

About 30% of farmers own their land, possibly through tribal sharing. The soil is good and the climate encourages growth but the government spend only about 5% of the budget on agriculture and other landlords spend almost nothing on development.

Three-quarters of the arable land is more than one day's walk away from the nearest road. One-third of the population live more than 30 km from the nearest road. More roads are needed but it is difficult to convince administrators that they should spend money on roads.

The social picture of Ethiopia is not attractive, and it is not difficult to understand why famine should exist in a country which could, with compassion and planning, be the granary of North-East Africa. It is not possible to forecast any significant protein development, either through agriculture or industry.

FIJI

Fiji is a nation of half a million people spread over at least 800 islands. It has a precarious economy based on sugar. It also has a mixture of races, recently tabulated as:

	Numbers
Indians	263 000
Fijians	220 000
Europeans	24 000 (part-European are counted as Europeans)
Pacific islanders	13 000
Chinese	5000

There is inevitable racial tension, particularly since foreign investment has encouraged inflation. The economy is in the hands of the non-agricultural Indians and Europeans, whilst 80% of land is owned by Fijians, frequently in extreme poverty. The races do not mix and there cannot be satisfactory development of agriculture because the land is owned by one defined sector whilst investment capital is owned by the other. Fijians are also moving into urban areas, creating a problem which is made worse by the lack of free education.

As the profitability of sugar production falls there could be protein production from sugar but this will be entirely in the hands of the Indian population. As things are, roughly half the population would not benefit from any such industrial protein. The problem is not a shortage of protein, or even of malnutrition, but a matter of social disorganisation which needs to be overcome before there can be any real progress. There are 15 000 sugar growers and one miller. Sugar accounts for two-thirds of exports, six times more important in export than the next crop which is coconut oil, and roughly 30 000 people depend on sugar for their income. The sugar industry owns half the freehold land and there is already a problem of inflated prices for land. Of the income from sugar, two-thirds goes to the farmer and one-third to the miller.

There is a significant tourist industry and it would seem sensible to build up a high-value agriculture based on expensive fresh vegetables and fruit. At present the number of tourists is of the order of 200 000 and it could climb to 600 000 by 1980. This has further increased the price of land and agriculture takes second place.

GREECE

Greece has the advantage of a history which encourages tourists but lacks the political and social stability to profit by its income. Whilst still classified as a developing country, Greece has reached a level of affluence in which sophisticated control is needed to prevent chaos. Invisible earnings are important to the economy from tourism, shipping and money sent home from workers abroad. Tourism could become less profitable as more warm sunny countries, notably those distant from Middle East tensions, compete for customers. There has been some effort to promote small industries but Greek industry is already fragmented and promotion of small-scale industry is unlikely to have influence.

In agriculture the government faces the common problem of giving producers a fair price in a period when consumers are resisting inflated retail prices. There has been rapid industrialisation, notably using foreign capital, at a time when population growth has been very slow. With the constant movement of workers into foreign countries where they can earn more, there has developed a labour shortage which has led to a general shift of labour from agriculture to industry. Currently, about 42% of labour is in agriculture but this proportion could reduce rapidly. There are, in fact, proposals to transfer underemployed farm labour into industry. Also, shipyards have sought labour in the countryside, although it must be mentioned that most of the recruits (92%) returned home after saving 10 000 drachmas.

Foreign investment in Greece covers a wide pattern with aluminium production as a major consideration. This is loosely related to Algerian liquid natural gas which is exchanged for Greek alumina, Algeria having low-cost electricity to refine the aluminium. Greece imports about three-quarters of its energy requirements and is unlikely therefore to become a dominating industrial power in world economics. The land is described as good but neglected and needing better communications if agriculture is to expand. At the time of writing a dozen Greek engineering companies are jointly involved in producing roads across very difficult terrain and other cooperative efforts are concerned with land improvement and reclamation.

General comment on Greece is that future protein developments could be by industrial routes using foreign instigation and capital, or by agricultural routes if labour can be found for agriculture in the future. Cultivated land now covers about one-third of the country and is responsible for half the export value. Roughly 80% of farms are less than 10 acres and investment in farming is calculated at below £1000/farm. One-third of the meat consumed is imported and there are efforts to promote pigs and poultry which can be produced on the small farms.

Government efforts in Greece follow the conventional pattern of increasing farm area, introducing mechanisation and, since the meat shortage, concentration on animals more than on arable crops. In theory, by the late 1980s, this policy should release half a million rural workers for industry to cut the proportion of total workers in agriculture to 20% (half the present proportion). The broad intention in agriculture is to reduce food imports by growing more wheat, white meat and sugar beet, and to increase exports of tobacco, cotton and fruits. Even so, the share of GNP held by agriculture is expected to drop by the late 1980s to below 10%.

GRENADA

In Grenada, agriculture is primitive and disliked as an occupation, probably because it can be associated with slavery but also because it holds no promise of early riches or comfortable retirement. Accordingly, the government is faced with a problem of finding work for ex-farm workers in industry or tourism. In theory the solution is to divide the 120 square miles into lots which can be owned by prospective farmers but such division would produce uneconomic units. Exports are mainly nutmegs, cocoa and bananas but these are expected to decline in value as tourism brings in more real money. Decline could be rapid since planters have been left to carry the cost of higher wages whilst selling prices are pegged low.

In terms of potential protein production Grenada is unlikely to be a major contributor. The indication is that available land will be subdivided and used either for accommodation or for growing luxury vegetables for tourists. Industrial routes to protein are not probable although there could be development of microbial protein if some manufacturer sought a location where he could be free from industrial pressures in large industrial countries. It could be very convenient for a small isolated community to have regular income from a foreign concern dealing in a product which does not require manual labour and which does not rely for survival on erratic world prices dictated by large estates elsewhere.

HONG KONG

Land in Hong Kong is far too valuable for it to be used for growing crops or carrying animals. Nor is it likely that most of the population would take kindly to agricultural conditions. In effect, Hong Kong is a synthetic society based on manufacture and trade. There could be manufacture of cultured protein, although this would mean importing the raw materials and the manufacture might as well be located with the raw materials. The population density is of the order of 750–1000/acre and the outstanding problem is designing a social structure.

HUNGARY

Amongst other things, Hungary produces economists. Some are exported but a significant number stay at home and have positions of authority. They operate in a mixture of central planning and decentralised marketing, with notable success in agricultural affairs. National income rose 40% in the 1966–1970 five-year plan, which was twice the rise expected. The economic manipulations of wages, materials and margins are remarkably simple, which is why they work when more sophisticated systems in other countries become inactivated by self-strangulation. Hungary is a good country for economic experiments, being small with an educated population but without racial or tribal conflict. It is doubted that such a simple approach could be applied in countries where every move is suspected and where one can always find some pressure group to object to any venture.

Although engineering is favoured as a subject for development, chemicals have led the growth. An early agricultural background led to mineral fertiliser industries but, even in 1970 some of the fertiliser used had to be imported. Typical of the simple economic approach, chemicals are examined to decide if they can be bought cheaper than they can be made, which is why Hungary will not be self-sufficient in fertilisers but will profit from fertilisers produced in Bulgaria using Hungarian capital.

Twenty-five years ago, Hungarian agriculture used hands and horses in a feudal system of land tenure. By 1970, about two-thirds of agricultural output was from large farms. Farming was forced into modern times by the injection of heavy capital, and tied increases in output to food processing industries. This directly relates agriculture to industry and includes marketing, although there is the opinion that the long-term target is an industrialised Hungary using agricultural raw material from less-expensive Balkan land. Non-agricultural protein is under examination by the economists and it may, or may not, be attractive. If found attractive it will be developed and fitted into the master plan.

IRAN

Iran has limited supplies of oil which it can use for economic development and as a foundation for capital-intensive projects. Almost certainly, Iran will become the strongest national unit in the area if military and political situations can be controlled with skill. Growth rates of GNP have been of the order of 11–15% and should continue if land reform intentions take power away from feudal landlords. The intention is to reorganise the social structure and remove the very large number of small and unprofitable agricultural holdings. In effect, the large oil revenue is being used to bring prosperity to the impoverished agricultural sector and this can only be through central planning. It is doubted that *per capita* spending power could increase at a rate which could support available industrial development and the capital is therefore being used for general welfare improvement and revitalisation of agriculture. Over 40% of GNP is state expenditure but there is considerable private investment.

Agriculture employs about 40% of the national labour force and output rises by about 6%/year, but wages in non-agricultural activity are high and there is an inevitable shift of labour out of agriculture. One particular problem is that education is growing in urban communities and part of the shift from agriculture to industry is due to people seeking education. Accordingly, high-school graduates are used to teach village children and to encourage the formation of rural schools. The retention of rural labour depends strongly on ability to increase this education programme, almost as much as on ability to increase *per capita* earnings of farm workers. Whilst only about 10% of advanced students come from rural backgrounds and very few university students come from agricultural homes there is little potential for agriculture in the country, at least during the period when oil revenue dominates the economy. At present the ratio of rural to urban incomes is of the order of 1:5 and, whilst rural incomes have grown they have not been supported by rural facilities.

Iran faces the very difficult problem of dividing its considerable income of low-labour content amongst its poorly educated population of which 40% are in rural communities and need labour-intensive occupations. The inevitable conclusion can only be reduction of agricultural activity and increased dependency on imports or industrial production of food. In this climate the development of protein from oil is unavoidable although protein from natural gas would be more in keeping with potential supplies of raw material. Such a development is encouraged by the peculiar military situation which demands self-sufficiency in food and ability to produce such food without imported fertiliser or other essential material or service.

ISRAEL

The misfortune of Israel is that it was created as a nation under circumstances which made expensive conflict inevitable. The structure is unique in that there is a constant absorption of foreign capital and people with ready-made skills. The statement that less than 10% of the total labour force is in agriculture has, therefore, little significance when one considers that yields in agriculture are very high and frequently are world records. Production is limited mainly by a shortage of land to process and a shortage of water. Hence, the dramatic increase in productivity in occupied territories was inevitable.

The first wave of immigrants were of European origin from countries with a fair level of agricultural development. Later came the wave of people from moslem countries, mainly uneducated and low in agricultural skill, bringing a need to establish agricultural villages to absorb the labour and increase food supplies. Later came a wave of immigrants who came by free choice, not under pressure. These people brought high levels of culture and standards of living, and were highly educated young people.

The limited areas of land available to Israel can be expected to be used for high output of food providing mechanisation and planning can reduce the labour content of productivity. On the other hand, Israel appears to have ideal conditions for the production of proteins by industrial routes, possibly from oil but also likely from bulk carbohydrate crops grown intensively for fermentation. Animal husbandry in general takes too much area but there is potential for poultry rearing, possibly associated with microbial protein feed.

Developments in traditional agriculture date back to the 1968 Jerusalem Economic Conference (Millionaires Conference) designed to introduce technology into Israel economic effort. As a result, new crops were planted and there was more planning for preservation and shipment. The emphasis was taken away from citrus and tomato and placed on high-value products and new forms of food, including SVP which is meat substitute from soya beans. The mixture of religions and prejudices in Israeli society helps to develop substitute foods and provides a domestic market for almost any food produced.

IVORY COAST

The Ivory Coast suffers from foreign control over the economy, and from differences in levels of welfare in various parts of the country. In the 1960s there was a healthy economic growth at 8%. Resources for industry are limited and the main business is agricultural, notably cocoa, coffee, fruit and timber. The stability of the country attracted many foreign workers. From a quarter to a third of the working Africans are from other countries and the French population is roughly double that before independence. Europeans own up to 90% of the modern sectors of the economy.

There is an inevitable subsidiary problem of urban unemployment, which is seen to be a possible nucleus for unrest. This sub-problem is indirectly related to that of the regions which have inferior standards of welfare, and are likely to provide more unemployed urbanites if conditions are not improved.

In effect, the country is divided into two by a stretch of virgin forest. On the east side are the rich cocoa farms, the timber concessions, most of the industry, all the roads and both big cities. In the south-west, which is 11% of the area, live a thin population of 130 000 at a density of three per square kilometre. There is a scheme to open up the coast for shipping, including moving into the area those who were displaced by the building of a dam in the north. In effect, this opening of the coast to deep-water traffic will allow inland development, based in the early stages on timber exports of 700 000 tons per year. There will also be settlement of new inhabitants on farms, and there are hopes of industry based on iron ore.

As far as protein is concerned there is a vast potential output of agricultural protein to be developed at a rate coincidental with that of new settlement. The climate is conducive to most agricultural adventures and there seems to be no point in developing industrial protein.

LEBANON

Lebanon is one of the many sites reputed to have been the garden of Eden. The land and climate is conducive to the production of excellent vegetables but the geographic location and traditional trading habits of the Lebanese, encourages capital in commerce more than in agriculture. The Gross Domestic Product contains only 10% for agriculture and 13% for industry. The rest is commerce or affiliated activities. Agriculture occupies about 45% of the labour force, which is said to be too high and if agriculture is to become economic it will evidently be necessary to reduce the labour content, which is fortunate for the merchants but not for the agricultural workers.

Farm income along the coastal strip, which is near to the tourists, is of the order of £L9700, whilst the income from inland farms is only £L1800. In many respects the inland land is better but irrigation is disorderly. The water from six main rivers is not used but it could increase inland output to exceed that along the coast. Part of the problem is financial, agricultural loans being given at interest rates from 15–70% and it is very difficult to find long-term credit.

The protein potential of Lebanon is vast but it cannot be realised until agriculture is given equal attention to that devoted to commerce and tourism and there is some danger that agricultural labour could meanwhile be lost and that industrialised systems of culture may be made necessary.

MALAYSIA

Malaysia has shown a steady rate of growth and improvement of welfare levels. The social structure is, however, delicate and includes a high level of unemployment. The problem is to promote light industry and improved agriculture in rural areas, and to encourage integration of the Malay and Chinese populations. The economy is based on primary materials and tropical products, notably rubber and later palm oil and it is now necessary, without reducing the valuable income from rubber and palm oil, to introduce diversification which is labour-intensive but which also pays high wages. The national structure and economic climate favours foreign investment but there is sufficient local capital if needed.

Good land is available for development in agriculture but the growing conditions are so good that emphasis is on higher yield per area more than on extending area, which brings more profit but does little for the unemployment situation.

The potential for protein is almost exclusively in traditional agriculture, not in routes which call for little direct labour. There are probably a quarter million rice farmers of which at least 80% are uneconomic, mainly because land is held and cropped under an archaic credit system. A change of crop is essential, with central fair buying facilities, to force a change in the agricultural structure.

MAURITIUS

From the moment of independence in 1968, Mauritius has had a stormy history. To some extent the projected image hides the fact that the population is energetic, relatively well provided, educated and not unduly aware of its racial mixture. The racial mixture is African, Indian, Chinese and European. The main problem is the number of unemployed. Over 90% of agricultural land and over 95% of exports are accounted by sugar, grown on efficient estates giving over 30 tons of cane/acre. Sugar factories have been reduced in number to twenty-two. Not all the sugar comes from efficient estates, however, and there are many 2-acre private holdings working at 50% efficiency and needing to be removed from the agricultural picture. More urgent is the need to introduce diversification. Tea is suited to the highlands and there are plans for 30 000 acres, although a third of this may prove unsuitable and much of the rest is far too wet and cold to attract workers. There are also plans for cattle and deer imported from Java, which could be useful in a country needing 3600 tons of meat but producing less than 100 tons. The deer population could expand to 60 000 head, equivalent to 900 tons of meat per year, and there are about 25 000 dairy cows which could add another 2000 tons of meat. The staple diet is rice but rice-suitable land is scarce and there is more potential in cash crops replacing sugar.

Tourism is being encouraged and could provide profit from expensive cash crops but the country is far from tourist markets. There is also reason for encouragement if industry could be found which is suitable for the location but it is doubtful whether industry could provide jobs for the anticipated very high unemployed proportion.

There would appear to be justification for protein production from sugar, if only to reduce the very high importation of food. With a low-cost protein feed from sugar it should be possible to build up an animal-rearing route to protein.

MEXICO

There has been comparatively little interest in agriculture in Mexico for at least twenty-five years. In 1972, agricultural ouput fell by at least 1% and cereal imports increased four-fold. Living conditions of agricultural workers have not improved for half a century and productivity continues to fall.

Agriculture is needed by Mexico to feed the growing population and to provide foreign exchange so that machinery can be bought for the intended industrial boom. Only about 15% of Mexico is fit for cultivation and the climate is not gentle. In fact a first requirement is water control to prevent damage by alternating floods and droughts. Most of the farming is on very small holdings which hardly produce sufficient to feed the tenants and as each farmer dies his land is divided amongst his sons to provide even smaller units. It is not remarkable that 400,000 people arrive each year at Mexico City from rural areas, or that there is a constant drift, legal and illegal, across borders into the USA. About 40% of the total population is classed as rural but they account for only 11.3% of GNP. In effect, the agricultural pattern comprises a few very large industrial farms and countless inefficient small units working at subsistence level. The large concerns are on the best land in the north-west, from whence come the export crops, the cattle also being found in this area. Four per cent of land plots account for 50% of agricultural production and agricultural exports rose 21% in value to $856 million in 1972 only because world prices inflated.

The main problem is that small farms cannot produce sufficient grain to feed local populations. Imports are of the order of half a million tons each of wheat and maize, 300 000 tons of sorghum and 200 000 tons of soya. Since the small farmers cannot deal with climatic problems their survival depends on good years. Private agricultural credit is inevitably lacking and most of the needed developments—roads and water control for example—are not the concern of the Ministry of Agriculture.

The social situation in Mexico can be illustrated by the experience of Nestle company, which had a project in Chiapas with local farmers. Nestle bought milk from farmers to supply a dairy complex some 370 miles away and introduced forty Holstein bulls—given free for breeding with Zebu cows—to improve the herds. Most farmers resented the implication that they could not produce good milk and regarded the introduction as an insult to their Zebu bulls, and where Holsteins were accepted there was no control over the breeding. Subsequently, Nestle imported milk cows from North America but sold them to the farmers and then supplied fodder at 40% below market prices, only to find that much of the fodder was being eaten by pigs and poultry, not cows. Now, Nestle sell the fodder at market prices and it is used for cows. Later, Nestle financed silos for the feed but found two years later that only 3% of the new silos were in use. They then supplied silos at cost to the farmer, or at least with cost shared, and found that 60% of the silos were then used.

Ultimately, Nestle issued grants to farmers to ensure supplies of milk to a new dairy complex but after one year it was discovered that most of the money had been spent on new cars or similar non-productive items. Being now familiar with the situation, grants were stopped and replaced by 6% loans tied to agricultural improvement. Now, Nestle finds itself acting as an agricultural bank lending money at 4% below common interest rates and the latest report was that farmers are improving pastures and herds and that milk, previously directed only at local cheese-making, is now supplied at regular prices in regular quantities to Nestle.

MOROCCO

The economy of Morocco grew at an impressive rate of 5.5% until 1973, when there was a crop failure. The world need to increase agricultural output was duly appreciated and Morocco sought economic recovery through a three-fold increase in the price of phosphate, the primary export. The major internal problem is that half the population is under twenty years of age and most of them are heading for the urban districts. The population is violently religious, which makes it fairly easy for the government, which is also the religious leader, to introduce plans and controls. Plans aim for agrarian reform and Morocconisation of key sectors, including taking over the remaining foreigner-owned land. So far, about half a million acres have been taken back from the French.

Phosphates dominate in the economy, with output of the order of 15 million tons/year. Sugar is important and Morocco is probably growing two-thirds of needs, which are high *per capita* with Moroccan diet. In

1973, about 1 million tons of grain had to be imported but there should be sufficient home-grown food in a normal year. The difficulty is to establish purchase power in the population, with probably half a million unemployed and 8 million unemployable out of the total of 16 million. Wealth distribution is also a problem, most of the wealth being held by a select few. Phosphates bring at least a quarter of national income and many of intended projects are capital-intensive, not labour-intensive, even though much of the population lives slightly above subsistence level. There are voiced plans for dams which will bring an extra million acres into agricultural production, and it is fully appreciated that EEC markets are within easy reach. There is a 7-mile limit set for fishing, with temporary permits for 200 Spanish boats to operate, and there could be development of sophisticated fishing but this will require long-term planning. To some extent, the main problem in Morocco is independence. Citrus output fell from 30–12 tons/hectare after the French left, and some cereal farms reduced output to 40% on an area basis. The Bour zone is not only the most important in terms of food outlet but is also the most backwards-looking and lacking in agricultural technology.

There is potential in microbial protein from citrus pulp and sugar beet waste but the main potential appears to be in conventional agriculture. In this, output could probably be doubled if the farmers could be educated, which means finding experts who can speak the Berber dialects.

NEW HEBRIDES

The land in New Hebrides is said to be so fertile that fences take root. Administration is French and British but the duality is of no concern to the natives, who can exist in comfort from their casual effort providing they are not forced into a cash economy. The intended future of the islands is a financial centre, which also need not concern the natives. The basic agricultural crop is copra, but the potential demand for coconut oil is suspect against oil from estate-grown oilseeds in other countries. There are intentions of producing beef and fish on a scale suitable for export and this has introduced some allied light industry, notably canning. In view of the richness of the land and the conducive climate the range of food imports is remarkable.

There is no doubt that agricultural output of protein could be increased by the introduction of modern methods but it is difficult to discover how such agricultural development could do more than substitute for imports.

There is justification for an industrial route to algae or microbial protein for export to Australia as production in New Hebrides could be far less complicated than production in countries where there is an influential cereal lobby.

NEW ZEALAND

New Zealand was damaged in economic terms by United Kingdom steps into Europe but was rescued by world inflation of food prices. In 1971–1972 farm incomes rose 40%, followed by another 26.5% in 1972–1973 and there was associated growth in other sectors. The bulk of the population did not, however, benefit from the growth and the country fell in terms of standard of living from about fourth to fourteenth on the world scale. Meat producers found it necessary to protest against price controls, the domestic market being important despite higher values of exports. There is need to develop new world markets for products based on grass as it is being realised that world buyers do not need to buy from New Zealand simply because production is efficient, since other countries can supply and can, where necessary, reduce prices to levels which New Zealanders consider uneconomic. Hence, there are efforts to escape from the grass-dominated economy or at least to upgrade the farm products by processing. The dairy industry is looking closely at dehydration, which upgrades notably by its reduction in freight cost, but it is difficult to find equivalent technologies for meat processing. Raw meat prices are high and processing is likely to reduce product value rather than offer more profit per ton exported.

Average wages increased by 13% in 1972 and 12% in 1973, and are likely to be increased by at least 8.5% in 1974. The New Zealand dollar was revalued by 10% when New Zealand had record overseas reserves but this did not benefit farmers who grew their own raw material and sold on home markets. Export earnings rose by 17% in 1972 and 28% in 1973, the biggest increase coming from wool and meat, which brought benefit to farmers selling into export markets. In fact, farm incomes were made too high for national comfort and part of income was frozen by agreement.

The dairy industry comprises 20 000 farmers with an average herd of 108 cows, mostly tended by one man and his family. Small farms are being eliminated because farmers consider up to 200 cows can be kept by a family without skilled additional labour. Milk is sold through cooperative companies who process for the New Zealand Dairy Board.

This system encourages the development of new products on a massive scale, as for example the shutting down of 14 cheese factories in the Taranaki dairy region for replacement by a single dairy complex. Diversification is essential when one considers that butter in New Zealand in 1973 was worth less than it was in 1970. The price to New Zealand of cheese sold into the United Kingdom is less than the ex-store price in Britain. Of a typical United Kingdom price ex-store in Britain of £480/ton, only £350 went to New Zealand and the rest was claimed by the EEC levy. The United Kingdom provides about 43% of earnings from dairy exports, against 70% ten years ago.

Diversification of dairy products has allowed the Dairy Board to show a surplus of $NZ100 million over three years, although much of this is from butter sales to South America and the USA with some credit to sales to Japan. It is thought that butter sales to Japan will rise to 4000 tons in 1973–1974 and there are talks towards substantial movement of dairy raw materials to Japan for processing. Sales to South America rose 50% to $NZ60 million in 1973 but sales to the USA are inhibited by restrictions.

The meat industry is showing profit from world inflation with 1973 exports showing a rise in value of about one-third. Sheep and cattle products other than dairy products account for one-third of export earnings, with almost equal division between sheep and cattle. Exports are to eighty countries but there is still domination by three main markets, North America taking most of the beef, Britain taking most of the lamb and Japan taking most of the mutton. The current problem concerns home prices but there is a pending problem arising from legislations in the export markets. New Zealand meat factories are geared to thousands of animals per day with organised job-allocation in which one man makes only one cut or trim. Thirty-two men can deal with 3000 lambs in a day and three such lines can process and freeze 10 000/day. To satisfy the USA demands in particular, extra inspection is necessary and the rate of output drops. Present output is about 25 million lambs in an eight-month season but it is thought that output will be reduced next year.

Wool is intimate with meat in sheep economics. New Zealand wool production fell to about 309 000 tons in 1972, the lowest clip in eight years' history. The clip could be lower for 1973 following slaughter of ewes in the 1972 drought. On the other hand, world prices have risen 112% within one year and the low clip has been profitable. However, prices are likely to drop sharply under pressure from synthetics and to some extent because sellers may lose their right to find private buyers outside the Wool Marketing Corporation. The main influence of wool prices on the meat market is its determination of the time, age and weight of slaughter of the animal. Early slaughter provides less wool but more young meat. Late slaughter for the sake of high wool prices provides more old meat but more carcase weight.

NORWAY

Norwegians are independent but have affinity to other Scandinavians and to the United Kingdom. For various reasons, more distant countries are regarded with suspicion and Western Europe is known as The Continent, a place to be visited only when selling aluminium or fish. In terms of statistics, fish are not important since it is only 1.5% of the gross national product but there is sentimental affinity to fish and 45 000 people depend entirely on fish, frequently in districts which could support no other activity. Their problem, notably with regard to EEC countries, is the danger of overfishing of local grounds.

There is a significant paper industry, developed around the waterfalls as small units. A typical unit may produce only 40 000 tons of pulp, although it has been calculated that units producing less than 250 000 tons are not economic anywhere in the world. The Norwegian small mills cannot afford pollution control without conversion of the effluent into yeast protein, and there is a market for yeast protein in agriculture.

The discovery of oil in the Ekofisk area has changed the attitudes to development. Energy-starved Europe can now regard Norway not only as a supplier of aluminium but also of oil or of piped energy as electricity. Ekofisk should supply twice the oil needs of Norway but it is doubtful if any surplus will be used for protein. The fermentation of papermill waste should provide sufficient microbial protein and there are developments of more fish meal.

PERU

Peru has a history of conquest and combat which has left a feudalistic society. There are many races and the main problem is to unite the various groups into a single nation and to remove the administrative obstacles to progress. When the government took over the sugar and sheep companies of respectable size, there was a marked increase of output which was maintained after the estates and ranches were given to the workers. Increased output is vital, since natural increases have not kept pace with population increases and more area needs to be cropped, and yields need to be improved. Half the population is in agriculture, which accounts for only 15% of the gross domestic product and about 20% of imports are food which could be grown in Peru if workers could be given more benefit from their labour. This is a slow process, made slower by the complications of legislation, but it does show signs of success. In terms of protein production, Peru has good agricultural land and rich fishing grounds. If the established social structures, laid down during a stormy history, can be replaced by effective cooperative schemes, then Peru should develop to be a major source of agricultural protein.

The fish off Peru have not been fully commercialised other than the anchovy for fish meal. One advantage of the Peruvian fish is said to be that schools are long-distance migratory, which means that they can be exhaustively caught when found but there is some danger that improved location equipment will enable boats to follow schools, and to extract too many fish for effective recovery.

RUMANIA

Rumania has a reputation of being independent but it is firmly a member of Comecon and the Warsaw Pact. The Soviet Union is its biggest trading partner but there has been considerable effort to establish trade elsewhere. Industrial output is dominated by mechanical engineering and chemicals, with considerable diversification of products to encourage growth and new market areas. There is a tourist industry but this concerns more East Europeans than West Europeans and there is doubt if Rumania can offer significant inducements for the tourist industry to develop fully. Distance is the problem, West Europeans finding similar facilities in Yugoslavia or Bulgaria or Turkey with less complication of travel.

Development plans favour capital-intensive heavy projects and neglect agriculture despite the high proportion of the population engaged in rural activities. Agricultural workers comprised some three-quarters of the population in the 1950s but now account for probably less than a half of the working population. This is high but it has to be appreciated that agricultural output accounts for only 25% of GNP and therefore warrants a minor share of investment. It took the 1970 floods, affecting 700 000 hectares, to bring attention to the low producer prices and therefore the low interest in farming. Since then there have been efforts to improve agriculture but it is doubted if agriculture will develop to the extent thought possible.

The protein potential is mainly through industrial routes and there is a project for protein from oil. It is probable that the protein from oil will be associated with developments of beef cattle. Arable sources of protein are not likely to be provided with sufficient capital for satisfactory development.

SARDINIA

Sardinia can be exampled as typical of places which have been targets for massive sums of investment capital with little improvement in the welfare of the local population. Self-generating industrial prosperity was not evident from the few giant complexes, and urbanisation produced more problems than benefits. The quality of land can best be described by reference to a local lore that when God had finished laying out the world he was left with a bag of stones which he dumped in the most convenient stretch of water. It was once thought that the rocks were rich in coal and copper, and 50 000 men were paid to be miners, but the minerals are not in fact of minable quality. There was also a plan to run a power station on the coal, which is lignite, but the plans failed and oil firing was introduced. In 1971, another plan arose concerning aluminium, but this too seems doomed to failure. To the majority of the population the plans and failures are of no interest.

Up to 1820, Sardinia held free-range sheep and had no other activity. The thousand miles of coast did not promote fishing and most Sardinians then regarded the coast as no more than a point of entry for Arabs, Romans, Spaniards, or anyone else looking for territory. In 1820 there was introduction of enclosure of land, which destroyed the sheep prospects although there are probably 2.5 million sheep still grazing. There could be 50 000 herdsmen, plus many so-called brigands. By 1980 there could be industrial development in the sheep area and both herdsmen and brigands will be no more than history.

There could be development of cattle but only with bought feed. A breed of cattle suited to the climate is identified and there could well be microbial protein feed from oil or from cultivated algae. In this, the problem is the fragmentation of the land into small lots and the refusal of farmers to unite.

There are probably 5 million acres of agricultural land but 700 000 acres are forest. Crop selection is difficult because soils are thin and the air is dry. Excellent wine is produced but only by selecting grapes from 50 cm above ground level. Nearer the ground the grapes are too sweet and may taste burned. Tourism has revived fishing but it is not probable that fish protein will develop to any significant extent. The future for protein in Sardinia appears to be in cattle fed on microbial or algae feed, not in the fish which carries its name.

SAUDI ARABIA

Saudi Arabia requires special mention for its climate, which is sufficiently inhospitable to send the few rich inhabitants on visits to Cairo or Alexandria when political relationships permit. The society is extreme Muslim and rightly claims to be the only true Arab group in an Arabic political front. Inside the country, legislation is defined and exacting, with drastic retribution for offenders but complete freedom within the law for those who obey. It is a police state with relatively little technology in high places.

Devotion to the tribe is strong and activity is within the restriction and liberty of Islam. Without oil, Saudi Arabia would endure for ever without change but oil has introduced technology, a factor not included by Mohammed in his writings, and this has created a reasonably progressive minority mainly in the eastern parts. It should be noted, however, that whilst most countries introduce development plans Saudi Arabia declared a development discipline in 1959.

Of the oil revenue much has been written. It has been directed into transport and communication, and into dealing with the accepted drift of people from rural to urban life. There is some effort to produce a broad national economy, with equal attention to agriculture and industry based on oil. Welcome as the oil revenue is, Saudi Arabia is aware that income cannot be maintained from one source, and is also aware that the outside world is actively seeking energy in systems other than the burning of oil.

The transformation is difficult. The religious, moral, social and political structure is inertly fixed in the Kuran and Sunnah. Whilst a Muslim might question the genuineness of an edict or saying, when proved the statement is unavoidable law and there are many books of such demanding statements from the prophet. Muslims do not worship Mohammed but devotedly respect his inspired comments, and they respect the words of Jesus. Jews are criticised for denying Christ and Christians are criticised for promoting Christ into a god.

In the Koran, animals stand on the same footing as humans in the sight of God—'There is no beast on earth nor bird which flieth with its wings, but the same is a people like unto you, and to the Lord shall they return.'

This can cause some complication in animal rearing. The problem is not that the statement could be variously translated, as it already is, but that future pressure groups could rightly expose animal projects as contrary to the Koran, bringing inevitable closure by failure of the market. The fervent Muslim is likely to object if he learns that his meat has been grown in restrictive boxes and with injections.

Hence, the emphasis has to be on arable crops and conventional meat, but with industrial development to provide spending money. It is relatively safe to manufacture microbial protein and such manufacture can in fact be claimed as providing livestock (if microbes are regarded as livestock) with pleasant conditions of rearing. From the ethical point of view, and from the economic point of view, there is logic in the development of microbial protein for human and animal diet. Oil is one obvious feedstock but microbial protein can also lead to profit from unpalatable crops which can thrive in the arid conditions.

Roughly 1 million of the 6 million inhabitants are fully urbanised and about half of the population enjoy the benefits of urban health and education facilities. About 45% of the people are concerned with agriculture, although agriculture accounts for probably no more than 6% of gross product. Vegetable growing is being developed and there is serious production of alfalfa and rice. Wheat yields are low, at about 0.5 tons/hectare. Livestock production is the main activity with fluctuating numbers of animals. At any time there could be roughly 2.5 million sheep, 2.0 million goats, 0.5 million camels and 0.25 million cattle. Goat numbers increase with drought and are favoured as the ideal animal for rearing whilst cattle do not appear to thrive outside the Red Sea coastal plains. The main problem, as might be expected, is water. Irrigation water is being brought up from depths of 2000 m, this water being some 30 000 years old and limited in quantity with no recharge possibility. Desalination is a possible source of water but this is expensive and the salt water is not where the crops are required to grow.

SINGAPORE

Singapore has the highest standard of living of countries in South-east Asia, mainly due to its provision of facilities for investors interested in trade or industry. The society is multi-racial but not integrated. There are only 224 square miles of land available and all this has potential value for profitable factories or offices. Future agriculture can be discounted, particularly with Malaysia in the background offering more area and cheaper labour.

It can be doubted that Singapore will contribute any protein to world food supplies, although it could possibly profit from an algae project designed to deal with the organic effluent of urban society. A tourist industry is intended and it is fully realised that a system of waste disposal must be introduced before the tourists arrive in number. If this can be related to industrial protein production there is a ready market for the animal feed in foreign poultry projects and, of course, in the many pig projects intended by societies based on Chinese. The relatively affluent Chinese element in the population is likely to be significant in any industrial protein development, and it would be sensible to site such a project within Singapore if only to take advantage of the existing trade structure.

SOLOMON ISLANDS

It is difficult to locate the Solomon Islands. There is a story that Mendana, after having found the islands, could not rediscover them when he returned to take up residence. The economy depends on copra and business is in the hands of ex-patriates. The natives live in primitive overcrowded villages but there are plans to develop a balanced agriculture. The main difficulty is the spread of the small population over a large area of ocean. Better domestic agriculture is needed to provide healthy diet but it is doubted if any agricultural project for export can succeed. The economy appears to demand some form of industrial development, which could come from the bauxite, and easier communication with the world outside. There is an oil palm development which could possibly be associated with microbial protein production which could at least provide a satisfactory basic diet for the local population.

Beef cattle are a possibility, arising from the habit of coconut growers of raising cattle to keep down grass under trees. By 1980 the islands should be self-sufficient in flesh protein, beef and fish, and there is a probability of fish meal production. The reason for fish meal production is not the usual one of needing a profitable outlet for fish. It is needed to dispose of fish waste which cannot be dumped at sea because sharks are thereby attracted inshore.

24—WPR * *

Overall, the Solomon Islands could become self-sufficient in protein but there is doubt that they could contribute to exports.

TANZANIA

To some extent, Tanzania has followed an unusual path of development. Other new nations have invested in familiar growth sectors of the economy whilst Tanzania has sought blanket development from rock bottom. Also, foreign aid has been discouraged and more emphasis placed on domestic ability regardless of its financial backing. There has been a genuine effort to generate income in the poor subsistence farmer. This has been mainly through rural socialism including village settlements entitled Ujamaa, Swahili for family, villages.

Obviously, the main target has to be import-substitution but it has been of equal importance to eliminate the layer of trading middlemen between the income from exports and the producers who provide the material to export. The State Trading Corporation has taken over distribution and made the Asian fraction obsolete. Many Asians simply carried boxes of cash into Kenya, probably to the extent of £7 million although no one will ever know.

The Ujamaa concept is sound. An isolated community will pool resources and develop an isolated structure including production by agriculture and industry, and taking care of social facilities. It differs little from the original African tribal structure, which proved effective before so-called improvements damaged communal attitudes.

With 90% of the population in agriculture it is obvious that the only significant route to more protein is through conventional agriculture, fragmented rather than intensive so that the Ujamaa concept can be shown to be good. The future depends on local improvements more than on new introductions.

TURKEY

The history of Turkey has been written frequently and from most points of view. Modernisation started in 1923 and the influence of Mustafa Kemal Attaturk is strong. His policy was to use local resources for local people, through efficient large state companies alongside private companies. Success has been mainly in industry and it has led to a split-level society. Overall growth rate has been a healthy 10%, but this has brought

15% inflation which is encouraged by a massive inflow of foreign money from Turks working overseas.

Cereals and livestock account for two-thirds of agricultural output. Both are showing reductions of yield and it may be necessary for Turkey to import significant food supplies in the future. Two-thirds of the population are in agriculture, and the level of education is low. Fresh vegetables are produced with excellent quality but wastage is high. Meat quality is not good and output is falling in terms of weight *per capita*. The livestock population is of the order of 72 million (or two/person in the country) but exports are impossible whilst foot-and-mouth is endemic.

The future protein situation in Turkey depends mainly on the rate at which drive and initiative can be introduced into agriculture. The facilities for agriculture are excellent, the labour is available and there is sufficient inflow of capital from non-agricultural exports (including exported labourers) for a rise in public purchase power. Unfamiliar sources of protein could have value, notably those concerned with the rescue of waste, but there is no need for urgency to escape from agricultural methods. In fact, Turkey could become a major supplier of processed meat and vegetables.

UGANDA

It has been claimed that Uganda is an ideal country with relaxed well-fed people enjoying the correct balance of sun and rain, providing that friction between the north and south can be avoided. In 1971, the potential paradise was disturbed by military government, supported by 98% of the population but not outstanding in administrative efficiency. Overspending on military activity and failure to handle the national economy correctly has left Uganda extremely short of capital and it is unavoidable that any protein projects must be from domestic resources and skill. It would, in fact, be wrong for Uganda to change from the existing agricultural economy which is stable and can survive a few years of administrative chaos. The removal of the Asian members of the society has made it impossible for local capital to be applied effectively, and has encouraged the movement of money out of the country by any available route, legal or otherwise.

Intentions are, therefore, related to agriculture or industries which are tied to agriculture, such as a new sugar refinery and a paper mill using sugarcane cellulose. One intention is a 1000-mile main road with 400 miles of feeder roads, all aimed at linking agriculture to markets. Increases of protein can be expected to come from new areas of land and the introduction of better seed.

The society is to some extent unusual in that it shows paid employment of only about one-third million out of 10 million population, with almost as many jobs available as recorded paid workers and only 50 000 workers on record in a country which is almost entirely agricultural. In fact, there are 1 million farmers producing a healthy balance of local food and a few export crops, namely:

	Thousand tons approximately per year
Coffee	180
Cotton	450 (thousand bales)
Tobacco	3–5
Sugar	150
Tea	20

The country is 10 000 sea miles from its markets but only 5000 air miles, bringing interest in air freighting. Most air cargo is high-value, not particularly high-protein, but there is an interesting development of seeds. With organisation Uganda could become a vital supplier of air-freighted seeds to world agriculture, although this is not likely to improve the lot of the average subsistence farmer.

Farm mechanisation schemes have a poor record. Large areas are cultivated using oxen and hand-hoes. There are plans for more animals, including dairy cattle, and there are intentions to integrate agricultural services such as transport. Farmers can listen to over an hour per day of radio programme about agriculture in five languages. Whether they will change their habits after the education and advice can be doubted. As they exist, they can feed the increasing population and live in comparative luxury, although statistics might not show the academic improvements needed by political persons. About 90% of the population rely on agriculture for their welfare and they might be well advised to concentrate on preservation of their welfare more than on export crops.

Coffee accounts for half the export revenue but could show lower earning value as freight costs rise and more instant coffee becomes demanded. Cotton could also show reduced value as synthetics develop. It could rapidly become necessary for the traditional export crops to be sold into domestic manufacture, as for instance into the production of instant coffee, which would leave waste for microbial protein manufacture, and cotton mills or other outlets for cotton cellulose. Industrial protein could be manufactured but it would appear pointless to develop industrial protein when agricultural protein can be produced with ease, and whilst other countries in Africa might be forced to use industrial routes because they lack agricultural facilities.

UNITED STATES OF AMERICA

During the 150 years of significant history the USA showed remarkable agricultural progress. The society benefited from a peculiar set of events and circumstances which are unlikely to be repeated elsewhere. There was a combination of vast virgin areas of good land with a spasmodic influx of agricultural labourers, bringing with them a varied pattern of cultures and skills. There were a number of economic stimulations including a major depression and a series of wars which encouraged development without draining national resources. Also, there was a plentiful supply of oil to encourage the introduction of machinery into farms and into the markets for agricultural products.

Up to 1900 most Americans were farmers and each produced sufficient to feed five people. By 1930 each farmer could probably feed ten people. In 1930, towards 30 million horses and mules became obsolete as tractors and combine harvesters took over. The number of satisfied consumers per farmer rose to fifteen in 1950 and to twenty-five in 1960. It is now probable that the American farmer feeds at least forty people. Over the past century the proportion of workers engaged by agriculture has fallen from 90% to 10%. The number of civil servants concerned with agriculture rose from 30 000 to 100 000 between 1930 and 1940.

There are about 1000 million acres of land available, much of which is in worse condition than when it was farmed by pioneers. Farmers seek high yields and rely on heavy-bearing crops with over-use of artificial fertilisers. Consequently, there is no sharp differentiation between agriculture and industry. A traditional farmer relying on nature might find it impossible to survive in the environment of mechanisation, synthetic feeding, chemical pest control, hybrid stock and business management techniques.

Even so, the structure of USA agriculture is based on one-family farms. There are a few massive multi-million-dollar operations but these have not impoverished the small farmers. This is fortunate since a revolution in American agriculture is forecast. It is thought probable that higher oil prices and more unemployment amongst low-skill workers will make it essential to encourage labour-intensive techniques in agriculture. Substantial increases in food prices are expected, with full realisation that Americans can benefit from a reduction in their intake of food.

Americans are diet-conscious, including the understanding that a meal is not complete without meat. Another understanding is that obesity is to be avoided, preferably by avoiding animal fats and refined sugar.

URUGUAY

Uruguay can be exampled as a classic example of synthetic urbanisation. Batlle went to Europe and returned to develop industrial workers and the bureaucracy which he felt was essential background to growth and industrial magnificence. After slightly more than half a century everybody in Uruguay is a product of the development and most are seeking a new society, either at home or abroad. At the height of the chaos one could borrow money from a bank, have 60% interest taken away at the time of borrowing, and still make a profit from the uncontrolled inflation. A house bought in the early 1950s might have a 6% interest on the mortgage and fifteen years later the interest and repayment would be a matter of pence. Half a century ago there was the ultimate in luxury, buildings with fittings shipped from Italy in solid mahogany chests, magnificent houses in extravagant settings, all the glories which could be displayed as money poured into the country from the sale of meat and wool. Batlle overspent on welfare and pensions, and ultimately created a way of life which could only end in national bankruptcy.

Of the 1 million workers, about a quarter are civil servants. At one time, the airline had 1000 workers and one flying aeroplane. There are countless grades of civil servant, most of which are created positions to hide the real unemployment problem. The unemployment problem is made worse by the need to make money, which forces everyone to seek two jobs—both urban because the created dream is of national wealth through urbanisation and industry. In fact, most of the industrial ventures are academic failures and Uruguay still relies on meat and wool for its survival. The future, as far as protein is concerned, is in traditional agriculture but whether the population can be returned to the land, after tasting the delights of city life and the benefits of affluence, remains to be seen.

VENEZUELA

Venezuela has a history of violent politics and the availability of oil has not helped to stabilise economic affairs. The country is trying to establish an economic structure based on the oil, instead of selling it to the point where 90% of foreign earnings rely on oil. The country has the highest average national income in South America but there are inevitable problems. For example, investment seeks higher and quicker returns than can be had for low-cost housing or agriculture. Although a quarter of the active population can be described as agricultural, agriculture accounts for only 7% of the national income, causing rural people to become urban people as soon as they can afford the urban houses.

The run-down of agriculture can be expected to continue whilst industry and oil offer more profit to the investors. There is a rich storehouse of raw material yet to be developed by industry quite apart from the oil as a petrochemical platform. In the midst of the raw materials there are massive rivers which can offer energy. For mainly political reasons the water control has been associated with agricultural schemes but there is doubt that labour will be available for the farms. More probable are the schemes for paper and pulp manufacture. The Guayana forests alone promise half a million hectares of high-grade timber within reach of the water needed for a pulp mill.

It can be doubted that conventional agriculture will advance, although profitable intensive farming could find investment. The economic climate is suitable for industrial protein manufacture, based on oil fractions perhaps but more probably based on pulpmill waste through fungi and yeasts. It can be forecast that such proteins, cheaper than agricultural products to produce in the Venezuelan situation, will be used for animal rearing to satisfy domestic demands for meat.

VIRGIN ISLANDS

Virgin islanders managed to remain hospitable and colour-blind during the troubled period of the Caribbean. There are sixty islands holding 10 000 people, 90% on the main island and the other thousand distributed widely. In the middle 1960s there was a tourist invasion, because the area gave peace and contentment, and the economy expanded at a rate of 30%/year. All indications are that the islands will develop into a holiday centre with full employment and no outstanding interest beyond the visitors. Subsistence agriculture and fishing have given way to tourism. The average islander owns a few acres of land, on which he intends to be buried after death and by which he claims status whilst alive.

There is a history of migration away from the islands and most families have many connections in other countries. Many have returned with ability to use owned property for profit production without working. The ultimate fate of the Virgin Islands could be no more than a holiday centre with the locals grown rich by property speculation, most of the work done by contracted imported labour, and all the protein imported.

YUGOSLAVIA

There are about 1 million Yugoslavs working abroad and the country relies on their money sent home for its balance of payments. The economic structure is unusual in that unearned income (money sent home by foreign workers) produced inflation whilst heavy internal debts between Yugoslav companies stagnated industry and agriculture. Consequently, agriculture has failed to the extent of making Yugoslavia an importer of basic food. There is a need for an agricultural surplus to support the confused economy, which would probably suffer if it had to include a heavy cost of imported industrial raw materials. As in any developing country the importing of heavy equipment drains resources. Up to the mid 1960s the balance was made up mainly by tourism but then money sent home by foreign workers took over.

Yugoslavia was a food producer of importance but production fell to a point where imports became necessary, particularly of wheat. The decline was mainly because capital was concentrated on industrial projects. Attempts to collectivise all land failed although the probable 15% of land which is nationalised accounts for two-thirds of the cereals produced. Recent increases in output have been absorbed by higher domestic consumption. The situation encouraged workers to seek urban life or to emigrate on a temporary basis. This left large areas of good land unproductive, particularly since private owners could not hold more than 25 acres, which is only productive if the land is good and the crops have high value. Money is not available for agricultural development because the early plans did not provide for raw material production and the country carries a high burden of raw material import cost.

Broadly, Yugloslavia has agricultural potential for most protein foods but it needs a massive development plan for which funds are not available. Despite the availability of the land and the conducive climate it is probable that industrial routes to protein would develop quicker than conventional agricultural routes.

Chapter 34

Future Proteins

The foregoing national situations in selected countries has concentrated on so-called developing countries because their need for protein is greater. They can either develop native skills and facilities within the existing social structure or introduce new protein routes which have proved profitable in other countries. As a general rule capital is severely limited and it is difficult for a country to finance comprehensive and localised schemes at the same time. Comprehensive schemes are more difficult because they have to include social and educational effort which, in terms of output statistics, is not visibly productive. There is little political glory in unrecorded improvements of output amongst the majority of a group of subsistence farmers. Localised schemes are attractive because they show visible benefits which can be treated in mathematical reports, although such schemes rarely benefit the majority of populations.

Examination of the list shows that very few countries need to be lacking protein. In almost every example there is some local inhibition to progress which has nothing to do with climate or capital or technology, and is frequently an influence from some foreign society. It is becoming increasingly obvious that the next generation will only be well fed if each pocket of humanity can be made self-sufficient, producing protein according to local circumstances. Whether the protein is animal or vegetable, agricultural or industrial, is of little importance. When the pockets of humanity are self-sufficient, then trade can be used to distribute surplus. The function of trade is not to satisfy needs, since the identification of need causes evil speculation. The function is to exchange goods which are not required for goods which are desirable, but which can be rejected if the quality or price is not satisfactory. The world protein gap will never be filled whilst men can make money from the misfortune of others, but it will be filled as soon as each social group can survive and thrive in isolation if need be.

The significance of microbial protein is in its ability to multiply outside the politics and restrictions of agriculture. Even if its contribution to world supplies is small, which is unlikely, the fact that it exists as economic competition to conventional agriculture makes its development worth while. This is particularly true of political climates in which there is conflict between agricultural and industrial interests.

The list of countries is by no means complete but it serves to illustrate the complexity of the protein supply and demand situation. Very rarely is a lack of protein due to inability of the country to provide a suitable area of land and conducive climate. The common cause of failure is inefficient administration of available capital, the emphasis being too frequently on short-term profit-making which benefits few of the populations. Much of this emphasis will need to be reduced following the increases in energy costs, and particularly since world inflation has made it advisable for local activity to be based on local materials and labour, and to be aimed at local markets. Most of the countries mentioned should now be able to develop domestic production of protein, either agricultural or industrial, because more capital should be available for internal activity.

Any statistical prediction relative to this world is not to be trusted. Predictions have been made impossible by the acceleration of trends. It took 10 000 years for agriculture to spread from a modest development in Asia Minor to a world activity. It has taken only 200 years for industry based on fossil fuel to become a major factor in social development and it could take less than 50 years for fossil fuels to be replaced by new energy sources. Even within living memory it could take half a century for an invention to become common reality. Under modern conditions of marketing, a new product can be on world supermarket shelves within six months of its conception.

Trends are synergistic, each one promoting and being promoted by all other trends. It is not practical to isolate any trend as a major influence in protein technology but it is possible to outline a number of trends which dictate the future. For example:

1. Overall population of the world is increasing constantly and the rate of increase is higher than the rate at which new agricultural facilities can be provided.
2. The proportion of young people in the population is increasing. One result of this is a decline in the importance of tradition in buying habits.
3. There is a continued drift of workers into urban areas, where they can earn more money and enjoy more of the material benefits. Associated with this is disfavour of agriculture as a main occupation, although the drift does encourage suburban horticulture.
4. Urban communities are becoming more complex and more congested, giving favour to processed foods more than fresh foods. Retail prices of processed foods should rise at a lower rate than retail prices of fresh food, despite the increased output from suburban horticulture.
5. Perpetuated groups are becoming less important in society. Notably, the family as a unit is declining in favour of loose aggregations. Alternatively expressed, social groups are becoming less mixed in terms of ages of members and they survive for shorter periods, but are becoming more mixed in terms of culture. At the same time, where groups of like characters are forming the formation is with more dogmatic identity and less sensitivity to external pressures. Associated with this is growing practical antagonism to authority.
6. Arising from the above, there is a trend towards impulse buying by individual consumers, mainly with complete disregard for actual value but with regard for instant satisfaction and rejection if the purchase does not provide instant convenience.
7. The development of personal wealth is uneven and the majority of consumers face inflation as represented by reduced purchase power. This is particularly serious in so-called developing countries, where welfare feeding programmes will have to be increased to prevent widespread starvation and world disease.
8. The quantity of official interference with all aspects of human activity is growing and the ability of the administrators is getting progressively lower.
9. Quite apart from official interference, there is growing complexity in human activity, inducing conservatism but at the same time making it essential for programmes to be revised at short notice and for people to accept activities and circumstances which are not as they would wish. Notably, traditional markets for output face

more varied competition, frequently from some remote and un-anticipated source.

10. Familiar species in agriculture are being replaced by versions which give higher yields or new analysis patterns. In theory, there should be unlimited increase in the range of hybrids and modifications but economic forces must put emphasis on selected individuals.

11. The rate of cash flow in all activity from initial planning to final retail purchase is increasing. Realisation periods, which are the periods between spending and finding benefit, become shorter and this means less long-term planning, more wasted cash in develop-ment and trial instead of research, and consequent inflation.

12. With higher costs and precipitated activity, production economics need to take more account of waste as a source of profit and pollution as an expensive loss. The growth area for development is in the processing of materials which have previously been discarded.

13. Associated with the above, raw materials become more expensive as labour and freight costs increase. It can be prophesied that there will be constant introductions of new materials, notably those which can replace petrochemicals or metals. Food components, notably sugar, can be expected to develop industrial non-food outlets. Also, fermentation can be expected to develop as a major industrial platform process.

14. There is progressive acceptance of new substances, including foods. Partly, this is encouraged by the greater mobility of consumers and more exposure to new cultures. Mainly, however, inflation induces experimentation if lower-priced alternatives are made available.

15. All costs which originate from energy, whether the energy is fossil, human or animal, are rising. This means expensive freight, hand-ling, insurance, housing, service, direct labour, etc. and a con-sequent increase in the cost of goods.

16. All costs which relate to area or space are rising. Notably, agricul-tural area and storage volume are becoming progressively more expensive. Future activities will have to be with minimum use of area or volume. Where large areas or volumes are available, as in Amazonia and Siberia, the cost of making the area and volume fit for use will prohibit free expansion.

17. Arising from the above, societies will have to develop closed-cycle operations in which they produce essential needs without reference to foreign authorities. Importation costs are making it uneconomic to buy any goods which can be home-produced and exportation

costs are making it uneconomic to ship any low-value goods. Hence, societies can be expected to produce and manufacture from their own resources, to some extent reverting to historic regional development. A new phase is developing in which regional resources and facilities will use international capital and technology for regional demands. In other words, the international movement of substances will decline in favour of international movement of money and experience.

18. Since protein is directly related to health, it is to be noted that there is a trend towards curing ill by early prevention, rather than taking active steps after the illness has been made obvious. The significance of protein in diet is being slowly realised, not only in terms of body energy and tissue replacement but in terms of body function and chemistry.

19. There is, despite statistics relative to meat, a trend towards vegetable proteins. Previously, vegetable proteins have been disfavoured as second-class but it is now being appreciated that they can be mixed to complete patterns and can be adjusted in their genetics. Meat can be expected to move entirely into processing in due course, particularly when the low productivity of large-animal production results in rejected retail prices for all fresh meat. White whole fish can also be expected to decline to a point where it becomes a luxury or specialty food.

Broadly, it can be forecast that most existing protein foods will become mainly raw materials for compounding, to be consumed alongside more fresh vegetables and luxury–specialty foods from increased suburban horticulture. The indication is of a rapid decline of agriculture which relies on low land prices and more use of intensification and scientific culture to save space and labour. The most important development appears to be the introduction of factory foods based on algae and various microbes, using wastes and effluents as raw materials, removing threats of pollution at the same time as making more profit from available space and feedstock.

The greatest potential source of protein is in the vast quantity of natural growth which is ignored. Of special interest is animal protein which is not only neglected as a source of food for humans, but is also a contributory factor in losses of existing protein supplies. There is no technical reason why unfamiliar animals should not become food for humans after they have become fat and plentiful on food supplies which man intended for himself.

Rodents and insect grubs need study as rapid breeders but the point may best be made by reference to the African Quelea. This bird is a member of the weaver family and is the world's most populous bird. It could number 1000 million million, or 2000 tons of first-class protein per person in the world. It is being destroyed at a rate of 1000 million/ year by sophisticated methods which include a special pesticide, Quelaetox. So far, control methods have failed and the bird now multiplies and ravages territory across most of tropical Africa. The largest roost is reported as covering 40 square miles with 25 million birds.

Quelea can breed three or four times every year, raising three young per hatch. It is not uncommon for farmers to lose a quarter of a crop of grain to the pest, and there are many records of total crop loss. Up to 90% of the diet of quelea is wild grass seed and they have 2 million square miles of Africa in which to find it. The other 10% is sown grain which the bird feeds on as it moves in front of rain belts. They are justly described as the modern version of biblical locusts but in fact they are worse than locusts. Locusts are occasional destructive visitors whilst the quelea is a regular annual pest. An average flight of quelea, numbering perhaps 3 million birds, can take 100 tons of grain/day for four days, after which they move on to richer fields. At present world prices this could mean a loss of about £60 000 for the unwelcome four-day visit.

Switching attention to the sea, it can be forecast that many new types of fish will be landed, ground to flakes and compounded, and then passed into distribution chains. Of the 20 000 or so species of fish available only a very few have so far been caught for human diet. It can also be forecast that human-grade fish meals will become common, with consequent reduction of meals for animal feed, and that plankton will be harvested directly. All indications are that the traditional fishing systems will become uneconomic as familiar fish become scarce and the new forms of marine life will become compulsory diet.

The decline of fish meal in animal feed is almost certain to be alongside a decline in soya for animals as techniques improve for making soya meal for humans. How far this will influence the development of simulated meat cannot be forecast but it has to be appreciated that textured imitation meat from vegetables is the most attractive form of soya, and can be a useful method of up-grading the value of concentrates from most pulses. It is, in fact, difficult to see how any bought feed can continue against the indicated economic probabilities. In the rearing of animals, feed costs have risen at twice the rate of increase of prices of finished protein, making it inevitable that other costs will rise to the point where operations using bought feed become non-profitable.

Quite apart from the problem of feed costs, animal rearing using familiar beasts is indicated as becoming impossible because area costs are not covered by output rates. In most countries, it is more profitable to use land for non-agricultural purposes than for the rearing of animals, which is itself an uneconomic sector when measured in terms of land value and utilisation. It can be forecast that beef and sheep meat will decline other than in undeveloped vast areas of grazing. Pig and poultry meat can be expected to increase because pigs and chickens can be intensively reared for short-term periods (short-term because future farmers will need a quick return on investment capital).

Broadly, human diet will in the future include more vegetable protein and less animal protein. It is fortunate for humanity that high-protein high-lysine cereals have been developed since more of the world population will be depending mainly on bread for their protein. The reasons for the swing to cereals is not only the inflated price of flesh protein, although this is a significant factor. A more effective reason is the change of habits which is found when consumers become affluent. They seek convenience and they disregard food values. The market is concerned with compounded foods, for which cereals are ideal as foundation materials, particularly if associated with human-grade soya and fish meal.

The rate, scale and direction of development of microbial protein is impossible to forecast. It is now doubted that mineral oil will be a favoured raw material outside the oil countries where use is sought for foreign money, but there is potential production from sugar, starches and cellulose products. The indication is that all three carbohydrate groups will be commercialised but for different reasons. Sugar can be expected to develop as food for microbes for the sake of economies in developing countries who need to up-grade products. Starches can be expected to develop because it will become essential for food manufacturing concerns to find higher-value markets for their reject and discard. Cellulose can be expected to develop because industry at large is faced with higher raw material costs, and must seek low-priced alternatives or upgrade a greater proportion of the raw materials purchased. Since cellulose is a common component in raw materials, notably in food production and processing, it can be expected that cellulose will develop as a material to be fermented to protein.

It is possible to extract a cellulose-destructive enzyme from certain organisms and use this to manufacture sugars from any cleaned cellulose. Alternatively, the cellulose can be cooked in acid to sugars. Either route will provide food for known fungi or yeasts. There is under development a perpetual system of conversion from cellulose to protein using a pipe construction, cellulose slurry in at one end and protein slurry out at the other end. It is probable that this will provide a fair proportion of future feed protein and the only problem is selection of the most convenient raw material. In this respect it is obvious to seek raw materials which need disposal and there is notable interest in excrement.

Intensive farming methods produce vast quantities of excrement slurry which is rich in nitrogen. Roughly 10% of United Kingdom excrement from chicken farms is already dried and fed to ruminants, furnishing about 2% nitrogen or 12–14% protein equivalent in rumens. The output of other livestock is too wet for simple dehydration, a cow for example producing 330 l/week of which only 27 kg is solids. In theory, 2.5 cows need one acre of arable land to absorb their slurry output. In the United Kingdom all the cows produce some 40 million tons of slurry/year and there is not the area to absorb this quantity. Pigs, which produce three times the excrement volume of humans, could possibly occupy land at a density of thirty-three to the acre without causing a disposal problem, although the metals content of pig excrement is likely to spoil any receptive land. There are already systems of processing pig excrement, at 3% nitrogen and 2–7% total solids, using thermophilic fungi under acid conditions to manufacture acceptable and economic protein. Cow excrement is less contaminated than pig excrement and will probably be needed for land improvements as synthetic fertilisers become more expensive. Human excrement, like pig excrement, is contaminated with metals and is better studied as a source of nitrogen and carbon for microbial growth.

The economic advantage of processing excrement is of course that both the raw material and the demand follow the same statistic—the number of people or animals involved.

PROTEIN FROM URBAN WASTE SOLIDS

Solid fractions in urban waste contain very little animal waste, the bulk being products of industry. Compositions of refuse vary over very small distances and there is a constant danger of occasional inclusion of undesirables such as tins of rat poison or damaged car batteries. The cellulose content can be broken down into sugars, which can be water-extracted for subsequent fermentation, although breaking down the cellulose does not overcome the economic problem of handling rubbish. As a source of cellulose, urban solid waste is less provident than agricultural waste and its cellulose is far from clean.

Many of the problems can be overcome by pyrolysis. For average urban solid refuse it should be possible to obtain a heat content equivalent to 1 ton of coal/10 tons of refuse. This heat content can be used to incinerate mixed urban waste including a fair proportion of wet waste. From such an incineration process it is not difficult to fractionate the clinker using fluidised bed techniques. A process which is tightly controlled could possibly convert 20–70% of the organic matter to gas, which would be more than sufficient to keep the pyrolysis fires burning. In addition, roughly 5% of the rubbish would convert to ill-defined oil. From 20–40% of the original weight would terminate as ash, including sufficient copper and aluminium for the ash to have a sales value. There is one claim that a controlled process resulted in a barrel of oil per ton of urban waste, 7.6 barrels being equal to 1 ton. In brief, pyrolysis in theory burns urban waste using its own gas content, meanwhile producing oil at a rate of up to about 13% of the original weight, and leaving a char which should have calorific value about half that of coal, plus a valuable mineral concentrate as a final residue.

There are a number of reasons why pyrolysis has more potential in waste disposal than has protein culture.

1. Pyrolysis is simple non-specific conversion in which output patterns vary after input patterns. Urban waste is variable and seasonal, calling for a flexible technique.
2. Pyrolysis overcomes any problems of occasional inclusion of concentrated toxins, although it is to be noted that organic metal compounds need not by necessity finish in the ash, but may travel with the oil.
3. The biological composition of urban solid waste has no significance in pyrolysis. For protein culture it would be essential to use an efficient sterilisation technique, which could be difficult with such large volumes of mixed rubbish.

Even so, the concept of producing protein from urban solid waste is attractive, particularly since the handling of such waste at present comprises a cost without profit.

The toxic content of urban solid waste depends mainly on the definition of toxic. Indisputable toxins account for less than 2% if recorded only when recognised in high concentration. As dilutions with other pollution the content is probably near 4%. If acids, alkalis and flammables are included, then the proportion of undesirables can exceed 14% but disposal may be by special treatment outside the common disposal system. In 1966 in the United Kingdom the pattern of undesirables (for protein culture) in urban solid waste was:

	Million tons
General factory rubbish	1.16
Inert process waste	9.17
Flammable process waste	0.13
Acid/alkali	0.43
Deadly toxins	0.20

This gave a total of about 12 million tons of industrial waste of no interest for biological reaction, to be noted alongside 14 million tons of household refuse, which is of partial interest for biological reaction. The industrial waste had a disposal pattern of:

	Million tons
Official tips	0.38
Private tips	2.71
Mineshafts	0.87
Incineration	0.12
Sea dumping	0.18
Lagoons for settlement	5.71 (including pumping water)
Unspecified	1.11

This disposal pattern is not accurate since the weight of added water needs to be taken out of the proportion dumped at sea or pumped either into lagoons or mineshafts. The table indicates, however, the relatively low proportion of undesirables which are mixed with household rubbish after urban collection. If a process can be shown to be effective and economic for the conversion of urban solid waste into microbial protein, there should be little trouble in confining contamination to that within normal household rubbish.

The costing of urban solid waste as a potential raw material is difficult, mainly because no disposal method is ever used at maximum economy. In land-in-fill it is necessary to hold unfilled volume against future deliveries. Incineration systems lack the necessary equipment for maximisation of input of rubbish and output of rescued energy. Composting has not proved to be a sophisticated technique, attractive as it may be to conservationists. In 1966–1967 in the United Kingdom, collection of 20 million tons of rubbish cost £45.5 million and the disposal thereof cost £13.5 million. It is reasonable to add 25% for inflation and other on-costs to give an early 1970s figure of about £3.75/ton, a late 1970s figure of nearer £5/ton.

The composition of a typical urban solid waste might be:

	%	
Dust/cinder	12	
Vegetable matter	17	Density—120 kg/m^3
Paper	43	
Metals	9	
Textiles	3	
Glass	9	
Plastics	5	
Unclassified	2	

Household refuse production is of the order of 0.7 kg/person. The analysis shows that the organic content of about 60% is mainly cellulose, which would need cleaning and hydrolysis before it could be used for cultured protein. It can be mixed with sewage to result in a relatively poor substitute for farmyard manure. The mixture is not outstanding in its nutrient value but it is excellent as a soil conditioner. Unfortunately, there is some evidence that urban waste is likely to contain metal contamination above that regarded as sensible for fertiliser or compost. All things considered, there does not yet appear to be a practical and economic route to protein from urban solid waste, either through conventional agriculture or microbial protein.

Cellulose products can be expected to develop in microbial protein because any community can find some waste cellulose, making it possible for any community, regardless of location or circumstance, to produce its own protein. The special case with regard to protein from carbohydrate is papermill waste, which is mixed sugar and higher carbohydrates and is already used for proteins as an alternative to dumping as pollution.

The inevitable protein route which concerns pollution is that starting from urban sewage and possibly solid waste. For psychological reasons it may be essential to use the sewage route only for animal feed protein, not for direct human consumption. The most economic and practical route from present analysis is sewage to algae or bacteria, through coarse fish to fish meal and thence to animal protein. Whichever route is used, protein from sewage and town waste, via microbial protein, will become essential for many urban communities within the coming decade. The problem of waste and effluent from humanity is considered to be the most serious yet experienced. The choices are:

1. Dumping, which will become impossible for major cities within five years.
2. Composting, which is possible for urban areas with available areas of rural land to be enriched, but not practical for most areas.
3. Mixing with dry waste and then incineration. This is an expensive process and it could prove unsuitable for large cities.
4. Dehydration, possibly by spray drying, for powder fertiliser. The economics of such a process are attractive but are not yet sufficiently detailed to compare spray-dried sewage against synthetics.
5. Microbial protein, as mentioned probably by a predator chain through algae or bacteria, fish, meal and livestock.

Looking forward to 1980, the final choice must be between incineration, dehydration and microbial protein. Incineration has economics which relate directly to fuel prices and there could be 1980 justification for using sewage and solid waste as fuel. Dehydration requires a significant energy input and present opinion is that sewage in 1980 will be too low in product value for energy-consuming dehydration processes. Overall economics favour microbial protein but exhaustive studies are needed to relate the input–output rates of factories. It is doubted if existing organic reactions would offer sufficient speed of conversion and initial treatment by boiling in sulphuric acid may be necessary so that more-energetic microbes can be employed.

The most important trend is probably introversion by social groups. Events during the 1970s have shown that it is not safe for a producer to rely on foreign sources of raw material. Future projects will need to be based on local materials, local energy, local labour, and most important on local markets. Although the pattern of familiar protein can be expected to continue, the routes whereby such protein is manufactured will change considerably. Notably, animal rearing will use less imported bought feed and will use more grazing and local feed. In general, arable farms can be expected to use less imported synthetic fertiliser and more natural fertiliser as sludge or dehydrated powder since the prices of most fertilisers must rise after the inflation of oil prices and increases in the wage rates where potash and phosphates are mined.

No country can escape the consequences of inflation during the early 1970s. It has presented new orders of costs for area, labour and raw materials, and introduced new marketing problems. Notably, it has encouraged rejection by consumers of high prices and, by inference, encouraged consumers to accept new standards and forms of food. It is probable that by 1985 most of the familiar foods will have become little more than memories and that new foods will have become standard diet. It is worth reflecting that future diet may differ little from the diet of early scavenging man—in terms of protein sources if not in the manner of presentation—and that the diet of scavenging man was of sufficient quality to allow him to develop above all animals. Further reflection on the 1970s may cast doubts on the extent of his superiority.

Index

A

Addiction, 45
Additives to feed, 86
Agricultural outputs, 275
  problems of, 276
Alanine, 11
Allergy, 43
Algae, 219
  industrial cultivation, 220
  production conditions, 221
  yields, 227
Amino acids, 8
  essential, 9
  non-essential, 9
Amino-acid contents in diet, 24
Amino-acid sweeteners, 29
Angola, 320
Animal proteins, 61
Autagonism, 44
Argentine, 321
Arginine, 10
Ascorbic acid, 32
Aspartic acid, 12
Aspergillus flavus, 111
Attisholz process, 233

B

Bacteria, 248
  industrial production, 248
Bacterial activity, 253
Bacterial protein, 250, 255
  amino-acid patterns, 250, 255
  feeding trials with, 251
  from fats, 255
Baker's yeast, 245
  amino-acid patterns, 245
Bananas, 164
Barley, 159, 198
Beet sugar production, 244
Bird meats
  fat content, 104
  mineral content, 104
  protein content, 104
Birds, 97
  orders of, 98
  protein from, 98
Blast, 201
Botswana, 322
Brazil, 323

C

Calcium, 37

Cans
  alternatives to tin, 59
  design, 55
Canning, 53, 55
  sequence, 56
Carbon dioxide
  use in freezing, 95
Carifta countries, 327
Carnivores, 17, 69
Cassava, 159, 165
  areas of production, 166
Cattle, 71
Cereals, 155
  amino-acid patterns, 156
  areas of growth, 158
  production, 156, 166, 316
  protein content, 155
  world output, 159, 194, 275
Cellulose, 224, 254
Cereals in feed, 189
Cheese, 110
  amino-acid patterns, 115
  natural, 111
  processed, 111
  protein content, 114
  ripening of, 112
Chlorella, 220
Chlorella Growth Factor, 222
Clostridium botulinum, 57
Coconut cake, 170
Coffee, 323
Coffee rust, 199
Cold shortening, 89
Comfrey, 215
Compounds, 47
Compound feeds, 186
  economics of, 187
Compounding, 47
Condensation reactions, 9
Corynebacteria, 256
Cottonseed, 171, 172
  flour, 175, 178
  fractionation, 175
  glandless, 176
  protein concentrate, 182
Cotton plants, 213
Crocodiles, 73
Cultivated crops, 211

Cured fish, 149
Cured meats, 86
Cyclamate, 28
Cyprus, 328
Cystine, 10

D

Dairy protein, 107
DDT, 207
Debarking, 237
Decay of food, 67
  of fish, 139
  of meat, 68
Deep freezing, 23, 92
Dehydration, 52
Diet, 17
  in Middle Ages, 18
  vegetarian 24
Dik-dik antelope, 71
Dried fish, 148
  spoilage, 152
Dubai, 328

E

East Germany, 329
EEC, 329
Egg
  dried egg composition, 110
Energy
  consumption *per capita*, 286
  from protein, 21, 284
  from fossils, 284
  nuclear, 284
Enzymes
  metal dependent, 40
Ethiopia, 333

F

Farming
  domestic birds, 101
  enclosed, 271
  fish, 145

Farming—*continued*
  free-range, 271
  intensive, 273
  mixed, 272
  mussel, 144
  reptiles, 73
  shellfish, 148
  turtles, 73
  wet, 145
  wild birds, 100
Fat
  in meat, 81
Feed
  for intensive rearing, 193
  mercury contamination, 86
  prices, 194
Feed components
  amino-acid patterns, 190
  protein content, 192
Fibre plants, 213
Fibre proteins, 14
  amino-acid patterns, 15
Fiji, 334
Fish, 119
  cured, 149
  dried, 148
  evolution, 128
  feeding habits, 25, 127
  influence of temperature, 126
  mercury levels, 146
  migration, 131
  protein, 120
  protein concentrates, 121
  reconstitution of, 120
  reproduction and survival, 129
  salt, 148
  society of, 123
Fish decay
  preventative techniques, 139
Fish farming
  problems of, 145
  projects, 146
Fishing
  available waters, 292
  cost, 119
  restrictions, 136
  size of catch, 293
  techniques, 133

  use of factory ships, 135
  world catch, 120
Fish meal, 141
  production, 295
Fish paste, 141
Fish spoilage, 137
Food chains, 290
Food decay, 67
Food preservation, 47, 48, 50
Food spoilage, 58, 59
Foot-and-mouth, 202, 321
Fowl pest, 202
Freezers
  economics, 93
  types, 94
  use of carbon dioxide, 95
Fuels, 286
Fungi, 223
  as parasites, 225
  protein, 224
  use in cellulose breakdown, 224
Future proteins, 362
  trends, 263

G

Gas oil, 260
  amino-acid pattern, 260
Glutamic acid, 12
Glycine, 9
Gossypol, 173
  extraction, 174
Grasses, 214
Greece, 335
Green leaf protein, 209, 212
  amino-acid pattern, 213
Green Revolution, 201
Grenada, 336
Groundnut cake, 170
Groundnuts, 171
  fractionation, 175

H

Halophilic bacteria, 151
Halotolerant bacteria, 151

Herbivores, 17
Herbs, 51
Histidine, 10
Hong Kong, 337
Hoofed mammals, 69
Hungary, 337
Hybrids, 198, 201

I

Imitation meats, 16, 88
Industrial protein, 280
    advantages, 283
    cost factors, 282
    disadvantages, 283
Industrial waste
    disposal pattern, 371
Infestation, 203
    control, 204
Insects, 204
    methods of control, 207, 208
    reproduction rates, 204, 206
Insecticides, 207
International sugar agreement, 243
Iran, 339
Iron, 38
    absorption, 39
Isoleucine, 11
Israel, 339
Ivory Coast, 340

K

Kefir, 116
Keratins, 14
Kesp, 83
Kwashiorkor, 36

L

Lactalbumin, 116
Lactobacillus bulgaricus, 116
Lactoglobulin, 116
Lebanon, 341
Lesotho, 322

Leucine, 11
Lizards, 73
Lysine, 11

M

Maize, 158, 159
Malaysia, 341
Mammals, 68
    breeding, 70
    feed requirements, 69
    hoofed, 69
    marine, 70
    social organisation, 71
Marketing techniques, 45
Mauritius, 342
Meat, 63
    annual output, 63
    compounding, 65
    cured, 84
    decay, 68
    demand, 75
    distribution, 67
    energy conversion factors, 64
    fat, 81
    imitation, 16, 88
    pre-packaging, 65
    price-demand relationship, 79
    production, 63, 316
    protein content, 78, 188
    simulated, 83
    variability, 80
    world output, 275
Mercury
    in feed, 87
    in fish, 146
Metals, 40
Methionine, 11
Mexico, 343
Microbial proteins, 217
    amino-acid patterns, 261
Microbes
    thermal death time, 58
Milk, 107
    amino-acid patterns, 115
    composition, 108
    liquid concentrates, 108

Milk—*continued*
  nutrients in, 88
  powder, 108
  production, 316
  proportions fed to stock, 109
  skim, 108, 117
  soured, 115
  vitamin content, 108
Minerals, 35
Mixtures, 47
Monoculture, 200
Monomers, 5
Morocco, 344
Moulds, 224
Mozambique, 320
Mushrooms, 226
Mustards, 211

N

National situations, 319
Natural gas, 288
New Hebrides, 345
New Zealand, 346
Nitrogen content in food, 27
Norway, 348
n-paraffins, 260
  amino-acid patterns, 260
Nucleoproteins, 13
Nutrition intakes, 279

O

Oats, 158
Oil, 257
  production, 287, 317
Oilseed cake, 168
Oilseeds, 167
  amino-acid content, 169
  isolates, 172
  production economics, 170
  world output, 275

P

Packaging
  of fish, 140
  of meat, 65
  vacuum, 66
Palm, 171
Paper pulp, 23
Pekilo process, 234
Peru, 348
Peruvian fish meal industry, 141, 310
Phenylalanin, 11
Phosphorus, 37, 39
Phytic-acid phosphorus, 37
Plankton, 125
Plant cells, 210
Plant development, 209
Plutonium, 41
Poisoning, 43
Pollution
  control, 240
  economics, 239
  in pulp manufacture, 235
  of waters, 131
Polymerisation 6
Polymers, 5, 6
Polysaccharides, 7
Population growth, 278
  rates, 299
Potassium, 36
Potatoes, 159
Poultry, 97
  consumption *per capita*, 102
Preference, 45
Prejudice, 46, 75, 77, 269
Preservation
  of food, 47, 48, 50
  of vegetables, 161
  techniques, 23
Price rises, 312, 314
  movements, 317
Proline, 12
Protein absorption, 22
Proteinates, 181
Protein chemistry, 5
Protein daily allowance, 22
Protein deficiency, 20, 305
Protein demand, 300

Protein demand—*continued*
  by affluent societies, 301
  by mixed societies, 306
  by poor societies, 304
Protein economics, 263
  consumption, 265
  distribution, 265
  production, 265, 270
Protein from urban waste solids, 367
  composition of, 372
Protein regeneration, 40
Protein requirements, 307
Protein sweeteners, 28, 243
  amino-acid patterns, 243
Protein world supply, 289
  factors which inhibit supply, 298
Protein yeasts, 244
Pulses, 183
  amino-acid patterns, 191
  dried, 184
  infestation, 184
  protein content, 184
  vitamin content, 184
  world output, 276
Pyrolysis, 370

Q

Quelea, 100

R

Radioactivity, 41
Rapeseed, 171
Red rust, 201
Refrigeration, 53
  of meat, 89
Reptiles, 72
  farming, 73
Rice production, 315
Rodents, 69
Rumania, 349
Rye, 158

S

Saccharine, 28
Salt fish, 148
Sardinia, 350
Saudi Arabia, 351
Scavengers, 63
Scenedesmus, 220
Serine, 12
Shellfish, 142
  farming, 148
  feeding, 143
  protein content, 144
Shrimp farming, 145
Simulated meat, 83
  market sectors, 84
  protein content, 88
Singapore, 352
Skim milk, 108, 117
  amino-acid patterns, 118
  composition, 117
Slimes, 224
Snakes, 73
Sodium, 35
Sodium-potassium balance, 36
Solomon Islands, 353
Southern Corn Blight, 199, 201
Soya, 83, 167
  fractions, 180
  protein analysis, 87, 179
Speculation, 309
Spices, 50
Spoilage of fish, 137
  of food 58, 59
Sugar
  extraction, 242
  mineral concentrations, 243
  world production, 243
Swaziland, 322

T

Tanzania, 354
Thermophilic bacteria, 59
Threonine, 11
Tilapia, 147
Torula yeast, 231, 245

Torula yeast—*continued*
  amino-acid patterns, 247
  composition, 245
Toxins, 40
Tryptophane, 12
Turkey, 354
Turtle farming, 73
Turtle grass, 215
Turtles, 72
  diet, 73
Tyrosine, 12

U

Uganda, 355
UNDP funds, 305
United States of America, 357
Uraguay, 358
Urea, 169, 252
  starch-bound, 252

V

Vacuum packaging, 66
Value, 12
Vegetable genetics, 197
Vegetable oils, 82
Vegetable protein, 83, 153
  high-protein vegetation 164
Vegetables
  dehydrated in feed, 186
  fresh, 161
  preservation techniques, 161
  protein content, 163
  yields, 162
Vegetarian diet, 24
Venezuela, 359
Vicia faba bean, 83, 184

Virgin Islands, 359
Vitamin A potency, 33
Vitamin D estimates, 34
Vitamins
  A, 31
  B, 32
  B6, 34,
  B12, 34, 216
  C, 32
  D, 32, 37
  E, 33
  K, 33

W

Waste paper
  fermentation of, 239
  recovery, 238
Water content of food, 27
Wet farming, 145
Wheat
  hard, 158
  soft, 158
  world output, 157
  yields, 198
Whey, 113
  amino-acid patterns, 118
  composition, 113
  protein content, 116
  vitamin content, 117

Y

Yeasts, 228
  Baker's, 245
  culture from paper waste, 232
  culture from sugar, 241
  fermentation, 228